The Practitioner's Path
in Speech-Language Pathology

The Art of School-Based Practice

The Practitioner's Path
in Speech-Language Pathology

The Art of School-Based Practice

Wendy Papir-Bernstein, MS, CCC-SLP

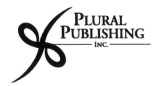

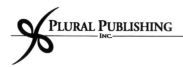
PLURAL PUBLISHING
INC.

5521 Ruffin Road
San Diego, CA 92123

e-mail: info@pluralpublishing.com
Website: http://www.pluralpublishing.com

Typeset in 11/13 Adobe Garamond by Flanagan's Publishing Services, Inc.
Printed in the United States of America by McNaughton & Gunn

Library of Congress Cataloging-in-Publication Data:

Names: Papir-Bernstein, Wendy, author.
Title: The practitioner's path in speech-language pathology : the art of
  school-based practice / Wendy Papir-Bernstein.
Description: San Diego, CA : Plural, [2018] | Includes bibliographical
  references and index.
Identifiers: LCCN 2017045293| ISBN 9781944883454 (alk. paper) | ISBN
  1944883452 (alk. paper)
Subjects: | MESH: Speech-Language Pathology | Evidence-Based Practice |
  Schools
Classification: LCC RC424.7 | NLM WL 21 | DDC 616.85/5--dc23
LC record available at https://lccn.loc.gov/2017045293

Contents

Preface

We are part of an immense field of practice, with new practitioner roles and client populations emerging as we speak. Technology has enabled us to change the way we think, and perhaps even the way we sometimes provide our services. As someone who has survived and thrived within decades of change in our field, and helped thousands of students and practitioners do the same, I offer up a new perspective. We are on the *practitioner's path*, and we must *build it, support it, follow it, and ultimately become it*. That is what this book is about.

In describing this textbook, I borrow a term from the field of architecture: *parti*. A *parti* is the overriding concept of a building, and the departure point for its design (Roth, 1992). It demands professing a particular belief that permeates every aspect of the design; however, it is far from being solely intellectual. Parti derives from understandings that are more transcendent than mere architecture, and must be cultivated before design can be born (Frederick, 2007). The parti manifests the true essence of a design, and the essence needs to be "felt" and experienced rather than intellectually figured out. It gives order, meaning, and rationale to an architectural project, and becomes the design philosophy.

This textbook has a definitive parti. Its purpose is to bridge the gap and lesson the divide between theoretical research and practice. It emphasizes the importance of integrating practice-based evidence along with evidence-based practice, and highlights the artistry of our field along with the science. It is built on *guiding principles and recurring themes* that flourished in different centuries and parts of the world, across fields and throughout the ages, and that seem to transcend time and culture. My hope for this book is to offer the reader a professionally balanced perspective, helping to neutralize the pendulum swings, and give greater functionality to the scientific practices we all must adhere to.

This book takes a critical look at areas related to our own professional wellness, and the necessity of sustaining both the personal self and the professional self. It challenges us to consider our own perceptions about the nature of professional practice, and facilitates the development of four necessary attitudes that can have a profound impact on both clinical success and professional satisfaction: *a scientific attitude, a therapeutic attitude, a professional attitude*, and *a leadership attitude* (Cornett & Chabon, 1988). It contains a blend of clinical evidence and research, practitioner views, common sense, philosophical stances, and historical overviews. It examines each area through a perspective of interdisciplinary research, in addition to personal stories or narratives illustrating key principles and strategies. The stories—emanating from years of field experience, academic leadership, and professional judgment—are used to investigate a variety of larger questions and clinical issues, with the goal being to encourage reflection about our choices and the reasons they make sense. The clinical principles are discussed through a multitude of experiential lenses: that of clinician, staff development specialist, educator, supervisor, and professor. They comprise the narratives or *autobiographical reflective tales* (A.R.T.) woven through most of the chapters, much like a mosaic of practice-based evidence.

The *first section* of the book takes us from data to wisdom. It helps us understand the importance of *building* a foundation for our *clinical path* through a discussion about the necessary *pillars of practice* and underpinnings of a *scientific attitude*—scientific and evidence-based principles, different types of knowledge systems, and development of *wisdom*. Some of the topics include translational research, knowledge management, the place of science, the significance of storytelling, the heart and soul of our work, and the value of intuition.

The *second section of the book* helps us understand the importance of *supporting* our foundation through an introduction to the *philosophical and therapeutic pillars of practice*: reflection, counsel and care, balance and harmony, growth and detachment. Each *pillar of practice* becomes the context for discussing specific principles that sometimes get overlooked in traditional academic textbooks, such as becoming a reflexive practitioner, mindfulness, nonverbal communication, counseling, using feedback, clinical reasoning, prompts, and termination from service. The *philosophical pillars of practice* provide the underpinnings of the *therapeutic attitude*.

The *third section of the book* helps us understand the importance of *follow*ing specific *guideposts and stepping-stones* on the path to clinical effectiveness and professional fulfillment. It serves as a kind of field-guide for the development of a *professional attitude*, and includes chapters that serve as *pillars of practice*: organizational frameworks, materials and activities, measuring progress, best practices, and the importance of community. Principles from assessment and intervention practices are highlighted, such as learning theories, activity analysis, the hidden curriculum, client adherence, ethnographic research, therapeutic alliances, and universal themes.

The *fourth and final section of the book* helps us understand the ultimate purpose of this path we have chosen, to sustain and grow our profession through an *attitude of leadership*. It includes discussions about *ownership and self-direction*, the creation and implementation of a *learning organization* and the development of *leadership practices*. This sec-tion highlights shared vision, clinical expertise, emotional intelligence, leadership trends, the scholarship of teaching and learning, and research dissemination.

This is a book with a particular philosophy about our field, and it contains concepts that may be ancient, but align well with current principles related to client-centered practices, holistic views, interdisciplinary practice, and inter-professional education. I believe that the path to an enlightened future in our field begins with understanding the wisdom of the past. One of my goals in writing this book is to make the *process and practice of therapy* more explicit so that we may sustain our personal self as well as our professional self. A second goal is to support and *engender the mindset and attitudes* necessary to become *reflective practitioners*.

This is a textbook designed for students and practitioners who are actively involved with the process of knowledge acquisition, and it targets issues related to the excellence behind and scholarship within teaching and learning. By weaving together personal stories and clinical narratives, I have created a compendium of experiences that narrate the arc of my career. It is my hope that this book, along with its real life scenarios, will help students, as well as new or seasoned practitioners assimilate, integrate, and synthesize knowledge into a more meaningful and integrative gestalt.

This book has many layers. It may send you searching for additional information about a particular topic, or entice you to rethink some prior knowledge. It is for students and practitioners alike. I think of myself as a weaver who loves to synthesize different textured threads into a single cloth. I have brought together ideas that may not traditionally appear in speech pathology textbooks, but those which are all related to the holistic nature of our work. As you consider the ideas from this book, I invite you to tap into your deeper experiences with life and academic knowledge. Slow down, reflect, listen to your inner wisdom, and attend to what emerges.

REFERENCES

Cornett, B. S., & Chabon, S. (1988). *The clinical practice of speech-language pathology.* Columbus, OH: Merrill.

Frederick, M. (2007). *101 things I learned in architecture school.* Cambridge, MA: The MIT Press.

Roth, L. M. (1992). *Understanding architecture.* New York, NY: HarperCollins.

Acknowledgments

I acknowledge the following people who inspired me on *The Practitioner's Path*:

My husband Peter, for his endless love and support; my *family and friends* for giving me the time and space to get this done.

Rhoda Ribner, for being my work mom, best mentor and most supportive speech therapy supervisor ever; *Joanna Doster,* for boosting my morale at every bend and fork in the road; and *Bob Goldfarb,* for inviting me to contribute to his book and then encouraging me to write my own.

New York City Department of Education (NYCDOE) District 75 *speech supervisors, staff developers,* and every *member of my curriculum, assessment, and intervention committees* for the opportunity to have worked together.

And finally, the *clients, students, and practitioners* with whom I have worked, taught, supervised, and who continue to be my muses and provide motivation for my life's work.

Reviewers

Plural Publishing, Inc. and the author would like to thank the following reviewers for taking the time to provide their valuable feedback during the development process:

Perry Flynn, MEd, CCC-SLP
Professor
Department of Communication Sciences
  and Disorders
University of North Carolina Greensboro
Greensboro, North Carolina

Stephanie Meehan, MA, CCC-SLP
Clinical Assistant Professor
Department of Speech-Language-Hearing
University of Kansas
Lawrence, Kansas

Introduction

WHO WE ARE AND WHERE WE NEED TO GO

The astounding complexity of our work entices one to truly appreciate the beauty of its ongoing process, from education through experience. We all begin with outstanding education, with coursework and practicum experiences as stipulated by national and state standards. However, where we go from there can be approached with broad diversity and a great deal of variation within professional latitude. Each one of us begins as a type of single-celled creature relative to our experiences, and evolves into something unique and original. Our training programs prepare us for many areas of clinical practice. Our knowledge base is diverse, and resources are plentiful. When we need information about an area of treatment, we know how to get it. We buy assessments and materials, and our professional associations supply us with legislative and research updates. As members of a booming profession, we are availed with endless opportunities for work.

Most professional courses and textbooks used in higher education are organized, (for reasons related to *professional necessity),* with a subject or disorder-based epistemology (Kamhi, 2011; Levittt, 2011; Procaccini, Carlino, & Joseph, 2016). External pressures for accountability drive this professional necessity, starting with accrediting bodies at the university level, through certification standards at the professional level (Scudder, 2016; Scudder & Apel, 2005). However, the architectural design of our field, or *signature pedagogy,* is in an ongoing process of change. As practitioners evolv-

ing and responding to society's needs, we are slowly transforming our therapy approaches from disorder and task-centered to person-centered. And so our course designs and textbooks should be similarly transformed.

Today especially, we have unlimited access to information about any subject. Nate Silver tells us that information is no longer a scarce commodity, and that we have more than we know what to do with. "We think we want information when we really want knowledge. Which is the signal, and which is the noise? The signal is the truth. The noise is what distracts us from the truth." (Silver, 2012, p. 17). What is our truth, and what detracts us from seeing it? Where does our present fit into our past and future? What do we do with all of this information, and how do we make it work for us, as well as our clients? The answers to these questions do not necessarily lie within our field, but rather take us on an interprofessional journey, where stories and narratives become the vehicles of flight. We look for the answers to these and other, "larger than life," questions in the "golden fields" of positive psychology, spiritual studies, sociology, medicine, philosophy, religion, architecture, and anthropology. I know I did.

GETTING BACK TO THE BASICS

As we journey to find the answers, let's begin with the works of Joseph Campbell, best known for his discussions regarding the importance of stories and mythologies. Myths are not simply fairy tales or false stories; in ancient times, they often encoded both pragmatic information and profound knowledge (Lukav, 2001). Joseph Campbell spent most of his life telling us we needed to get back to our stories, our mythology. When a friend of his asked him about the relevance of mythology and ancient themes to modern life, Campbell replied that the laws of the ancients are not only applicable to modern society, but that they drive much of what we still hold sacred today (Campbell, 1988).

How can we get back to remembering those basic principles we once knew, or that most of us were brought up knowing? A major premise of this book is that much of what we need to know about achieving success and satisfaction in our clinical practice is what we learn from our life experiences. In our training programs, we have learned about the science behind evidence-based practice (EBP): collecting data, hypothesizing, phasing out prompts and assists, varying materials and activities. This is a book about *why* they are important. The principles are embedded in life's lessons, and are exemplified throughout history. They are certainly not new, just oft-times forgotten.

We examine principles from our own practice that have origins in ancient works, and the connection of these professional principles with historical themes can infuse new life into our practice. We understand why certain themes simply make sense, and are therefore important to follow. Like the ocean, these principles are enduring because they carry the life-blood of our profession. These larger truths show themselves throughout our field, appearing again and again in a variety of contexts. They are addressed in historical writings around the world and throughout the ages, confirmed with translational research from a variety of disciplines, and communicated through my own personal narratives.

When our work is viewed as part of a greater context, the scope of our study must also be broadened. Our *artistry* becomes

ingrained within a continuum of practice, and we must question ourselves and our methods in order to push deeper and further into our work. We find those lessons in life that transform our everyday work events into an experience of artistry. As we do this, through the stories and professional folklores we tell, and the metaphors we use to highlight experience and meaning, we are learning to "artify" and "storify" our work experiences (Zeitlin, 2016).

TAKING OFF OUR BLINDERS

Most of us are comfortable when dealing with patterns and trends. They represent a type of continuity, and enhance our feelings of safety and security as we come to more easily recognize and predict what is expected to happen. Although it is true that our training programs help us become pattern seekers, especially in the area of human behavior, the overabundance of papers, budgetary laws, and other bureaucratic compliances sometimes *blind us* to simple and basic truths. Therefore, we miss the often hidden or disguised commonalities of universal principles and deeper themes that run through our work, much the way they run through all that we experience. The organization of this book helps bring those basic truths and principles back to life.

Our blinders sometimes prevent us from developing a type of wisdom, the final step in the clinical learning process and the ultimate level of understanding as described in the fields of information design and knowledge management. Wisdom is achieved when we see enough patterns in our knowledge base so that we can now synthesize information and use it in novel ways. We are able to predict, see what is missing, and create something new. Wisdom, in this sense, implies a larger vision, and the ability to holistically connect that vision with the well- being of the larger community. Wisdom enables us to travel along the path, and ultimately become it (Allee, 1997; Papir-Bernstein, 2012a; Shedroff, 2000).

ACKNOWLEDGING OUR STORIES

How is this achieved? Wisdom involves tacit knowledge, knowledge that often cannot be directly taught, but is rather acquired or inferred through a range of life experiences in a variety of contexts (Haidt, 2006). We need to begin with an understanding of the different types of knowledge frameworks, which help explain how we get into this quandary to begin with. One framework distinguishes between *tacit* or personal knowledge and *explicit* or formal knowledge.

Tacit knowledge is deeply personal and communicated best through shared experiences. It consists of perceptions, insights, and know-how that are more easily implied than directly expressed. It is often deeply internalized and even unconscious. Most of what we learn through formal education is of the explicit type—information that can easily be communicated to others. If explicit knowledge is the know-what (the facts), the know-why (the science), and the know-who (the networking), then tacit knowledge is the know-how (Alavi & Leidner, 2001; Nonako & Hirotaka, 1995; Papir-Bernstein, 2012a).

A shift is happening in academic conversations as we yearn to share stories of professional adventures and create opportunities to learn from each other's experiences. This has become an *age of epic storytelling*, in part, due to the revolution created by social networking and reality shows. Because narratives and stories help us explore our own internal experience, they become tools for sharing our deeply personal tacit knowledge. Stories lift us to higher ground, and move us from *knowing in our head* to *knowing in our heart*. They model beliefs, convictions, and values while providing inspiration and motivation to make a change.

ENHANCING PROFESSIONAL SATISFACTION

One of my ongoing interests has been to read books from diverse fields of study, and to integrate that information within my own work. About five years ago, I picked up a book called *The Happiness Hypothesis by* J. Haidt (2006), and began to think about the concept of "professional happiness" as it relates to the art and science behind the development of clinical wisdom in our field.

Although our knowledge of what comprises clinical success comes in part from explicit academic sources outside of ourselves, the ability to experience it as satisfactory and pleasurable comes from within. And ultimately, that ability is a key component in the phenomenon called "professional happiness" (Haidt, 2006). We learn most and best when learning gives us pleasure and inspires us. Is it not surprising that what provides inspiration for us in our personal lives can do the same in our professional world? Happiness, whether personal or professional, is driven by the same themes: we want to make a difference, we want to be useful, we want to connect with something greater than ourselves, we want to feel passion, we want community.

As we continue on the path to enhancing professional satisfaction, perhaps we need to begin by taking an information break. Let's follow the lead of Joseph Campbell who talks about arriving at a place where the information stops, and then, in order to proceed, we look for something else. He calls it "a plane of invisible support" (Campbell, 1988, p. 71). Others call it *invoking spirit*. I call it *finding the glue*.

FINDING THE GLUE

Professional glue is the stuff that holds it all together and helps us feel connected to the larger picture. My first memory of glue or paste takes me back to my childhood, sitting on the floor with my mother and mixing flour with water. I remember my amazement with the knowledge that ordinary, everyday ingredients might be transformed into something so totally different. It felt like magic. Several years ago, when Bob Goldfarb asked me to contribute to his textbook about translational research in our field, I had an opportunity to reexamine this as one my personal and professional "drivers" (Goldfarb, 2012). This is how I began my explanation:

> We all have preferences, ways of thinking and patterns of behavior that generate self-comfort, and which dominate our professional lives as well as our personal ones. One of my beliefs is that *everything is connected.* Information is all around me, and my job is simply to look for, receive, and translate it toward some practical purpose in my life. This "information" comes to us at the most unexpected times, from the most unexpected sources, and crosses over from one field to another (Papir-Bernstein, 2012a, p. 51).

When we do believe that everything is connected, we know we cannot talk about something without simultaneously talking about ourselves. In this new age, we must now talk about the *common experience* of practitioner and client, mutual possibilities that set in motion reciprocal acts of therapeutic relationship building. We must talk about con-structing knowledge networks by converging professional actions with other professional communities (Sampaio, 2014). We must reexamine the way we see ourselves in relationship to our work. We must figure out how to reach deep down inside of ourselves to the unknown, and go below the surface of what we *must do* to examine what we believe, and what we *need to do* to stay on path (Zeitlin, 2016).

Two people have the same experience. To one, it is neither noteworthy nor exceptional, and to the other it is something quite magical and mystical. That fact that sometimes something seemingly quite mundane has startling significance is what motivated me to write this book. It is the story of a client, 5 years old and severely language impaired, who asked me if I was blind when I kept prompting her to tell me what she saw in the picture. It is about the student who taught me the best practice principles of "functional and naturalistic" in a restaurant, unable to order her food from a menu. It is the story of a parent, who, when asked by the SLP, what she wanted her non-verbal daughter to be able to say to her with a new and very expensive AAC device, replied, "I just want to hear her say 'I love you mom.'" And most recently, it is the story of the undergraduate student who startled me one day in class, by suggesting that we had a profound responsibility to share the information that was being received in my courses with other professionals. In many of the chapters of this book, content of that type is communicated through my narratives, which I have coined as A.R.T., *autobiographical reflective tales.*

Carl Jung, when asked about the creative spark for his immense body of work, explained that his quest for the meaning of life had been addressed through the posing of professional questions, which he ultimately was able to answer through his life's work (Kerr, 1993). It is those same types of questions that directed me to write this book. I ask, "What is clinical wisdom and how do we find it?" What qualities define the practitioners who excel at their work, communicate through their passion and enthusiasm, and are generally happy and fulfilled in their daily practices? As professors, how do we grow them; as supervisors, how do we encourage them; and as practitioners, how do we become them?

HOW MY PATH BEGAN

As a practitioner, supervisor, staff developer, and professor, I have spent more than 45 years conveying the experience of our work. Joseph Campbell refers to this experience as a kind of "interior road map," a map that is best drawn by the traveler himself (Campbell, 1988, p. 71). Throughout my career, my journeys on this map usually took place on "the blue highways." Westfall, Mold, and Fagnan (2007) use this term to denote the back roads on a map, the places where most people live.

In the field of medicine, the blue highways are the clinics and hospitals where health care is delivered. In the field of education, the highways lead us to the schools and institutions of higher learning. The distance between blue highways and research/funding institutions is long and arduous, which helps explain the relationship between Evidence-Based Practice (EBP) and Practice-Based Evidence (PBE), and why PBE is such an essential component of the translational process (Papir-Bernstein, 2012a). This is especially true when working with low-incidence populations, which are largely underrepresented in research.

Such was the case in the early 1970s, when I was the speech-language therapist in a New York City Department of Education school program called, School for Language and Hearing Impaired Children (SLHIC).

Many of the students were quite unique, having been born of mothers who contracted German measles in their first trimester of pregnancy. As fascinating as this population was to work with, research was sorely lacking and what we now call evidence-based practice was just a glimmer in our eyes and had yet to be born. So, we hypothesized, and engaged with professional practices in areas of assessment and intervention that made sense to us —even though the research or evidence had not yet been generated. And so, we created the path (Papir-Bernstein, 2012a, 2012b).

WHAT THIS BOOK IS ABOUT

What is *the practitioner's path*? It is a way of creating a sense of passage within our professional lives, highlighted by developmental phases and the attitudes that help them manifest. Our travels are not necessarily linear. Although we may backtrack or even remain dormant, new knowledge, new practices and new clients fuel our momentum along the path.

This book is part of many things: textbook, field guide, memoir, and narrative. It is filled with encounters. It focuses on experiences and expertise, as well as research and evidence, and reminds us that the primary and most important element in the definition of evidence-based practice is now, and has always been, the practitioner (Sackett, Rosenberg, Gray, Haynes, & Richardson, 1996). Personal skills and attitudes have been and continue to be identified as an integral component of clinical expertise (Kamhi, 1994; 2011). However, personal qualities have recently been expanded in both ASHA's 2014 clinical competency standards as *interaction and personal qualities*, and to the 2015 revision of standards for accreditation of graduate programs as *professional practice competencies* (ASHA, 2014; 2015).

There is a newly acknowledged type of pedagogical scholarship in our field referred to as *wisdom of practice*, largely based upon professional experiences. Such experiences may include personal accounts of change resulting from implementation of new instructional practices, policies, and personal narratives (Papir-Bernstein, 2012b; Weimer, 2011). What is the nature of professional practice in our field? What types of knowledge, qualities, and competencies are required for exceptional practice? What attitudes exemplify excellence in our field? The first three types of attitudes have been identified by Cornett and Chabon as central to the provision of high quality therapeutic services (1988). To these three, I have added a fourth. The first is a *scientific* attitude, relating to theoretical and scientific knowledge (covered largely in Part I). The second is a *therapeutic* attitude, relating to interpersonal skills, such as care and compassion (covered largely in Part II). The third is a *professional* attitude, relating to values about the work setting (covered largely in Part III). The fourth is a *leadership* attitude, relating to self-direction and the creation of a learning organization (covered largely in Part IV).

HOW THIS BOOK IS DIFFERENT

- It identifies the *guiding principles, recurring themes, and enduring truths* that continue to drive our field.
- It explains why *tried and true clinical principles* simply make sense.
- It melds *ancient wisdom* with modern scientific methodology to forge new approaches for practice in our field.
- It emphasizes the importance of developing and trusting *tacit or personal knowledge* in addition to explicit or formal academic knowledge.

- It reacquaints us with the *heart, soul, and spirit* of our work, and reminds us why many of us were attracted to this field in the first place.
- It illustrates and exemplifies *clinical stepping-stones* through the use of personal narratives and practice-altering clinical stories.
- It presents a theoretical framework and rationale for the development of clinical wisdom: *building* our path, *supporting* our path, *following* our path, and *becoming* our path.
- It elucidates the necessity of integrating our fund of knowledge with sprinklings of *translational research* from a variety of diverse fields.
- It validates the importance of incorporating principles from *practice-based evidence*, in addition to evidence-based practice.
- It facilitates our identification of the *recurring motifs*, themes, qualities, and properties that define our practice.
- It exemplifies much of the chapter content with A.R.T.©, autobiographical reflective tales that illustrate implementation of the targeted principles of practice.
- It targets *art* plus the *science* of our field, the *know-how* plus the *know-what*.
- It creates a context of practice that is older, larger, and more universal than the classroom or the therapy room.
- It introduces the concept of earning your "Ps" in addition to your "Cs": *The Pillars of Practice* ©, which are needed to support and reinforce *The Practitioner's Path* ©.

For this adventure, and in the spirit of embracing the best thinkers of work that has gone before, I have examined and studied the works of others in this and many other fields. I have attempted to create an alchemy of science, philosophy, and experiential narratives by integrating concepts and relationships that have been described across a variety of disciplines, as well as centuries. I hope to build a solid foundation on our common wisdom and reach a new synthesis of information and knowledge for facilitating the artistry of our practice.

This textbook is written from the inside out, as a reflection of my life's work. I have approached it with courage and patience, and hope it is utilized in much the same way. The stories contained within have unfolded as part of my day-to-day work over the decades of my career. Steve Sabol, filmmaker, founder, and president of NFL Films said, "Tell me a fact and I'll learn, tell me a truth and I'll believe, tell me a story and it will live in my heart forever." (Barron, 2013). These stories have journeyed with me from information through wisdom, research through practice, science through art—and back again. They have been my teachers and my mentors along the *practitioner's path*.

As Jake Silverstein points out in an editor's letter in the *New York Times Magazine* several days after our 2016 presidential election, one current theme that seems to be infiltrating all we do in politics, industry, health care, and education is our obsession with "redesigning" (Silverstein, 2016). We can call it optimizing, improving, tweaking, refreshing, modernizing, or simply updating—it all points to our belief that *change* is the flavor of the day. Let us remember that, as Silverstein eloquently states, "No design is every permanent but merely a way station between what a thing used to be and what it might yet become . . . " (p. 22).

The same might be said about signature pedagogy and textbooks. I like to think that this book provides a *way station* for students and practitioners. As defined by Merriam-Webster, a way station is *a place where people can stop for rest or supplies during a long journey*. Perhaps you discovered this book at a conference, perhaps online, or maybe as a requirement for a course. As you read, you may at times wonder how a particular piece of information connects with speech-language pathology, or how this relates to practice in the school setting. Please know that you are not alone as you wonder. Wonder often begins with a thought or question, and transforms to amazement, surprise, and the pleasurable state of *wonderment*. Use this book as a tool of wonderment, and it may help you find your "professional glue."

REFERENCES

Alavi, M., Leidner, D. (2001). Review: Knowledge management and knowledge management systems: Conceptual foundations and research issues. *MIS Quarterly, 25*(1), 107–136.

Allee, V. (1997). *The knowledge evolution: Expanding organizational intelligence.* Newton, MA: Butterworth-Heinemann Press.

American Speech-Language-Hearing Association. (2014). *Standards for the Certificate of Clinical Competence in Speech-Language Pathology.* Retrieved from http://www.asha.org/Certification/2014-Speech-Language-Pathology-Certification-Standards/

American Speech-Language-Hearing Association. (2015). *Proposed revised standards for accreditation of graduate education programs in audiology and speech-language pathology.* Retrieved from http://caa.asha.org/wp-content/uploads/Accreditation-Standards-for-Graduate-Programs.pdf

Barron, D. (2013). NFL Films stages a fitting tribute to Steve Sabol. *Houston Chronicle.* Retrieved February 14, 2013 from: http://blog.chron.com/sportsupdate/2013/02/nfl-films-stages-a-fitting-tribute-to-steve-sabol/

Campbell, J. with Moyer, B. (1988). *The power of myth.* New York, NY: Doubleday.

Cornett, B. S., & Chabon, S. (1988). *The clinical practice of speech-language pathology.* Columbus, OH: Merrill.

Goldfarb, R. (Ed.). (2012). *Translational speech-language pathology and audiology.* San Diego, CA: Plural.

Haidt, J. (2006). *The happiness hypothesis.* New York, NY: Basic Books.

Lukav, G. (2001). *The dancing wu li masters: Overview of the new physics.* New York, NY: Harper One.

Kamhi, A. (1994). Toward a theory of clinical expertise in speech-language pathology. *Language, Speech, and Hearing Services in Schools, 25,* 115–118.

Kamhi, A. G. (2011). Balancing certainty and uncertainty in clinical practice. *Language, Speech, and Hearing Services in Schools, 42,* 59–64.

Kerr, J. (1993). *A most dangerous method: The story of Jung, Freud, and Spielrein.* New York, NY: Knopf.

Levitt, H. (2011, November). *Principles of change used by expert therapists.* Presented at ASHA Convention: San Diego, CA.

Merriam-Webster. (2015). Available from https://www.merriam-webster.com/dictionary/way station

Nonako, I., & Hirotaka, T. (1995). *The knowledge creating company: How Japanese companies create the dynamics of innovation.* New York, NY: Oxford University Press.

Papir-Bernstein, W. (2012a). The artistry of practice-based evidence (PBE): One practitioner's path —Part I. In R. Goldfarb (Ed.), *Translational speech-language pathology and audiology* (pp. 51–57). San Diego, CA: Plural.

Papir-Bernstein, W. (2012b). The artistry of practice-based evidence (PBE): One practitioner's path —Part II. In R. Goldfarb (Ed.), *Translational speech-language pathology and audiology* (pp. 83–89). San Diego, CA: Plural.

Procaccini, S., Carlino, N., & Joseph, D. (2016). Clinical teaching methods for stimulating students' critical thinking. *ASHA Perspectives SIG 11, 1,* 3–17.

Sackett, D. L., Rosenberg, W. M. C., Gray, J. A. M., Haynes, R. B., & Richardson, W. S. (1996). Evidence-based medicine: What it is and what it isn't. *British Medical Journal, 312,* 711–712.

Sampaio, T. M. M. (2014). The afterthought of speech language and hearing science therapy in the contemporary scientific epistemology. *Revista CEFAC, 16*(6), 2029–2033. https://doi.org/10.1590/1982-0216201411513

Scudder, R. R., & Apel, K. (2005). *Assessing learning: Classroom assessment techniques.* Rockville, MD: American Speech-Language-Hearing Association, Perspectives on Issues in Higher Education, Special Interest Group 10.

Scudder, R. (2016). *The pedagogy of university teaching.* Retrieved from http://www.asha.org/academic/teach-tools/scudder/

Shedroff, N. (2000). Information interaction design: A unified field theory of design. In R. Jacobson (Ed.), *Information design* (pp. 267–293). Cambridge, MA: First MIT Press.

Silver, N. (2012). *The signal and the noise: Why so many predictions fail—but some don't.* New York, NY: The Penguin Press.

Silverstein, J. (2016, November 13). Make it new. *New York Times Magazine,* MM22. Retrieved from https://www.nytimes.com/2016/11/13/magazine/design-issue-editors-letter.html

Weimer, M. A. (2011). A primer on pedagogical scholarship. *ASHA Perspectives on Issues in Higher Education, 14*(1), 5–10.

Westfall, J., Mold, J., & Fagnan, L. (2007). Practice-based research: blue highways on the NIH road map. *Journal of the American Medical Association, 297*(4), 403–406.

Zeitlin, S. (2016). *The poetry of everyday life: Storytelling and the art of awareness.* Ithaca, NY: Cornell University Press.

PART I

Building Our Path:
From Data to Wisdom

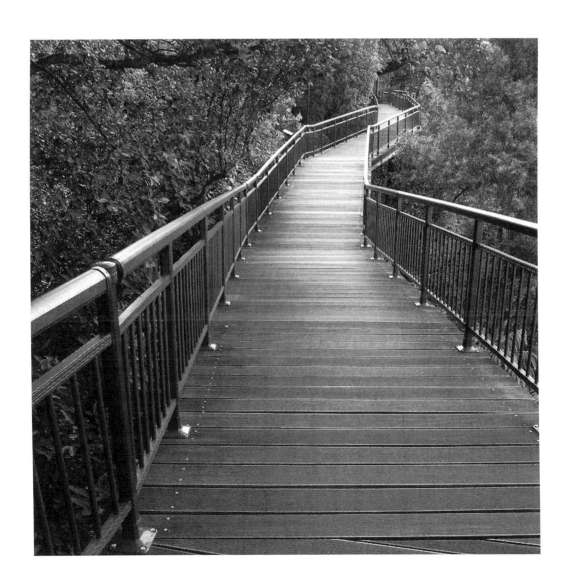

INTRODUCTION

Years ago, I came across the Tao quotation, "Find the path, enter the path, travel the path, become the path." In her book about knowledge evolution, Verna Allee refers to this quotation and explains the complexity of wisdom development. We must first find and build on the data, develop the information from the data, isolate the knowledge as we travel through it, and sift through it all as we ultimately model those enduring truths and become the wisdom (Allee, 1997; Papir-Bernstein, 2012). It is this very quotation that provides the structure for the four parts of my book (building our path, supporting our path, following our path, and becoming our path), as well as the first three chapters in Part I (development of information, acquisition of knowledge, obtainment of wisdom).

Part I begins our discussion about building the practitioner's path in speech-language pathology. There are three chapters in Part I that lead the way by helping us develop the _scientific attitude_ that informs the framework for our path (using the acronym DAO, which is the Chinese term for _way_ or _path_). As we begin this building process, we are introduced to the following _pillars of practice_: the **d**evelopment of information, the **a**dvancement of knowledge, and the **o**btainment of wisdom. Part I introduces the _heart, soul, and spirit_ of our work, and reminds us of reasons why we may have been _attracted_ to this field in the first place. Much of this information is intended to serve as a source of enlightenment, and may help you uncover some new and expansive perspectives or lenses through which to ponder and learn about our field of practice.

Part I sets the stage for the context of this book. All of our work begins with information and knowledge. _Building our path_ involves the transformation of data to wisdom as we learn to integrate our scientific attitude with our heart, soul, and spirit. Stanley Goldberg reminds us that complicated behaviors, activities, and thoughts are all built on a foundation of knowledge (1997). No human behaviors are more complicated than _speech, language, and communication_ with their intricately precise balance of motor, cognitive, and emotional systems. British novelist Arnold Bennett stated, "There can be no knowledge without emotion. We may be aware of a truth, yet until we have felt its force, it is not ours. To the cognition of the brain must be added the experience of the soul." (Swinnerton, 1932, p. 510)

Aristotle describes three approaches to knowledge: episteme, techné, and phronesis. Episteme translates from Greek as "to know," as in scientific knowledge. Techné translates as "craft or art," and phronesis as "practical wisdom." It is not surprising that we acknowledge how essential the bridge-building process is between science, art, and clinical wisdom as part of the therapeutic process in any setting (Smith, 2012).

Academic culture is in a slow process of transformation, fueled by a core group of professionals who understand the importance of merging a pedagogy of heart and soul with the existent pedagogy of intellect (Palmer, 2003). Our training teaches us so much about the science of our field; however, it may also be teaching us to ignore the "secrets" that are hidden in plain sight. We tend to ignore the powers of the human heart that can only evolve from within. Many of us have lost something important in the mass of professional training and practice. We are blinded by the bright light of science. We are like the person who looks for his lost watch in a place he knows it is not, but looks there because the light is brighter. Sometimes, just perhaps sometimes, we may be looking in the wrong places.

A number of years ago, I read The Alchemist (Coelho, 1993). There is a beautiful description of that "aha" moment, and how that moment is communicated:

> . . . he knew that any given thing on the face of the earth could reveal the history of all things. One could open a book to any page, or look at a person's hand; one could turn a card or watch the flight of the birds . . . whatever the thing observed, one could find a connection with his experience of the moment. (p. 101)

We have chosen this field because of our love for mankind, and our belief that nothing is more important than communication. We try to unravel the truths behind some of the most important clinical questions, but sometimes our studies take us to a point beyond which we cannot seem to go. Coehlo would say that the person who learns to read the signs, interpret the omens, and learn the universal language is an alchemist. Al Stewart has said it in his song, "Time Passages," "I know you're in there you're just out of sight . . . " (Stewart & White, 1978).

So let us begin our journey on building the path, as we learn about the design of information in our field, the advancement of knowledge, and the obtainment of clinical wisdom.

REFERENCES

Alee, V. (1997). *The Knowledge evolution: Expanding organizational intelligence.* Oxford, UK: Butterworth-Heinemann Press.

Coelho, P. (1993). *The alchemist.* New York, NY: HarperCollins.

Goldberg, S. (1997). *Clinical skills for speech-language pathologists.* San Diego, CA: Singular.

Palmer, P. J. (2003, Nov/Dec). Teaching with heart and soul: Reflections on spirituality in teacher education. *Journal of Teacher Education, 54*(5), 376–385.

Papir-Bernstein, W. (2012). The artistry of practice-based evidence (PBE): One practitioner's path —Part I. In R. Goldfarb (Ed.), *Translational speech-language pathology and audiology* (pp. 51–57). San Diego, CA: Plural.

Smith, H. (2012). *The spaces in-between: How the art of intuition informs the science of evidence based practice in psychotherapy.* Master of Social Work Clinical Research Papers. Paper 93. Retrieved from http://sophia.stkate.edu/msw_papers/93

Stewart, A. I., & White, P. H. (1978). "Time Passages" [Lyrics]. Retrieved from http://www.az lyrics.com/lyrics/alstewart/timepassages.html

Swinnerton, F. (Ed.). (1932). *The journals of Arnold Bennett.* New York, NY: PenguinBooks.

CHAPTER 1

Development and Design of Information

1. THE PLACE OF SCIENCE

Science Is Sometimes Debated, But Never Trivialized

Science and research provide the foundation for our profession, and we need them to advance our knowledge base as we learn to understand the importance of becoming critical consumers of scientific research. We, as practitioners, must make informed clinical decisions based in part on the evidence that exists. Research has even been called *the heart and soul of the professions* (Meline & Wang, 2004). There is no question that research is an integral and foundational member of our professional society. We depend on research to facilitate the delivery of best services as research justifies both the effectiveness and efficiency of the services we provide to our clients. We use science to seek knowledge and guide our discoveries of patterns and meaning from the research (Meline & Paradiso, 2003). But, what's the inside scoop on science? Let's talk a bit from a historical perspective.

Sixty-five years ago, Beveridge wrote a book that served as an orientation to scientific investigation and research. In the introduction, he begins by stating,

> Elaborate apparatus plays an important part in the science of today, but I sometimes wonder if we are not inclined to forget that the most important instrument in research must always be the mind of man. It is true that much time and effort is devoted to training and equipping the scientist's mind, but little attention is paid to the technicalities of making the best use of it. There is no satisfactory book which systematizes the knowledge available on the practice and mental skills—the art—of scientific investigation. (Beveridge, 1950, p. vii)

Fifty years ago, faith gave way to the scientific method as we looked for a better understanding of what was real. Science was key. However, what we used to consider "the best available science" is no longer an accepted truth. Our concept of scientific truths seems to be shifting to become interpretations of competing ideologies as a type of epistemological warfare (Johnson, 1995; Yong, 2012). Everything becomes a version of the truth. Science is now expected to accommodate personal beliefs fueled by the Internet and special interest groups. As we continue to study complex entities, such as animals and humans, results that appear robust in the lab and valid to editors of journals do not always stand the test of further studies (Russell, 2013). Science changes so quickly, it is not necessarily perceived as the final word.

Nate Silver discusses research from a broader and more controversial perspective as it relates to medical advances. He tells us that medical researcher John Ioannidis provides an opinion about why so many scientists believe that many published research findings are false, or at best, pointless. He studied findings documented in peer-reviewed journals, and concluded that when hypotheses are applied to the real world, most findings could not be replicated and were, therefore, likely to fail (Ioannidis, 2005; Silver, 2015).

Silver tells us that data-driven predictions can succeed or fail, but that the odds of failure rise when we deny our role in the process. He reminds us that before we demand more of our data, we need to demand more of ourselves (2015). In the field of medicine, the stethoscope is a tool used by doctors to listen to internal sounds coming from the lungs, heart, the stomach, and even the intestines. Although it is one of the most important additions to the medical world, physicians remind themselves that the most important medical tool is the part of the stethoscope that lies between their ears (Weinberg, 1993).

One of the most perplexing tasks for science is to understand individuality. Scientists generally study individual events to discover general principles, which can then be applied to other events. Validity is established by replicating findings under controlled conditions (Galland, 1997). Medical scientists are most often analyzing similarities and differences between groups of patients. Galland tells us that artists, on the other hand, use general principles (pertaining to things such as light, perspective, shape) to create unique works of art that derive their value from being one of a kind. Galland talks about his vision for the *art of medicine* in his medical textbook about healing, and within the art of practice, each patient is viewed and treated as biologically and psychologically unique. Principles of science would be applied for the purpose of better understanding the unique characteristics of each patient, not the disease.

The place of science in our field is sometimes debated, sometimes questioned, but it is never trivialized. The same is true about the relationships between practitioners and scientists. Discussions about clinician and researcher relationships are not new to the field of communication disorders, and over 40 years ago these relationships had been sometimes described as *discordant and dichotomous* (Costello, 1979; Ringel, 1972). In later years, however, the *collaborative promise* has led to these partnerships being described as necessary and complementary, rather than contradictory (Goldstein & Washington, 2001; Tavris, 2003). Perhaps we have finally come to our senses.

The Connection Between Science and Speech-Language Pathology

The role of science in our profession has been investigated and written about for at least 35 years (Siegel & Ingham, 1987). Although our field is founded from science, Siegel states that there are limits to the reach of science, and that not all problems have scientific solutions. There are questions of values, beliefs, and logic within our field that fall outside the purview of science and not conducive to scientific study (Medawar, 1984; Siegel, 1987). In those formative years in our profession, science had been described as:

- An approximation of truth, but not a system of well-established statements (Popper, 1968)
- Testing experimentally the logical implications of hypotheses (Medawar, 1984)
- A collection of human activities that culminate in certain kinds of verbal statements about contingencies that allow for prediction and control (Johnson & Pennypacker, 1980)

When the question was asked whether the field of speech-language pathology even constitutes a science, researchers concluded that what was needed to qualify it as a science was " . . . a dominant paradigm that provides a unifying conceptual or methodological structure" (Siegel & Ingham, 1987, p. 100). It was proposed that there were two possible explanations to help us understand "the science" of our field. One, communication sciences may be in a *preparadigm stage*, as were other behavioral and social sciences of the day. Two, we do not need to generate our own methodologies, theories, or models to be considered a science. We can share them with related disciplines such as linguistics, psychology, philosophy, sociology, and education (Siegel & Ingham, 1987). We are members within a much larger scientific community or family structure, and together we share in the testing of these theories. Substantive areas overlap, and when they do, there are no "privileged theories, concepts, or methods" (Siegel & Ingham, 1987, p. 100). We see ourselves "as partners in behavioral science, with equal access to the paradigms, theories, methods, and controversies that plague and energize all behavioral sciences" (Siegel & Ingham, 1987, p. 101).

Does Science Always Help Us?

While science is an essential component of information gathering, it does not always help us with our decisions as much as we would like it to. Sometimes, our clinical decisions are simply value driven. Our values can be influenced by many factors, and changing laws is only one of them. This has certainly been the case with how we think about our caseloads, and the clients we serve. Once upon a time, and prior to Education for All Handicapped Children's Act of 1975 (PL 94–142), many of the students we now have on our caseloads would not have been entitled to our services.

As a result of World Health Organization (WHO) and the Americans with Disabilities Act (ADA), our entire educational, health care, and vocational worlds have become more inclusive of people with disabilities. Education is justified because it benefits the individual, whether or not that person is perceived as having the capabilities of becoming an independent and contributing member of society (Siegel, 1987).

In an article in 1986, Perkins stated that theories provide imperfect guides to therapy, and the sessions themselves provided the insights. Yes, a theory is one very useful source for important research ideas, but by no means the only one. Another useful source is, "*I wonder what would happen if . . . ,*" which can later evolve into that theoretical explanation (Johnston & Pannypacker, 1980). Perkins further suggested that clinicians use clinical sessions experimentally to determine effectiveness of clinical procedures. A client's response to experimental procedures is one source of information, but the practitioner's common sense is another. Sometimes, the research really does lag behind the practice (Perkins, 1986; Siegel & Ingram, 1987).

There are times when a simple logical analysis of a clinical question is more useful than a program of research and experimentation. Through that analysis, perhaps a restatement of the question and the definitions will suffice. The first question we need to ask is, "Does a therapy make sense" rather than "Does it work" (Perkins, 1986). Regardless of the research behind it, our task as clinicians is to tailor or individualize general therapy techniques. The bottom line is what works for one client may not work for another (Siegel, 1987; Sudsawad, 2005). However, if the therapy makes conceptual sense, we are off to a good start.

There is another reason that the question "does therapy work" may not be the best question to ask. Most therapy works sometimes, with some clients. All human behavior is potentially malleable through a therapeutic approach, but the question is—do the gains justify the expenses? Science may not be always designed to answer this (Siegel, 1987). Scientific inquiry alone will not necessarily address ethical, political, and administrative issues. We discuss this in more detail in later chapters.

2. EVIDENCE-BASED PRACTICE

What Is Evidence-Based Practice (EBP)?

This section may serve as a review, expansion, or an introduction to evidence-based practice. The concept of EBP sprung from the world of public health and epidemiology. Public health agencies examine the way diseases affect entire populations and consider cost-effective ways to maximize health for the greatest number of people. Most fields in health care are grappling with, as well as shaping, the EBP movement. This is a public health agenda that calls on practitioners to use the best available scientific evidence as the basis for formulating client interventions (DeAngelis, 2005). The challenges facing most professions include the need to demonstrate that its practices are well backed by data and improved outcomes. Any discipline that regards itself as a scientific discipline, and a member of the scientific community, will be meeting this challenge.

It is interesting to note that *evidence-based health care designs (EBHD)* are now being used to create therapeutic and supportive environments for clients, families, and health care workers. Let's see what we can learn from urban planners, architects, engineers, industrial designers, and art consultants—all of who work together for unique solutions because each client is unique (Malkin, 1992; Sommer, 1969). A number of design professionals have continued to express concern that EBHD represents a challenge that limits their creativity and freedom or choice, or might lead to a "cookbook" approach to architecture (Hamilton, 2003).

Evidence-based practice is one of the most important developments for helping, health and human service professions (Gilgun, 2005; Sackett, Straus, Richardson, Rosenberg, & Haynes, 2000). The EBP represents many things. First, it represents the ideology that evolves from the ethical principle that all clients deserve to be provided with the most effective interventions possible. It also represents the method related to the way we go about finding and implementing those interventions. For us, the students and practitioners, it represents a commitment to use all means possible to locate the best and most effective evidence (Fischer, 2009). In an article from Healthcare Design Academy, five levels of evidence-based practice are proposed to identify commitments and practices by architects and their clients (Hamilton, 2003). We may have something to learn from looking at these levels.

1. *Level-zero practitioners:* Individuals who seem to grasp the concept that there is evidence out there, but they rarely read original research. They might take isolated comments from an article or conference presentation, and made a personal interpretation that fits with their design bias, and claim they are using evidence-based principles.

2. *Level-one practitioners:* An effort is made to stay current with literature in the field, interpret the evidence as it relates to the project, and make judgments as to best design for specific circumstances. These designers are advancing the state of their art, learning from others, and delivering better designs to their clients

3. *Level-two practitioners:* Based on research, they hypothesize expected outcomes of

design interventions and measure the results.

4. *Level-three practitioners:* In addition to following the literature, hypothesizing the intended outcomes of their design interventions, and measuring the results, these professionals report their results in the public arena.

5. *Level-four practitioners:* They take the next step by publishing in quality journals that require review by qualified peers, and collaborate with scientists in academic settings who contribute to the formal literature.

Evidence-based practice began in the field of medicine during the 1990s, and met with such success in improving services that the procedures became integrated (or translated) into an increasing number of disciplines. The definition most of us are familiar with is an approach that includes the integration of *high-quality research evidence* with *clinical expertise* and *client/caregiver values and preferences.*

High quality clinical research is often referred to as best evidence, and provides the foundation of evidence-based practice (EBP). EBP helps us solve clinical problems, keep up with the abundance of clinical literature, and provide opportunities for lifelong learning and improvements in one's clinical expertise (Meline & Paradiso, 2003; Self & Apel, 2002). There are three overriding reasons why EBP is so important: accountability, professional responsibility, and ethics (Apel & Scudder, 2005). The American Speech-Language-Hearing Association (ASHA) provides a position statement on the use of EBP, and its role in the clinical decision making process (ASHA, 2005). The implementation of EBP is rarely perceived as an all or nothing endeavor, but rather as a matter of degree. Every clinician can and must accomplish some degree of EBP within their everyday practice.

The use of research methods is an integral component of clinical practice. One of our roles is to determine the effectiveness of clinical treatments that we provide. We cannot simply infer that treatment has had an impact because we observe measurable changes in behavior. Research tells us that those changes are a direct result of the treatment, rather than because of developmental changes or spontaneous recovery (Holland, 1998; Wambaugh & Bain, 2002).

The Evolution of EBP

Although research ultimately guides intervention by transforming science into practice, most practitioners perform certain professional activities before they are in vogue or even have a name (Papir-Bernstein, 2012a). At best, professional practices should make sense prior to having become legally mandated or professionally sanctioned as best practices. In much the same way, assessment and intervention practices would hopefully make sense before the research and evidence has been generated.

Evidence-based practice can be perceived as relatively new or ancient, dependent upon definitions, interpretations of terminology, field of search, and depth of investigation. In our profession of speech-language pathology, the notion of basing practice on research evidence can be traced back to the early 20th century (Bothe, 2010; Duchan, 2002). However, in clinical psychology that same notion is traceable to the 1890s and centuries earlier in medicine (Hayes, S. C., Barlow, & Crilly, 2001; Nelson-Gray, 1999). In its most current and recognizable form, EBP was not introduced until 1992 and was adapted by the American Speech-Language-Hearing Association in 2004 (ASHA, 2010; Bothe, 2010; Evidence-Based Medicine Working Group 1992; Sackett et al., 2000).

EBP evolved from the field of medicine as a means of providing care that results in desirable outcomes. Evidence-based approaches to practice are being applied to most health care professions, including speech-language pathology. EBP, the conscious use of current and best evidence, helps answer the basic question that we must ask before we begin treatment: how do I know that what I am doing has a high likelihood of being effective? EBP offers a framework, flow chart, and set of tools that we can use to become better practitioners and researchers (ASHA, 2006; Bury & Mead, 1998; Dollaghan, 2004).

What Is Best Evidence?

On paper and through explanation, all three components of the triangular model are equally weighted, however, in everyday real practice this is not always the case. Although these principles are often depicted as the three points on a triangle, the weight or clinical significance of each point changes depending on perspective. For example, universities and clinical training institutions will emphasize best research evidence, while practitioners working in schools will cite the importance of clinical expertise and student/caregiver values when making decisions about assessment and intervention approaches (Papir-Bernstein, 2012a).

When we consider the EBP triad, or the EBP triangle, on the ASHA website, research evidence does not necessarily serve as the base of the triangle, as one might expect (ASHA, 2010). The only suggestion offered is that all three sources of information be represented. We have many ways of knowing: tradition, experience, introspection, and sometimes just lucky guesses (Bothe, 2010). EPB simply suggests that the most defensible way of knowing is to build a complete triangle.

On the surface, the EBP framework emphasizes all three aspects of clinical decisions that are evidence-based: best evidence, clinical expertise, and client preferences (ASHA, n.d.). However, as we examine the procedural steps for EBP, it becomes apparent that empirical research is often emphasized as the most important step in the process. On the ASHA website (http://www.asha.org/members/epb), a four-step process is outlined (ASHA, n.d.). It is not until the final step, that factors, such as client preferences, come into play in directing the treatment decision.

1. Framing the clinical question
2. Finding the evidence
3. Assessing the evidence
4. Making the clinical decision

The Gold Standard of Research: Randomized Controlled Trial (RCT)

The Randomized Controlled Trial (RCT), although considered the "gold standard" of research evidence, is limited in applicability for individualized clinical decision-making (Lemoncello & Ness, 2013; Malec, 2009; Ylvisaker et al., 2002). The RCT is considered of the highest quality because it reduces the potential for bias and control threats to internal validity of a study (such as spontaneous recovery or learning effect linked to repeated testing) (Meline, 2010). However, there are limitations of the RCT design, one of which is the ethical implication of withholding treatment for randomized or nonrandomized members of a control group (Malec, 2009).

Research-oriented professionals believe that only those services that have been supported by the most rigorous methodology for testing treatment efficacy, such as randomized controlled trials (RCT), should be offered. Practice-oriented professionals, on the other hand, would like to see greater attention paid to contextual, observational, qualitative research that captures the nature of the therapeutic experience (DeAngelis, 2005). The primary function of RCTs is to ensure that changes in the behavior under study are caused by the treatment, as opposed to determining the best treatment for individual patents (Berguer, 2004; Wambaugh, 2007). Other types of experimental designs can contribute to research evidence.

An Alternative to RCT

One alternative to RCT is the *single-case experimental designs (SCED)*, which establish evidence of efficacy when your client matches the client in a study based upon similarity of key features (Lemoncello & Ness, 2013). The SCED is different from a case study. Although a case study may provide in-depth (quantitative or qualitative) analysis of response to intervention, because there is no research control, a case study is considered non-experimental. Through SCED, we can collect and analyze data at the individual level, such as repeated measurement of a target behavior over time (Lemoncello & Ness, 2013; Richards, Taylor, Ramasamy, & Richards, 1999). A more thorough explanation of SCED may be found Craig Kennedy's book about single case designs for educational research (2004).

One type of SCED that allow practitioners to examine intervention effects is the *multiple baselines (MBL)*. Richards and his colleagues explain that interventionists are able to examine treatment effects on a target behavior by varying the timing of intervention across different conditions (1999). Lemoncello and Hess (2013) describe three variations of the MBL:

- *Across participants*—evaluate the efficacy of an intervention on three or more clients with similar profiles on the same-targeted outcome;
- *Across behaviors*—evaluate the efficacy of an intervention on three or more related targeted goals for a single client;

- *Across contexts*—evaluate the efficacy of an intervention on the same- targeted outcome in three or more specific contexts for a single client.

Wambaugh and Bain (2002) discuss two single-subject designs that provide a means for the practitioners to organize data in an ongoing process: the *alternating treatments* (AT) design and the *multiple baselines across behaviors* (MBAB) design. With the AT design, we are able to compare effects of two or more treatments by selecting two behaviors and submitting each to a different treatment. The behaviors should be of comparable difficulty. The MBAB design allows us to determine the treatment responsible for the change. For a more complete discussion, please see Wambaugh and Bain.

What Are the Steps in the EBP Process?

We learn about EBP in graduate school, and the process often begins with the PICO question (Straus, Richardson, Glasziou, & Haynes, 2005). We ask, on behalf of the *patient*, if this *intervention* or a *comparative* intervention will likely result in the desired *outcome*. This first step in the EBP process might yield some uncomfortable answers related to what we have been doing and what needs to be changed (prior to incorporating principles of EBP). Bothe suggests that rather than chastising ourselves, we keep in mind that we must always be seeking new and more current means of practicing (2010). The following are some suggested affirmations that may help:

- I do the best I can with the information I have.
- As my knowledge changes, my practices change.

- It's about being better tomorrow rather than defending what I do today. (Bothe, 2010)

The EBP is a continuous process within which we must reevaluate and adjust practices accordingly when new evidence presents itself, and when working with new clients. Think of the process as circular rather than linear. The steps can be summarized in the following way (ASHA, 2006; Dollagan, 2004; Robey, 2004):

1. Ask the *clinical question* that we refer to as PICO (population, intervention, comparison intervention, outcome)
2. Search for *best evidence* available:
   - *Level I:* meta-analysis of more than one well-designed randomized controlled trial (RCT) *or* just one well-designed RCT
   - *Level II:* One well-designed controlled study without randomization *or* one well designed, quasi-experimental study
   - *Level III:* well-designed, nonexperimental studies, such as case studies
   - *Level IV:* expert reporting, consensus, and clinical experience of respected authorities
3. *Evaluate* evidence
4. *Make clinical decisions with input* of client and family members
5. *Implement* clinical decisions
6. *Document* outcomes and evaluate

Where Do We Find the Evidence?

We no longer have to find and read hundreds of articles that are published each year. We currently have infrastructures developed that provide practitioners with high quality systems of information in the form of evidence maps, compendiums of EBP guidelines, and systemic reviews right on the ASHA website (ASHA, 2010).

Systematic reviews form the basis for evidence-based clinical practice guidelines. They are formal assessments of the body of scientific evidence related to a clinical question, and describe the extent to which various diagnostic or treatment approaches are supported by the evidence, but stop short of making specific recommendations for clinical practice. They are useful in helping clinicians make treatment decisions in that, when done properly, they have pulled together and in a systematic way characterized the available evidence on a clinical question. Where do we find systematic reviews?

1. ASHA's Evidence Maps (2015)
2. ASHA/N-CEP's Compendium of Guidelines and Systemic Reviews (2015)
3. Cochrane Collaboration (2015)
4. Campbell Collaboration (2015)
5. What Works Clearinghouse (U.S. Department of Education) (2015)
6. Psychological Database for Brain Impairment Treatment Efficacy
7. speechBITE: Speech Pathology Database for Best Interventions and Treatment Efficacy (2015)
8. Evidence-Based Communication Assessment & Intervention Journal (2015)

When clinical practice guidelines or systematic reviews are not available, current, trustworthy, and/or relevant, one can turn to individual studies to seek evidence to help make treatment decisions. The first place to find individual studies would be an online bibliographic database. For health care studies, the best place to start would be MEDLINE (2015), the world's largest online bibliographic database of health related studies. MEDLINE cites over 12 million articles from 4,000 peer-reviewed journals. ASHA also supplies web tutorials about finding the evidence on their website (http://www.asha.org/Members/ebp/Finding-Evidence-Tutorials/).

Thoughtful and purposeful consideration of evidence that supports specific clinical activities and interventions is just one part of the clinical decision making process (Apel & Scudder, 2005; Lemoncello & Fanning, 2011). These are the evidence questions we can use to support or refute treatments (Lemoncello & Fanning, 2011):

- Efficacy: Is the treatment responsible for the observed outcomes?
- Effectiveness: Are the outcomes robust in the real world?
- Efficiency: Is this the best treatment option for the client?

How Has EBP Changed and Expanded Over the Years?

The most broadly accepted definition of EBP was set by an influential 2001 Institute of Medicine (IOM) report. It reads, EPB is "the integration of best research evidence with clinical expertise and client values" (Institute of Medicine, 2001). The definition has expanded, and we now:

- Consider a broad range of evidence—everything from randomized controlled trials (RCTs) to clinicians' expert observations
- Expand the role of clinical expertise in treatment decision-making, including how practitioners should consider multiple streams of evidence
- Examine how patient values, sociocultural factors, and other patient characteristics influence treatment acceptability and consumer choice, and should inform treatment decisions.

Clinical expertise and client values must play strong roles in EBP because the best-researched treatments will not be work unless clinicians apply them effectively and clients openly accept them (DeAngelis, 2005). Clinical expertise cannot be dismissed. We do have data that show that seasoned clinicians are better equipped than emerging clinicians at choosing and individualizing treatments, not simply choose a treatment because research says it is effective. Client values are the area that still needs a bit of refinement because the term "values" does not necessarily represent cultural variables (De Angelis, 2005).

In an editorial by Hasnain-Wynia (2006), the goals of EBM and patient-centered care are discussed as being sometimes contradictory. Although they both appear to have goals to improve medical practice, they can be at odds with each other. Patient-centered care gained the medical spotlight, with an initial focus on cultural differences. It began by acknowledging and understanding cultural diversity in the clinical setting, as well as validating the beliefs, values, and behaviors of individual patients (Betancourt, 2004). This was termed cultural competence in medicine (CCM). Initially, both EBM and CCM suffered backlash over fears of either clinical stereotyping or cultural stereotyping, and a "cookbook" approach to treatment (Hasnain-Wynia, 2006). Cultural competence in medicine (CCM) has evolved into something more akin to patient-centered care, and uses the foundations of narrative medicine to better understand "the stories" that define each of us. It is these narratives that direct decisions and provide underlying reasons for choosing one course of treatment over another.

The EBP is challenging for both clinicians and researchers. As researchers, we struggle with bridging the gap between research and clinical practice. We need to know how clinicians use research to solve clinical problems and further their own expertise. As clinicians, we struggle to find the research apropos to our specific clients. When we do, the bureaucratic pressures of increased caseloads and paperwork demands compete for time. Some of the barriers to using EBP include time limitations, lack of knowledge, and inadequate administrative support (Chabon & Lemoncello, 2010; Lemoncello & Fanning, 2011).

Using EBP in School-Based Practice

Moore-Brown suggests a variety of reasons for incorporating EBP in our speech therapy programs (2005). First, *accountability* is important for helping students meet instructional standards. *Due process* is met by using evidence that helps make our work legally defensible. In addition, *administrative challenges, satisfaction levels of teachers, and concerns of home caregivers* can best be met with evidence. Finally, following standards in the field enhances our own sense of *professionalism.*

Here are some common-sense recommendations for gathering evidence and implementing EBP:

1. Collect journal articles, clinical studies, and testimonials from other experts and organize this information by therapy approach.
2. Gather your own evidence by writing task analyses, measuring outcomes after specific periods of time, and analyzing progress.
3. Be very specific about behaviors to be measured and treatment variables such as stimuli, trials, feedback, prompts, and so forth.
4. Present your findings at state and national conferences, as well as staff development meetings at the local level.
5. Create networking groups for gathering evidence

3. PRACTICE-BASED EVIDENCE (PBE)

What Is PBE?

PBE is a procedure for gathering good-quality data from everyday, routine clinical practice. It has been described as high-quality scientific evidence that is refined and implemented in a variety of real-world settings (Wambaugh, 2007). The practitioner becomes the active scientist who poses the clinical questions and collects the data (Apel, 1999). The PBE has also been referred to as *internal evidence,* or clinical expertise (Coppens & Hungerford, 2011). The PBE complements, and does not compete with EBP. It is rational and theory driven. Two of the most important components of PBE are to evaluate outcomes and share the findings (Lemoncello & Fanning, 2011). Public policy continues to urge the improvement of measurement techniques as they relate to pressures about increased accountability with medicine and all other areas of clinical practice.

Although EBP was adopted and is required as a method for enhancing clinical and research practices, significant challenges remain unmet as they relate to infusion of these practices into daily practices (ASHA, 2005; Chabon et al., 2011). The intention of EBP is to guide all clinical decisions, from assessment through intervention; however, most often EBP research emphasizes treatment evaluation data (Lemoncello & Ness, 2013). Practice-based evidence complements EBP by focusing on methods to evaluate and document treatment outcomes. Practice-based evidence is a reasonable complement, and not a replacement, to evidence-based practice. It encourages practitioners, within their role as clinical scientist, to pose questions and collect data for the purpose of evaluative decision-making of intervention techniques (Apel, 1999).

One model for PBE was proposed by Lemoncello and Fanning (2011), and is called the PBE 1-2-3 Model.

1. Develop and formulate the clinical question, long-term goals, short-term objectives, and the data collection plan.
2. Implement the targets, and collect data.
3. Evaluate client progress, make necessary changes, and answer the clinical question.

Why We Use PBE

EBP movements have become associated with an awareness of the need to develop more practice-based evidence. PBE encourages us to design, implement, and evaluate our own clinical practices. When we gather, analyze, and share high-quality data, we offer additional support through PBE to complement and support EBP (Lomoncello & Ness, 2013). Until recently, our work has focused on how to get evidence into practice—to address a perceived evidence-to-practice gap and encourage practitioners to use evidence. This discussion recognizes an alternative problem—a gap between the practice and the science, with a need to develop practice-based evidence (Green, 2008).

Its use is recommended when high-quality research evidence that pertains to an individual client is lacking or conflicting. We use all methods to guide our practice decisions, including levels of evidence that may not provide empirical support, but do provide theoretical and rational support. Ultimately, we are following EBP guidelines when we use our clinical expertise to guide our treatment decisions by balancing client values and preferences with a theoretically based intervention approach (Lemoncello & Ness, 2013; Ylvisaker et al., 2002).

Within the field of medicine, generalism is a type of complex intervention, as well as a professional philosophy of practice described as expertise in whole person treatment (Reeve J., Irving G., & Dowrick C. , 2011). It is not surprising to learn that generalism often lacks the evidence base, and so practice-based evidence is suggested for filling the practice-to-research gap.

What Are PBE Methodologies?

Lemoncello and Ness propose two PBE methodologies to evaluate our everyday practices:

SCED using the multiple baseline design, and case studies with control data. Both of these methods may be used to systematically develop, implement, and evaluate treatment (Lemoncello & Fanning, 2011).

We begin our assessment process using our clinical expertise to ultimately align individualized and functional goals with our client's values and preferences. Treatment plans should be selected with the highest quality available evidence. When evidence to support practices is not available, the clinician needs to engage in PBE and consider using both quantitative and qualitative methods to collect multiple *layers of data,* and thus provide the answers to the three essential clinical questions (Chabon, Morris, & Lemoncello, 2011; Lemoncello and Ness, 2013).

- *Treatment data:* behavioral response tracking, representing immediate response to intervention (Is the client responding to intervention?)
- *Generalization data:* application of learning to a variety of untrained examples or contexts (Is the change functional?)
- *Control data:* behavior that is not expected to change as a result of intervention (Is the treatment responsible for the observed change?)

The first two layers of data, treatment data and generalization data, are critical for demonstrating the real and functional impact of our therapy programs and intervention choices (Lemoncello & Ness, 2013). The third level of data, control data, will strengthen the evidence within PBE. However, it represents the most difficult aspect of data collection in our clinical settings. For a more detailed discussion, please refer to Olswang and Bain's abstract about clinical data collection (1994).

Research in our field that is conducted with single-subject experimental designs has gained popularity because it incorporates *repeated measurement,* which is more easily implemented within the confines of clinical practice (Wambaugh, 2007). Repeated or on-going measurement is an essential component of our practice routines, because it becomes part of our treatment accountability, as well as the documentation of treatment effects. Assessment is not something that happens merely at the beginning and end of a treatment protocol, but occurs throughout. It becomes the evidence that our work is making a difference. We sometimes collect this evidence through the use of *probes,* specific behaviors that are measured periodically at the beginning or end of our treatment session. During probes, no feedback or cues are given, which is the essential difference between treatment and probing.

Our role as clinical scientist is not complete until we share the data with clients, families, peers, and administrators. As we do that, we are validating the importance of the evidence we have created, and reinforcing the efficacy of our chosen interventions. We need to present our findings in articles or presentations at the local, state, and national levels (Lemoncello & Ness, 2013; Rosenbaum, 2005).

The Practice-Based Arena

One of the best explanations about the importance of practice-based arenas is stated by Westfall, Mold, and Fagnan (2007), who refer to the *blue highway,* and the need to increase the use of practice-based research and evidence to better serve the people living on those highways. Education and health care are tightly knit. They share legislation, similar problems, and solutions, and are both closely related to economic development and growth of a country (Blakemore & Herrendorf, 2009; Psacharopoulos & Patrinos, 2004)

The transfer of new knowledge to the clinical/educational arena has the potential to be translational, as well as transformational.

A translational school-based speech/language therapy program is, in fact, a practice-based educational arena. As such, it becomes the ideal platform for the identification, dissemination, and integration of new knowledge to take place. In order for the educational context to be considered translational, application vehicles need to be developed for transferring knowledge to practice, increasing accessibility through information-dissemination, helping professionals develop into active recipients of staff development, and developing strategies that will ultimately benefit students (Papir-Bernstein, 1995, 2012b). Staff development is one application vehicle, the success of which is influenced by individual and organizational variables such as attitudes about leadership, learning, and commitment (Westfall, Mold, & Fagnan, 2007).

4. TRANSLATIONAL RESEARCH (TR)

A.R.T.: Before It Had a Name

Several years ago, and following decades of discussions and debates related to the state of our profession, my lifelong friend and colleague Robert Goldfarb invited me to contribute to his book about translational research in our field (Goldfarb, 2012). My subsequent research for the two essays I contributed uncovered some interesting findings about my life's work. I was amazed to discover that so much of what I had been doing years earlier was now driven by science, had a strong research presence, and actually had names: translational research, the practice-based educational arena, knowledge management, information design, tacit versus explicit knowledge, and the Scholarship of Teaching and Learning (SoTL).

Definition of TR

One of the most comprehensive definitions of translational research states that it seeks to improve the health of the public by integrating the research that starts in the laboratory with patient needs and population-based research (Kent, 2012; Rubio et al., 2010). For that reason, TR is considered multidirectional and dynamic. In 2006, the question, "what is translational research" was asked and answered in one of ASHA's Academics & Research E-newsletters. Although translational research *does* refer to the process of research moving from lab to practice, it also refers to the process of current treatment stimulating new investigations (ASHA, 2006; Papir-Bernstein, 2012a).

According to the Center for Clinical and Translational Sciences, translational research includes two areas of translation (The University of Texas Health Science Center at Houston, 2008). One is the process of applying discoveries generated from lab research to the development of studies in humans. The second concerns research directed at enhancing the adoption of best practices in the community. Different stakeholders look at distinct aspects of the translational process, which is why the definition of translational research (TR) remains somewhat controversial and unclear. In academia, TR represents a desire to test novel ideas and hopefully turn them into useful clinical applications. For practitioners, TR will hopefully accelerate the capture of research benefits and close the gap between what we know and how we practice (Parks & Disis, 2004). In spite of the differences, the definition should unify the expectations of all involved, but especially the ultimate beneficiaries—the clients, and their medical or clinical outcomes.

How Did Translational Research Evolve?

Translational research (sometimes called outcomes research or clinical research) has evolved over the years as a result of time, practice, and the expansion of the translational continuum. The types or phases of translation are usually represented as *T-phases*, and research institutions have described these phases as interacting on a linear as well as circular plane. Woolf describes why the term itself conjures up different meanings to different professionals (Papir-Bernstein, 2012a; Woolf, 2008). Initially, the term "translational research" was thought of as movement in one direction (from bench to bedside). The newer model expands the number of T-phases from two to four, or sometimes five, and emphasizes the importance of bidirectionality and overall interaction throughout the phases (Papir-Bernstein, 2012a).

The Clinical Research Roundtable at the Institute of Medicine convened for the first time in June 2000. As a result of those deliberations, two major categories of obstacles or *translational blocks* (Sung et al., 2003) relating to the clinical research environment were identified. The first block impeded the translation of a scientific discovery into a clinical study (T1), and the second impeded the translation of a clinical study into clinical practice and decision making about patient care (T2) (Papir-Bernstein, 2012a). At that time, additional challenges were identified, and these included enhancing public participation in clinical research, as well as increasing staff development efforts and workforce training (Sung et al., 2003).

What This All Means

Traditionally, research and practice have coexisted in independent spheres with practitioners focused on the implementation of programs that affect individual behavior, and researchers focused on the development and testing of theory. Evidence-based practice (EBP), practice-based evidence, and translational research have attempted to unite these three worlds. Although advances have been made, there is a continued need to find mechanisms that enable a seamless connection between knowledge generation and application. In the next chapter, I propose methodologies that build on the traditions of knowledge systems, information design, narratives, and intuition, as necessary, bridging mechanisms between research and practice.

REFLECTIVE SUMMATIVE QUESTIONS

1. How has science impacted your thoughts about research in our field?
2. How comfortable are you with the process of researching and evaluating evidence?
3. What might be some implications if EBP levels, similar to those from Healthcare Design Academy, were implemented in our field?
4. How do you experience the PICO process in your clinical studies or practice?
5. What recommendations might you offer to ASHA for improving their compendiums of EBP guidelines and systemic reviews on their website?
6. Which aspects of PBE can potentially create the most challenging barriers to implementation?

REFERENCES

American Speech-Language-Hearing Association. (n.d.). *Evidenced-based practice.* Retrieved October 3, 2015, from https://www.asha.org/members/ebp

American Speech-Language-Hearing Association. (n.d.). *Web tutorials about finding the evidence.* Retrieved November 2, 2015, from http://www.asha.org/Members/ebp/Finding-Evidence-Tutorials/

American Speech-Language-Hearing Association. (2005). *Evidence-based practice in communication disorders* [Position statement]. Retrieved October 15, 2012, from http://www.asha.org/policy doi:10.1044/policy.PS2005-00221

American Speech-Language-Hearing Association. (2006). *Introduction to evidence-based practice.* Available from http://www.asha.org

American Speech-Language-Hearing Association. (2006). What is translational research? *Access Academics and Research.* Retrieved from http://www.asha.org/academic/questions/translational-research.htm

American Speech-Language-Hearing Association. (2010). *Introduction to evidence-based practice.* Retrieved from http://www.asha.org/Members/ebp/intro.htm

ASHA's Evidence Maps. (2011–2015). Retrieved from http://www.ncepmaps.org

ASHA/N-CEP's Compendium of guidelines and systematic reviews. (2015). Retrieved from http://www.asha.org/members/ebp/compendium

Apel, K. (1999). Checks and balances: Keeping the science in our profession. *Language, Speech, and Hearing Services in Schools, 30,* 98–107.

Apel, K., & Scudder, R. (March, 2005). *Evidence-based practice.* Excerpts from a presentation to the 2005 Annual CAPSCD Conference, Scottsdale AZ.

Bain, B. A., & Dollaghan, C. A. (1991). Treatment efficacy forum: The notion of clinically significant change. *Language, Speech, and Hearing Services in Schools, 22,* 264–270

Berguer, R. (2004). The evidence thing. *Annals of Vascular Surgery, 18,* 265–270.

Betancourt, J.R. (2004). Cultural competence-marginal or mainstream movement. *New England Journal of Medicine, 351*(10), 951–953.

Beveridge, W.I.B. (1950). *The art of science.* New York, NY: WW Norton.

Blakemore, A., & Herrendorf, B. (2009). Economic growth: The importance of education and technological development. *Productivity and Prosperity Project,* 1–31. Retrieved from http://wpcarey.asu.edu/sites/default/files/uploads/research/competitiveness-prosperity-research/Blakemore.pdf

Bothe, A.K. (2010). Evidence-based practice for the real world: Thoughts on clinical education in communication disorders. ASHA *Perspectives on Administration and Supervision, 20*, 100–105.

Bury, T., & Mead, J. (1998). *Evidence-based health-care: A practice guide for therapists*. Newton, MA: Butterworth-Heinemann.

Campbell Collaboration online library. (2015). Retrieved from http://www.campbellcollaboration.org/library.php

Chabon, S., Morris, J., & Lemoncello, R. (2011). An ethical context for evidence-based decision making: Obligation not an option. *Seminars in Speech and Language, 32*, 298–308.

Cochrane Collaboration. (2015). Retrieved from http://www.thecochranelibrary.com

Coppens, P., & Hungerford, S. (2011, November). *(Re-)conceptualizing the "clinical expertise" component of evidence-based practice*. Poster session presented at ASHA Convention, San Diego, CA.

Costello, J. M. (1979). Clinician and researchers: A necessary dichotomy? *Journal of the National Student Speech and Hearing Association, 7*, 6–26.

Crilly, M. (2001). Evidence based bloodletting. *British Medical Journal, 322*, 854.

DeAngelis, T. (2005, March). Shaping evidence-based practice. *American Psychological Association Monitor on Psychology, 36*(3), 26–27. Retrieved from http://www.apa.org/monitor/mar05/shaping.aspx

Dollaghan, C. (2004). Evidence-based practice: Not all evidence is created equal. *The Newsletter of the Illinois Speech-Language Hearing Association*, pp. 8–9. Retrieved from http://www.ishail.org/evidence-based-practice

Duchan, J. (2002). What do you know about your profession's history? And why is it important? *The ASHA Leader*. Retrieved from http://www.asha.org/Publications/leader/2002/021224/021224a.htm

Education for All Handicapped Children's Act of 1975 (PL 94-142). Retrieved from https://www2.ed.gov/about/offices/list/osers/idea35/history/index_pg10.html

Evidence-Based Communication Assessment and Intervention (EBCAI) Journal. (2015). Retrieved from http://www.informaworld.com/EBCAI

Evidence-Based Medicine Working Group. (1992). Evidence-based medicine: A new approach to teaching the practice of medicine. *Journal of the American Medical Association, 268*, 2420–2425.

Fischer, J. (2009). *Toward evidence-based practice: Variations on a theme*. Chicago, IL: Lyceum Books.

Galland, L. (1997). *The four pillars of healing*. New York, NY: Random House.

Gilgun, J. F. (2005). The four cornerstones of evidence-based practice in social work. *Research on Social Work Practice, 15*, 52–61.

Goldfarb, R. (Ed.). (2012). *Translational speech-language pathology and audiology*. San Diego, CA: Plural.

Goldstein, B., & Washington, P. S. (2001). An initial investigation of phonological patterns in typically developing 4-year-old Spanish–English bilingual children. *Language, Speech, and Hearing Services in Schools, 32*, 153–164.

Green L.W. (2008). Making research relevant: If it is an evidence-based practice, where's the practice-based evidence? *Family Practice, 14*, 20–24.

Hamilton, D.K. (2003). The four levels of evidence-based practice. *Healthcare Design*. Retrieved from https://www.healthcaredesignmagazine.com/article/four-levels-evidence-based-practice

Hasnain-Wynia, R. (2006). Is evidence-based medicine patient-centered and is patient-centered care evidence-based? *Health Services Research, 41*(1), 1–8.

Hayes, S. C., Barlow, D. H., & Nelson-Gray, R. O. (1999). *The scientist practitioner: Research and accountability in the age of managed care* (2nd ed.). Needham Heights, MA: Allyn & Bacon.

Holland, A. L. (1998). Some guidelines for bridging the research-practice gap in adult communication disorders. *Topics in Language Disorders, 18*(2), 49–57.

Institute of Medicine. (2001). *Crossing the quality chasm: A new health system for the 21st century*. Washington DC: Institute of Medicine. Retrieved from http://www.nationalacademies.org/hmd/~/media/Files/ReportFiles/2001/Crossing-the-Quality-Chasm/QualityChasm2001report brief.pdf

Ioannidis, J. (2005). Why most research findings are false. *PLOS Medicine, 2*(8), 124. Retrieved from http://journals.plos.org/plosmedicine/article?id=10.1371/journal.pmed.0020124

Johnson, G. (1995). *Fire in the mind: Science, faith and the search for order*. New York, NY: Knopf.

Johnston, J., & Pennypacker, H. (1980). *Strategies and tactics of human behavioral research*. Hillsdale, NJ: Lawrence Erlbaum Associates.

Kennedy, C. (2004). *Single-case designs for educational research*. New York, NY: Pearson.

Kent, R. (2012). Models and concepts of translational research. In R. Goldfarb (Ed.), *Translational Speech-Language Pathology and Audiology*. San Diego, CA: Plural.

Lemoncello, R., & Fanning, J. L. (2011, November). *Practice-based evidence: Strategies for generating your own evidence*. Paper presented at the Annual Convention of the American Speech-Language-Hearing Association, San Diego, CA.

Lemoncello, R., & Ness, B. (2013). Evidence-based practice and practice-based evidence applied to adult, medical speech-language pathology. *ASHA SIG 15 Perspectives on Gerontology, 18*, 14–26.

Malec, J. F. (2009). Ethical and evidence-based practice in brain injury rehabilitation. *Neuropsychological Rehabilitation, 19*, 790–806.

Malkin J. (1992). *Creating healing environments for special patient populations*. New York, NY: Van Nostrand Reinhold.

Medawar, P. (1984). *The limits of science*. New York, NY: Harper & Row.

Medline (National Institutes of Health). (2015). Retrieved from http://www.nim.nih.gov

Meline, T. (2010). *A research primer for communication sciences and disorders*. New York, NY: Pearson.

Meline, T., & Paradiso, T. (2003). Evidence-based practice in schools: Evaluating research and reducing barriers. *Language, Speech, and Hearing Services in Schools, 34*, 273–283.

Meline, T., & Wang, B. (2004). Effect-size reporting practices in AJSLP and other ASHA journals 1999 to 2003. *American Journal of Speech-Language Pathology, 13*, 202.

Moore-Brown, B. (2005). How evidence-based practice is impacting school services. California *Speech-Language-Hearing Association (CSHA) Magazine, 34*(3), 14.

Olswang, L. B., & Bain, B. (1994). Data collection: Monitoring children's treatment program. *American Journal of Speech-Language Pathology, 3*(3), 55–66.

Papir-Bernstein, W. (1995, November). *Supervision for the 21st century: Facilitating self-directed professional growth*. Presented at ASHA Mini-Seminar, Los Angeles, CA.

Papir-Bernstein, W. (2012a). The artistry of practice-based evidence (PBE): One practitioner's path—Part I. In R. Goldfarb (Ed.), *Translational speech-language pathology and audiology* (pp. 51–57). San Diego, CA: Plural.

Papir-Bernstein, W. (2012b). The artistry of practice-based evidence (PBE): One practitioner's path—Part II. In R. Goldfarb (Ed.), *Translational speech-language pathology and audiology* (pp. 83–89). San Diego, CA: Plural.

Parks, M., & Disis, M. (2004). Conflicts of interest in translational research. *Journal of Translational Medicine, 2*, 28. Retrieved from https://translational-medicine.biomedcentral.com/articles/10.1186/1479-5876-2-28

Perkins, W. (1986). Functions and malfunctions of theories. *ASHA, 28*, 31–33.

Popper, K. (1968). *The logic of scientific discovery*. New York, NY: Harper & Row.

Psacharopoulos, G., & Patrinos, H. (2004). Returns to investment in education: A further update. *Education Economics. 12*(2), 111–134.

Psychological Database for Brain Impairment Treatment Efficacy. (2015). Retrieved from http://www.psycbite.com

Reeve J., Irving G., & Dowrick C. (2011). Can generalism help revive the primary healthcare vision? *Journal of the Royal Society of Medicine, 14*, 395–400.

Richards, S. B., Taylor, R. L., Ramasamy, R., & Richards, R. Y. (1999). *Single-subject research: Applications in educational and clinical settings*. Belmont, CA: Wadsworth Group/Thomson Learning.

Ringel, R. L. (1972). The clinician and the researcher: An artificial dichotomy. *Asha, 14*, 351–353.

Robey, R. (2004). A five-phase model for clinical outcome research. *Journal of Communication. Disorders, 37*(5), 401–411.

Rosenbaum, P. (2005). From research to clinical practice: Considerations in moving research into people's hands. Personal reflections that may be useful to others. *Pediatric Rehabilitation, 8*, 165–171.

Rubio, D., Schoenbaum, E., Lee, L., Schteingart, D., Marantz, P. R., Anderson, K. E., . . . Esposito, K. (2010). Defining translational research: Implications for training. *Academic Medicine, 85,* 470–475.

Russell, J. F. (2013). If a job is worth doing, it is worth doing twice. *Nature. 496,* 7.

Sackett, D. L., Straus, S. E., Richardson, W. S., Rosenberg, W., & Haynes, R. B. (2000). *Evidence-based medicine: How to practice and teach EBM* (2nd ed.). Edinburgh, UK: Churchill Livingstone.

Self, T., & Apel, K. (2002, November). *Evidence-based practices: Backing up clinical services with research.* Presentation at the ASHA Convention, Atlanta, GA.

Siegel, G., & Ingham, R. (1987). Theory and science in communication disorders. *Journal of Speech and Hearing Disorders, 52,* 99–104.

Silver, N. (2015). *The signal and the noise.* New York, NY: The Penguin Group.

Sommer R. (1969). *Personal space: The behavioral basis of design.* Englewood Cliffs N.J.: Prentice-Hall.

speechBITE: Speech Pathology Database for Best Interventions and Treatment Efficacy. (2015). Retrieved from http://www.speechbite.com

Straus, S. E., Richardson, W. S., Glasziou, P., & Haynes, R. B. (2005). *Evidence-based medicine: How to practice and teach EBM* (3rd ed.). Edinburgh, UK: Churchill Livingstone.

Sudsawad, P. (2005). Concepts in clinical scholarship —A conceptual framework to increase usability of outcome research for evidence-based practice. *American Journal of Occupational Therapy, 59,* 351–355.

Sung, N., Crowley, W., Genel, M., Salber, P., Sandy, L., Sherwood, L. M., . . . Rimoin, D.

(2003). Central challenges facing the national clinical research enterprise. *Journal of the American Medical Association, 289*(10), 1278–1287.

Tavris, C. (2003). Mind games: Psychological warfare between therapists and scientists. *Chronicle Review, 49,* B7–B9.

The University of Texas Health Science Center at Houston. (2008). Retrieved October 3, 2015, from https://www.uth.edu/ccts/translational-research.htm

Wambaugh, J. (2007). Improved effects of word-retrieval treatments subsequent to the addition of the orthographic form. *Aphasiology, 21*(6), 632–642.

Wambaugh, J., & Bain, B. (2002). Make research methods an integral part of your clinical practice. *The ASHA Leader, 7*(21), 1, 10–12.

Weinberg, F. (1993). The history of the stethoscope. *Canadian Physician. 39,* 2223–2224.

Westfall, J., Mold, J., & Fagnan, L. (2007). Practice-based research: Blue highways on the NIH road map. *Journal of the American Medical Association, 297*(4), 403–406.

What Works Clearinghouse (U.S. Department of Education). (2015). Retrieved from http://www.ies.ed,.gov/ncee/wwc

Woolf, S. (2008). The meaning of translational research and why it matters. *Journal of the American Medical Association, 299*(2), 211–213.

Ylvisaker, M., Coelho, C., Kennedy, M., Sohlberg, M. M., Turkstra, L., Avery, J., & Yorkston, K. (2002). Reflections on evidence-based practice and rational clinical decision making. *Journal of Medical Speech-Language Pathology, 10*(3), 15–33.

Yong, E. (2012). Replication studies: Bad copy. *Nature, 485,* 298–300.

CHAPTER 2

Acquisition and Advancement of Knowledge

1. KNOWLEDGE SYSTEMS

What Is Knowledge?

As students and practitioners of speech-language pathology, we are inundated with professional information and strategies for facilitating knowledge acquisition. Much has been written in our field, as well as in the fields of education and psychology, about dimensions of knowledge and knowledge frameworks. The study of knowledge dates back to Plato and Aristotle, but modern day credit is given to cognitive explorers such as management expert Peter Drucker (1993), philosopher Michael Polanyi (1958), and organizational learning guru Ikujiro Nonaka (1994).

Knowledge is dynamic and ever changing, but how does knowledge differ from information? Until people use information, it is not knowledge. Knowledge is information-in-action. We are overloaded with information, but rarely do we feel that way about knowledge. Information overload can leave us feeling overwhelmed and paralyzed. Knowledge, on the other hand, enables and facilitates motivation and confidence (O'Dell & Grayson, 1998).

One knowledge framework categorizes knowledge into three states: individual, organizational, and structural. *Individual knowledge* is in the minds of the employees, whereas *organizational knowledge* is the learning that occurs within a group or a division of the company. The *structural knowledge* relates to the manuals and codes that are embedded in the bricks and mortar of an organization (Edvinsson & Malone, 1997; Silver, 2012).

Knowledge Creation and Knowledge Action

One conceptual framework that is useful for facilitating the implementation of research knowledge is *The Knowledge-to-Action* (KTA) Process Framework (Graham et al., 2006). The two components within the KTA framework are *knowledge creation* and *knowledge action,* and each component can be represented by several phases (Sudsawad, 2007). Graham et al. (2006) states the following about the model:

- The KTA process is complex and dynamic, with no finite boundaries between components or phases.
- Phases may occur sequentially or simultaneously.
- Knowledge is both research-based and experiential.
- The framework emphasizes the collaboration between knowledge producers and knowledge users.

- The framework is useful for facilitating the implementation of research knowledge by practitioners, clients, policymakers, and the public.

Knowledge creation consists of three phases: *inquiry, synthesis,* and the *creation of tools/products.* The action cycle begins with identification of a problem and relevant knowledge needed to solve it. Barriers need to be assessed, knowledge must be adapted to local context, and a strategy plan is then developed and executed. The impact and effectiveness of the strategies must be monitored and evaluated so that new needs can be anticipated and knowledge continues to be used in changing environments as time passes (Graham et al., 2006; Sudsawad, 2007).

A second conceptual framework for knowledge implementation used in health services is called *The Promoting Action on Research Implementation in Health Services* (PARIHS) (Rycroft-Malone, 2004). According to this model, there are three core elements that will facilitate the implementation of research into practice: the *nature of evidence,* the *context* in which the research is used, and the *facilitation of research implementation.* Whereas each element has equal importance in predicting implementation success, each one is positioned on a continuum from low to high based upon a range of conditions.

Evidence is a combination of research, practitioner experience, client experience, and local information. *Context* refers to the setting or environment and is often the most complex to evaluate because it can include many variables, such as, decision-making processes, patterns of leadership and authority, organizational culture and attitudes, physical environment, operational boundaries, vehicles for monitoring and feedback, and various types of resources and supports. The purpose of *facilitation* is to ease the research implementation process. Facilitation is accomplished through sharing and influencing attitudes, habits, skills, ways of working, and ways of thinking (Rycroft-Malone et al., 2002; Stetler, 2001).

The investigation of knowledge and its components may help to identify training and information needs, as well as help us gain a better understand of its application and management in clinical practice. Although knowledge classifications and their management are studied in fields such as philosophy and anthropology, we receive little formal training in this area. Yet, it is expected that we would develop sophisticated knowledge management skills—for example, within the obvious application of evidence-based practice—in order to practice effectively. The very process of evidence-based practice (EBP) closely mirrors the steps in the knowledge management process, because EBP is simply a systematic method of identifying and managing specific gaps in knowledge (Sensky, 2002).

2. KNOWLEDGE MANAGEMENT AND INFORMATION DESIGN

How Did Knowledge Management Get Started?

Knowledge Management (KM) is the quest to understand how organizations can derive value from the knowledge base that exists throughout their organizational practices. The scientific discipline called Knowledge Management (KM) has existed since the early 1990s and is currently utilized in fields of public health, information sciences, and business administration. Knowledge management efforts lead to successful knowledge creation, dissemination, and application, improvement of performance, an increase in innovative thinking, and greater integration of newly learned information (Addicott, McGivern, & Ferlie, 2006).

In 1999, the term *personal knowledge management* was introduced, (as distinguished from *organizational knowledge management*), which refers to the management of knowledge at the individual level (Papir-Bernstein, 2012). KM is the systemic process of identifying, capturing, and transferring knowledge that people can use in order to improve. With good knowledge, we can make better decisions faster, take action that is more intelligent, energize innovation, and improve motivation (O'Dell & Grayson, 1998).

Knowledge, in any of its manifestations, *is one of the most valuable commodities* that we have. The knowledge systems of local communities are sometimes referred to as Indigenous Knowledge systems (IK). The IK systems are dynamic, and encompass the skills, experiences, and insights of individual community members, as influenced by internal creativity and experimentation on the part of those individuals. The IK contrasts with the knowledge systems generated by universities and research institutions, and yet is often the basis for local-level decision-making in agriculture, health care, food preparation, and education. In fact, our Western thought process about the scientific method sometimes results in IK being undervalued, because it lacks scientific validation (Papir-Bernstein, 2012; Sahai, 1998).

More recently, there has been a trend toward acknowledging aspects of knowledge that are less structured, "softer," and cannot easily be captured and codified. The KM has gone through a major shift as it has become recognized as both a *people* as well as *object* process (Swan, Newell, Scarborough, & Hislop 1999). There are numerous viewing lenses, and most result in the viewpoint that knowledge contains duality of meanings (Hildreth & Kimble, 2002). The terms *formal and informal* have been used, with formal knowledge found in books and training courses. Informal knowledge is used to describe the process for creating those books, documents, or courses (Conklin, 1996). Another distinction is between the *know-how* and the *know-what*. Both may be considered core competencies, but the more elusive *know-how* is a particular ability to put the *know-what* into practice (Seely Brown & Duguid, 1998). *Soft knowledge and hard knowledge* is yet another distinction. Hard knowledge is codifiable into tools and techniques, whereas soft knowledge includes internalized experiences and cultural knowledge embedded in practice (Hildreth, Wright, & Kimble, 1999; vonKrogh, 1998). Soft knowledge is communicated through "war stories" (Orr, 1997).

Information Design: From Data to Wisdom

The process of structuring data, presenting information, and leading to integrative knowledge and eventual evaluative wisdom is called Information Design (Shedroff, 2000). Information Design specialists focus on four areas: data, information, knowledge, and wisdom. *We are all involved with the process of information design, because we all move information from data to wisdom.* Data are discovered, researched, and gathered. They involve sensory input without much reflection. The problem is that data easily overwhelm us, and most users of information are not terribly interested in seeing the raw data. One model has been proposed by organization systems experts Bellinger, Castro, and Mills (2010). They explain it with the following four steps:

1. *Data* are represented by a number, a fact, or a statement with no relationship to anything else.
2. *Information* contains an implicit understanding that a *relationship* of some sort exists. We build with information, much the same way we do with legos.

3. *Knowledge* contains *patterns* of understanding
4. *Wisdom* embodies a complete system for understanding the fundamental concepts and *principles* embodied within the knowledge system, which actually define the knowledge being what it is.

How can we translate this into something meaningful for us, as speech-language pathologists? Knowledge begins life as data, which ultimately must get transformed to information, then to knowledge and ultimately to wisdom. Raw data, when given relevance, purpose, or context, become informational. Unless information is used on the job to increase levels of competence, it has little value (Pascarella, 1997). Some type of intervention program (staff and program development) is usually needed to interpret and "mine" the information, to shape it to knowledge and eventually to wisdom, or to intuition based on experience (Tobin, 1997). Bellinger summarized it beautifully when he drew an analogy to data-information-knowledge-wisdom from the Tao quotation, "Find the path, enter the path, travel the path, become the path." We must first find and build on the data, develop the information from the data, isolate the knowledge as we travel through it, and sift through it all, as we ultimately model those enduring truths and become the wisdom (Bellinger et al., 2010; Papir-Bernstein, 2012).

Organization Is Key

Although data can be the building blocks of meaning, there is no context aside from a relationship to other bits of data. In isolation, data can float disconnected and meaningless to the user. In order to make sense, data must be connected and contextualized, made to assume a form, and become converted to information

(Papir-Bernstein, 2012). Its purpose is to change and/or impact someone's perception, behavior, or judgment. *Information* is there to be learned, and learning is a change in behavior due to our experience with information (Ormrod, 1999). The change can be internal or external, but must be observable in some fashion.

Because the amount of information available to us is enormous, information needs to be organized and presented in ways that make sense and can be connected to what is already known. The LATCH principle for organizing information is represented by the following group of organizational strategies: location, alphabet, time, category, and hierarchy (Papir-Bernstein, 2012; Wurman, 1996).

In addition to using organizational strategies, another role that the information design specialist assumes is to structure the information to facilitate its share-ability. *Share-ability*, a term used in experimental psychology, refers to the extent to which information can be communicated to others (Freyd, 1993). Share-ability is highest when there is little loss of fidelity as information moves from person to person. According to Freyd's research, external or written information has the highest level of share-ability.

Barriers and Implementation Strategies

The greatest challenge of *information design* is for the manager or director to build a meaningful experience for the user, and that can only happen if the information is organized, translated /transformed, and presented in a way that gives it meaning. It must make sense. Organization knowledge must in some way be used to accomplish the mission of the organization. The management of such knowledge is the strategies that are utilized to "get the right knowledge to the right people at the right time and helping people share and put information in to action in ways that strive to improve organizational performance" (O'Dell & Grayson, 1998, p. 6).

Most organizations have experienced managing knowledge through their use of organizational strategies. Some of those strategies include organizational websites, communities of practice (CoP), social learning networks, storytelling, expert directories, knowledge fairs, mentors, knowledge repositories, cross-project learning, and after-action reviews, and debriefing sessions (Gupta & Sharma, 2004).

3. TACIT KNOWLEDGE VERSUS EXPLICIT KNOWLEDGE

Two Varieties of Knowledge

One of the key variables we must consider when we think about "the information revolution" relates to knowledge, and how to access and obtain the right information from a variety of resources, and transform it into useful knowledge. Some types of knowledge are more easily communicated than others. One type of knowledge framework distinguishes between *tacit* or *personal knowledge* and *explicit* or *formal knowledge.*

Although many terms have been used to describe knowledge, perhaps the greatest explanations have been made when comparing tacit knowledge and explicit knowledge. Knowledge comes in two varieties, *explicit* and *tacit.* This type of knowledge distinction is viewed on a continuum rather than as a dichotomy. Tacit knowledge lacks conscious awareness. It is held within the minds of individuals, and is difficult to access. Explicit

knowledge is easily structured and is accessible to many. Whereas explicit elements are objective and rational, tacit elements are subjective and experiential (Hildreth & Kimble, 2002; Leonard & Sensiper, 1998).

Explicit knowledge, usually formal and more easily codified, comes in the form of books, papers, written media, and policy manuals. *Tacit knowledge,* more informal and uncodified, can be found in people's heads, experiences, and memories. It is communicated best through shared or described experiences. Tacit knowledge is deeply personal and consists more of experience, perceptions, insights, and know-how that can be more easily implied than directly expressed. Because tacit knowledge is so individualized and experiential, it is more difficult to document (O'Dell & Grayson, 1998).

Most *explicit knowledge is technical and academic.* It is information that is formally shared through teaching and in textbooks, and requires a level of academic understanding that is acquired through formal education and structured study. The vast majority of information shared through our academic culture is formal, technical, and explicit. Whereas *tacit knowledge* represents internalized and often unconscious knowledge, *explicit knowledge* represents information that is consciously held in mental focus, and can be easily communicated to others (Alavi & Leidner 2001). Tacit knowledge, which is difficult to quantify, is thought of as *know-how,* as opposed to *know-what* (the facts), *know-why* (the science), or *know-who* (the networking) (Papir-Bernstein, 2012).

Nonaka has said that learning is created at the intersection between tacit knowledge and explicit knowledge (1994). Nonaka and Hirotaka (1995) describe a detailed relationship between these two types of knowledge systems. Whereas both explicit and tacit knowledge are valuable to any organization, one of the most vital responsibilities is to protect and enhance the sources of tacit knowledge by creating a culture of knowledge sharing, knowledge exchanges, and knowledge conversion (Nonaka & Hirotaka, 1995; Papir-Bernstein, 2012).

Tacit knowledge is based more upon common sense, intuition, and wisdom, and explicit knowledge is based on academic learning. Our goal is to become a knowledge-enabled professional who is able to acquire, measure, teach, share, and apply both types of knowledge.

Knowledge Conversion

Nonaka offers another explanation of tacit and explicit knowledge (1991). He says they interact with each other in a complementary way to form the *knowledge conversion* process. The sharing of tacit knowledge can take place only through joint activities, interpersonal interactions, and physical proximity (Leonard & Sensiper, 1998; Nonaka, 1991). This process consists of four stages: socialization, externalization, combination, and internalization (Hildreth & Kimble, 2002; Nonaka, 1991).

1. *Socialization* is the first step, and transfers tacit knowledge between individuals through observation, imitation, and practice. This process is sometimes referred to as brainstorming.
2. *Externalization* translates tacit knowledge into explicit procedures and documents via dialogue, collecting reflection, and the use of analogy and metaphor.
3. *Combination* reconfigures explicit knowledge through combining, sorting and categorizing information, and spreading it throughout the organization. This is sometimes referred to as "best practices."
4. *Internalization* is the final step, and links explicit knowledge with individual tacit

knowledge, as knowledge creation and sharing have become part of the organization's culture.

Consider the master craftsman with years of experience who cannot explain the principles behind what he knows. He can, however, teach someone by taking them through a period of apprenticeship. Tacit knowledge is like that: it is rarely articulated directly; however, the learner develops his tacit knowledge by becoming immersed in practice under guidance of a mentor.

It is apparent that learning occurs through interaction and experience with our environment, and involves both harder explicit and softer tacit aspects of knowledge. One of the key attributes of knowledge is that it exists in people's heads, and only becomes information once it has been translated to paper or the digital world. We still struggle with ways to share the softer or tacit type of knowledge.

The Application of Tacit Knowledge

There is little question that tacit knowledge does augment a person's academic learning, allowing her or him to integrate and implement into everyday functional situations (Wagner & Sternberg, 1987). Tacit learning is experiential, but not necessarily based upon experience of that field. It is reported that close to 90% of the knowledge in any organization is embedded within the minds of the individual workers, and has not been recorded into official training or professional development documents. It stays largely invisible, and is lost to the organization when these people move on, unless better use is made of these largely under-tapped resources of creative, and often unchallenged, workers who are eager to apply their knowledge (Bonner, 2000; Lee, 2000; Wah, 1999).

Tacit knowledge plays a key role in the overall quality of commitment and knowledge application within an organization. The value of knowledge is increased when it has a focus on core values. Our tacit knowledge is a combination of our use of resources and information, as well as our skills and experiences (Goffee & Jones, 2000; Quinn, Anderson & Finkelstein, 1996).

Tacit knowledge is acquired and applied in unique ways. We all use different perspectives to problem-solve, and have different ways of thinking about information and its connection to our lives. Smith defines tacit knowledge as practical know-how based on practice, and acquired by personal experience and individual expertise (2001). Explicit knowledge is academic knowledge or "know-what." Tacit knowledge tends to involve more creative, insightful, and divergent thinking, whereas explicit knowledge is logical, fact based, probable, and primarily based on convergent thinking. Knowledge-sharing strategies are also different—explicit knowledge is more easily shared through formal structures, and tacit knowledge through storytelling, narratives, and use of metaphors.

Integrating Tacit with Explicit Knowledge

Nonaka and Smith described four patterns of knowledge integration within organizations (Nonaka, 1991; Smith, 2001):

1. *Moving from tacit to tacit:* learn from mentors and peers by observing, imitating and practicing with others
2. *Moving from explicit to explicit:* transforming one type of explicit knowledge into another new one, like using data to write reports
3. *Moving from tacit to explicit:* recording brainstorming discussions and innovations into a manual, and then creating a new product from the content

4. *Moving from explicit to tacit:* reframing explicit knowledge using another person's lens or perspective so that knowledge can be understood and internalized by others.

Knowledge gets transformed and utilized most efficiently when people trust and cooperate with each other. Knowledge assets must be recognized, acknowledged, and rewarded when shared (Wah, 1999). Whereas technology plays a key role in collecting and codifying knowledge for distribution, it does not get knowledge out of someone's head (Smith, 2001; Wah, 1999). Only people can do that. One proposed strategy has been called *action research*. Kurt Lewin, a professor at MIT, first coined the term *action research* in 1944 (Lewin, 1946). He described it as a reflective process of progressive problem solving by teams of people as a way of improving how problems were solved or issues addressed. Action research involves participation in the research process as part of an existing organization for the purpose of improving the knowledge of the environments within which they practice, or the *community of practice*.

Through our intervention and the process of *action research*, we begin to generate *practice-based evidence*. Action research is simple a process whereby people work collaboratively while learning and tackling a clinical problem. We acquire new knowledge through actual practice, critical reflection on the process, and evaluation of outcomes (Edmondstone, 2011). Action research is a dynamic model, involving critical reflection and continual learning that translates tacit knowledge into explicit learning. It offers an approach that enables us to develop evidence from everyday practice, which we know is called practice-based evidence (Green, 2008). We can use *action research* principles to assess impact of care, to identify opportunities to enhance expertise, to evaluate impact of change, and to generate practice-based evidence.

4. KNOWLEDGE TRANSLATION AND RESEARCH UTILIZATION

Knowledge Translation Strategies and Barriers

Knowledge translation (KT) is defined as the exchange, syntheses, and application of knowledge from the researchers through the users (Sudsawad, 2007). KT was coined by the Canadian Institutes of Health Research (CIHR) in 2000 and has gone through a number of expansions and elaborations since that time (Canadian Institutes of Health Research, 2005). One of the significant adaptations was by the World Health Organization (WHO). The WHO defined KT as the synthesis, exchange, and application of knowledge by relevant stakeholders to accelerate the benefits of global and local innovation in strengthening health systems and improving people's health (World Health Organization, 2005).

How does the knowledge translation process begin? It usually begins with a focus to *create, identify, collect*, and *organize* internal knowledge and best practices. The final stages in the process continue with the ultimate target to *share, adapt*, and *use* those practices to new situations (O'Dell & Grayson, 1998). The KT encompasses all steps between the creation of new knowledge and its application for the purpose of yielding positive outcomes for society, and attempts to bring together the creators and the users of knowledge (Grimshaw Eccles, Lavis, Hill, & Squires, 2012; Sudsawad, 2007).

The growing interest in KT coincides with our engagement with the evidence-based practice (EBP) approach. The KT is one of the latest attempts to integrate research into practice, with six levels of interactions and collaborations that facilitate the process (Canadian Istitutes of Health Research, 2005; World Health Organization, 2005).

1. Defining research questions and methodologies
2. Conducting research
3. Publishing research
4. Placing research findings within other knowledge bases
5. Making decisions and taking action informed by research
6. Influencing other research based upon knowledge use

The ultimate goal of knowledge translation is the application and utilization of research knowledge, resulting in positive outcomes for the health and well-being of the public (Canadian Institutes of Health Research, 2004; National Institute on Disability and Rehabilitation Research, 2005; Sudsawad, 2007). The area of knowledge utilization embraces a number of subtopics such as information dissemination, research utilization, innovation diffusion, and organizational change (Backer, 1993). The interest in these topics has intensified in recent years as a result of increased recognition of the difficulties in moving research to implementation, and theory to practice (Sudsawad, 2007). How do we bridge that theory-practice gap? It begins with research reviews and ends with a change in the practitioner's beliefs and behaviors about implementing this new knowledge (Cook & Odon, 2013).

What are the *barriers to transfer of knowledge and thus implementation of best practices*? There are three overwhelming barriers that showed up time and time again in the research. The number one biggest barrier to the transfer was *ignorance* on the part of both ends, the *source* and the *recipient* (Szulanski, 1994). Neither one knew that the other had knowledge he needed, or even that he needed it. The second biggest barrier was the *absorptive capacity of the recipient*, which related to time or money resources and practical details for implementation. Interestingly enough, this second barrier emerged even if the manager knew a better practice existed. The third barrier was the *lack of a relationship* between the source and recipient of the knowledge. This manifested as absence of personal connection that impacted credibility and the justification of listening to or helping one another (O'Dell & Grayson, 1998).

The Implementation of Research

We need a conceptual framework to guide the design, implementation, and diffusion of research-based evidence. In order for an evidence-based practice approach to be successfully implemented, information (evidence) from research must be utilized by practitioners to support their practice. There are barriers that prevent this from happening, such as relevance of research studies to practice, and the meaningfulness of clinical questions that are studied in the research (Morrow-Bradley & Elliot, 1986; Sudsawed, 2005). Research in the fields of physical therapy, occupational therapy, and nursing confirmed that research findings can be difficult to interpret and understand as they relate to implications for practice (Law & Baum, 1998; Sudsawed, 2005).

How can we increase utilization of research? One approach that has been suggested is by Sudsawad in an article written for the practice of occupational therapy (2005). The Diffusion of Innovations Theory was presented as a means for specifying desirable characteristics of research information that may increase utilization for evidence-based practice. Research may be viewed as an innovation simply because it conveys new ideas through its findings (Sudsawed, 2005).

Diffusion of Innovations (DOI) is a theory that seeks to explain how, why, and, at what rate new ideas and technology spread through cultures. Everett Rogers, a professor of communication studies, popularized the theory in his book *Diffusion of Innovations*, The book was first published in 1962, and is now in its fifth edition (2003). Diffusion of Innovation is one of the oldest social science theories. According to the theory, characteristics of an innovation can either facilitate or impede its adoption rate.

There are five main factors that influence adoption of an innovation (Rogers, 2003).

1. *Relative Advantage*, or the degree to which the innovation is seen as better (more desirable and favorable) than what came before
2. *Compatibility*, or how consistent the innovation is with the values, needs, and past experiences of the potential adopters
3. *Complexity*, or how difficult the innovation is to understand and use
4. *Triability*, or the extent to which the innovation can be tested before a commitment to use it is made
5. *Observability*, or the extent to which the innovation provides tangible and visible results

According to this theory, utilization of research for EBP should increase if it represents better evidence than before, is consistent with practitioners needs and values, is easy to understand, can be easily implemented, and demonstrates outcomes (Sudsawed, 2005). The consideration of *social validity, ecological validity, and clinical significance* will facilitate the potential for creating a relative advantage through an increase of desirable characteristics.

All three types of validity originated within the field of psychology. The *social validity* relates to society and consumers of a service (Wolf, 1978). Social validity is a broad concept that includes anyone who is affected by the intervention process and outcome. *Ecological validity* is the functional relationship between performance on a test and performance in a variety of real-world settings (Sbordone, 1996). *Clinical significance* is the magnitude of change that impacts the client's life, and must extend past trivial changes or merely statistically significant changes to those that are practical and meaningful (Kazdin & Kendall, 1998).

Transferring Research Into Practice

Evidence for practice is still dominated by experimental designs, yet a number of sources are challenging this model of knowledge translation as sometimes simply a way of informing policy makers (and thus practitioners) what "should" be done (Gabbay & le May, 2011). As we critically examine our practice based on the principles of participatory research and action learning, we are addressing the practice-evidence gap and supporting the translation of practice into an evidence base (Montgomery, 2006). Perhaps the very term evidence-based might be changed to *evidence-informed plus a touch of wisdom* (Glasziou, 2005).

One of the overriding challenges still facing clinicians today is finding a model that facilitates transfer of research results directly into their practice to solve a clinical problem. One such no-nonsense model was proposed by Law in 2000.

1. Clearly identify the clinical problem.
2. Ensure that you have adequate knowledge to read and critically analyze the research studies.
3. Gather information from research studies about this problem.

4. Decide if a research article or review is relevant to the clinical problem.
5. Summarize the information so that it can be easily used in your practice.
6. Define the expected outcomes for the children and their families.
7. Provide education and training to implement the suggested change in practice.
8. Evaluate the practice change and modify if necessary.

Valuing Knowledge

Knowledge matters, and the internal transfer of best practices in organizations from one part to another matters even more. We need to build value in the transfer of knowledge, and this is done via benchmarking. External benchmarking involves looking outside of your organization; however, the most powerful scenario happens with *internal benchmarking*—looking inside of your own organization and transferring best practices (O'Dell & Grayson, 1998). Only then can we be certain that sharing of knowledge is valued within your organization. Benchmarking is the process of finding and adapting best practices, and then through a knowledge management system, we are able to spread and generalize the practices. Without a KM system, the spread of best practices may only happen through a stroke of luck, or casual communications.

We are more familiar with using "benchmark" as a noun, meaning some type of measure of performance. We know that the developments of short-term objectives or benchmarks are a step in the process of developing Individualized Education Programs (IEPs) for school-aged students with special education needs (Blosser, 2011; Moore & Montgomery, 2008). However "benchmark" used as a verb means " . . . to systematically identify and learn from best practices, internal or external, in order to improve your own performance" (O'Dell & Grayson, 1998, p. xiv).

---

5. THE SIGNIFICANCE OF NARRATIVES AND EXPERIENTIAL STORIES

What Are Stories?

Throughout history, people have passed their accumulated experiences, knowledge, and wisdom on to future generations by telling stories. We have come to learn that this type of "know-how" and experiential knowledge is our *tacit knowledge*. Most of our "know-what" is more easily communicated through written means, because it is more explicit and easier to communicate that way. Our pursuits of ways to communicate our self-knowledge, both tacit and explicit, "are timeless, endless, and relentless" (Smith, 2001, p. 311).

Storytelling is one of the oldest healing and teaching practices found in cultures throughout time. Our stories braid together imagination and memory, and define us. They remind us that we are of this world both individually and collectively. Stories connect us. They serve as a mirror, and we hold them up to reflect what we believe. You recognize your story in my story. Our stories shape and dissect us, and finally piece us back together again. Stories make us whole. They connect us with the world and describe our relationships (Bausch, 1984).

Stories create an *emotional transformation*, a type of *alchemical reaction* to a described circumstance. We identify and are stirred, sometimes even stirred, to action or to change.

It is not surprising that historical societies and university library collections now house personal diaries and journals as part of their archives (http://www.storycatcher.net). *The Legacy Project* was created as a national volunteer effort to preserve the letters and emails of active duty soldiers so that their stories will continue to be honored.

Since the beginning of recorded time, telling stories, listening to stories, and creating stories together, has been part of who we are and what we do within our professional context. The performance space for each story is created by the story's context, the storyteller's context, and the story's audience. Stories come to life through engagement and interaction with the listener (Wilson, 2007). A story is a type of map that helps people steer and navigate. A story belongs to all of us, but sometimes only those of us who have the courage to listen will be moved (Shlain, 1998). We need imagination to tell a story, and empathy to receive it. It can take us anywhere we want to go, and as we listen, we remember. They help us imagine the kind of world we would like to bring into being. Stories provide invitations for others to enter the world as we see it, to experience life as we have, to connect with moments that have shaped us (Atkinson, 1995). Stories provide the path for us to ride our experiences to a place of *wisdom.*

A story can articulate a vision and *create a compelling sense of community*. When you talk in "stories" you are talking in a person's "native language" (Denning, 2011). Whereas crafting a good story is one thing, getting people to listen is another. Other mediums may present nothing more than *background noise* (Silver, 2012). Nora Ephron (2006) has her own unique way of explaining why we like to tell stories. In the chapter called, "Everything Is Copy," she explained that when you slip on a banana peel, people laugh at you, but when you tell people you slipped on a banana peel, it's your laugh, and you become the hero rather than the victim of the joke (p.102).

Stories Give Life to Our Tacit Knowledge

> ### A.R.T.: Universal Feedback
>
> Years ago, I read a book entitled, *The New American Spirituality,* by Elizabeth Lesser (1999). Lesser talks about *The World Bank,* a brilliant universal feedback system that is working at all times and offering information about how we should and should not function in the world. We get little messages about our wisdom or folly, and all we have to do is pay attention and listen. When we use this feedback, we feel happy and confident, and the world begins to seem like a bank or reservoir of richness that never runs out of messages (Lesser, 1999; Trungpa, 2004).

That is how I think about the stories through which I communicate tacit knowledge to students and practitioners. I know when a story is born, and I know when it needs to be told. When a story pops into my head, I recount that experience as it relates to the content I am covering in one of my courses. Quite recently, one of my students surprised me by insisting on the importance of telling these stories to others who might not be in my classes—an inspiring moment for sure.

Clarissa Pinkola Estes, internationally recognized scholar and Jungian psychoanalyst, implores us to revisit the importance of communicating tacit knowledge by reawakening our natural instincts and deeply personal channels of ageless wisdom that have been put to sleep by our compliancy to the drone of society's demands. She does this through stories and her masterful storytelling style. Estes (1995) explains that stories and myths connect us more closely with our instinctual nature, or our "inner hearing," especially when we are able to get inside of the stories rather than letting them remain outside of ourselves (p. 20). She tells us that the ancients believed the ear had three separate pathways of hearing. The first pathway heard the mundane conversations of the world, and the second was responsive to learning and art. The third pathway exists, she says, " . . . so the soul itself might hear guidance and gain knowledge while here on earth" (p. 22).

Narrative Competence

Narrative is considered a form of discourse used for retelling past stories, whether recalled or imagined (Nelson, Moskowitz, & Steiner, 2008). It develops throughout childhood and is part of all adult language speakers' linguistic competence. Stories have the ability to transfer the experience of the narrator to the audience as if they are being experienced for the first time, as a type of *time travel* (Clark, 1996; Labov, 1997). Stories and the telling of narratives are of ancient origin, and were used to communicate myths and illustrate historical points. Over the centuries, they serve as entertainment, self-identify, memory, and meaning-making (Bell, 2002; Conle, 2000). One of the reasons that narratives are so powerful is due to the fact that it is easier for the human mind to remember and make decisions on the basis of stories with meaning, than to remember strings of data (Lakoff, 2004).

Jacqueline Hinckley, in her groundbreaking book about the use of narratives in our field, describes narratives as a technique for exploring "the difficult-to-define moments of interaction within the clinical process that have the power to become incorporated into our life stories" (Hinckley, 2008, p. x). Within these moments are the lessons, that when shared, become unique learning opportunities for others. Oprah Winfrey so beautifully described how stories impact hearts and spirits as they connect people by dropping threads of light into a person's consciousness (Winfrey, 2014). Ephron also talks about the "deep rapture" moment when an image turns from ordinary to fantastic, as seemingly ordinary events transform into the fantastic and magical (2006, p.122; Chabon, 2000).

Despite the technological advances in our field, we can sometimes lack the capacities to recognize our clients' plights, and to extend empathy, honor their stories, and join their journey with honesty and courage (Charon, 2001; Morris, 1998). Narrative competence enables us to practice with empathy, reflection, professionalism, and trustworthiness (Charon, 1993). Our narrative abilities help us to absorb, interpret, and respond to stories told by our clients, as well as facilitate the development of telling our own. After all the science that underpins clinical practice is said and done, practitioners and their clients make sense of the world by way of the narratives they recite and hear (Elwyn & Gwyn, 1999). Communication styles have a profound impact on both client satisfaction and clinical outcomes (Levenstein, 1984; Stewart, Brown, Weston, McWhinney, McWilliam, & Freeman., 1995).

Other fields, as well, have embraced the integration of narrative knowledge, such as nursing, history, philosophy, sociology, law, and government (Polkinghorne, 1988; Swenson & Sims, 2000). We use narrative knowledge to understand the significance of stories through cognitive, symbolic, and affective means (Charon, 2001). Narratives deal with experiences rather than propositions, and lead to local understandings about one situation between two persons. Narrative knowledge (NK) is different than logico-scientific (LSK) knowledge. Whereas LSK illuminates the universally true by transcending the particular, NK illuminates the universally true by revealing the particular (Charon, 2001). Reflective narration illuminates aspects of the client's story as well as your own.

Narrative discourse has been described as "someone telling someone else that something has happened" (Smith, 1981, p. 228). There are three questions that should be asked and answered: Who is telling it? Who is hearing it? and Why is it being told? With narrative competence, local authority often replaces master authority. The meaning is extracted collaboratively by both storyteller and story receiver, and both are involved with doing the work.

Narrative practices require active and authentic engagement of one person with another. Through narrative practice, our most potent therapeutic instrument is the self, which is attuned to the client through active engagement, on the side of our client through compassion, and available to the client through reflection (Charon, 2001; Novack et al., 1997). As reflective practitioners, we can identify and interpret our own emotional responses to our clients and make sense of their journeys. This ability requires disciplined and consistent reflection on one's practice (Connelly, 1999). To profess is, in and of itself, a narrative act (Charon, 2001).

Narrative Medicine

Narrative competence in medicine has been described as "the ability to acknowledge, absorb, interpret, and act on the stories and plights of others" (Charon, 2001, p. 1897). Narrative competence allows for reflection and exploration, and bridges the divide within four central situations: patient, self, colleagues, and society. It allows for the professional to more easily reach and join their patients in their struggles, acknowledge kinship with other professionals, recognize their own personal journeys, and provide information to the public.

Narrative medicine is informed by patient-centered care, and directs us to look broadly at the client and the disorder for the purpose of working effectively with patients, colleagues, and the public (Laine & Davidoff, 1996). Narrative medicine suggests that research, teaching, and practice can be made more effective with narrative competence (Charon, 2001; Hurwitz, 2000). Narrative mastery teaches us about client experience and gives us insight into our own interior development, and strengthens reflection, self-awareness, and perspective taking (Hunter, Charon, & Coulehan, 1995; Winckler, 2000).

Why Incorporate Narratives?

That which we preserve in our stories determines what we believe is possible in the world (Baldwin, 2005). Something happens with the power and practice of story—its voice calls us to remember our true selves, and we invite the "Storycatchers" (Baldwin, 2005). What is a Storycatcher? Baldwin tells us:

> It is the time of the Storycatcher. It is the time when those who understand the value of story and practice the art of connection have an essential role to play. Storycatchers come whenever we are in crisis to remind us who we are. Storycatchers entice our best tales out of us: they turn with a leading question, a waiting ear, and their full attention. In return, we speak . . . we write . . . and we are heart. Storycatchers invite the stories we most need to come forward into the community. Storycatchers know that the mix of wisdom and wit and wonder that spills into the room in story space will reconnect us. Come into these stories and listen for what will connect your life, and mine, and ours. (p. xii)

In her book, Baldwin (2005) discusses aspects of stories that honor the importance of telling them.

1. Stories mark generational reference points for millions of personal experiences.

2. Stories both reveal and conceal information.
3. Stories create social networks and social spaces that allow us to experience us as more similar than different.
4. Stories are as independent as their tellers, and come with a will to survive.
5. Stories can change the words, so if we don't like something we need to put our stories into place.
6. Stories can turn strangers into friends, and are our real legacy.
7. Stories are about ordinary people who are offering extraordinary gifts.

As we operationalize storytelling, we are bridging the gap between the data and the people who need to understand it. Stories convey the most important information to the intended audience, to the people who need the knowledge. The telling of personal stories enhances engagement and accelerates the use of innovation. It has been described as a moral imperative to share our stories and request the stories of others, and to elicit stories any way that we can in order to learn what they mean and their clinical implications (Holland et al., 2016).

Wisdom involves tacit knowledge, knowledge that often cannot be directly taught, but is rather acquired or inferred through a range of life experiences in a variety of contexts (Haidt, 2006). Tacit knowledge is deeply personal and communicated best through shared experiences. It consists of perceptions, insights, and know-how that are more easily implied than directly expressed. It is often deeply internalized and even unconscious. Stories avail the tacit knowledge, and provide an accessible path. They are concerned with feelings, not simply with actions. They are absorbing, engaging, and encouraging of a holistic approach to practice by facilitating reflection and discussion.

REFLECTIVE SUMMATIVE QUESTIONS

1. Describe one of your most productive contexts for knowledge-creation.
2. How has tacit knowledge been conveyed through your training program or work setting?
3. What strategies have helped you avoid becoming a *knowledge junkyard* when you have felt *information overload?*
4. What is the most valuable knowledge, explicit and tacit, that you have acquired about our field?
5. In your training or professional life, when do you feel wise?
6. Describe your "mindlines" and how they have developed.
7. Think of a story from your life that holds significance with regard to your career choice.

REFERENCES

Addicott, R., McGivern, G., & Ferlie, E. (2006). Networks, organizational learning and knowledge management. *Public Money and Management, 26*(2), 87–94.

Alavi, M., & Leidner, D. (2001). Review: Knowledge management and knowledge management systems: Conceptual foundations and research issues. *MIS Quarterly, 25*(1), 107–136.

Atkinson, R. (1995). *The gift of stories: Practical and spiritual applications of autobiography, life stories, and personal mythmaking.* Westport, CT: Bergin & Garvey.

Backer, T. E. (1993). Information alchemy: Transforming information through knowledge utilization. *Journal of the American Society for Information Science, 44,* 217–221.

Baldwin, C. (2005). *Storycatcher: Making sense of our lives through the power and practice of story.* Novato, CA: The New World Library.

Bausch, W. J. (1984). *Storytelling: Imagination and faith.* Mystic, CT: Twenty-Third Publications.

Bell, J. S. (2002). Narrative inquiry: More than just telling stories. *TESOL Quarterly, 36*(2), 207–213.

Bellinger G, Castro, D., & Mills, A. (2010). *Data, information, knowledge, and wisdom.* Retrieved from http://www.systems-thinking.org

Blosser, J. (2011). *School programs in speech-language pathology: Organization and service delivery.* San Diego, CA: Plural.

Bonner, D. (2000). Knowledge: From theory to practice to golden opportunity. *American Society for Training and Development,* 12–13.

Canadian Institutes of Health Research. (2005). *About knowledge translation.* Retrieved September 9, 2012, from http://www.cihr-irsc.gc.ca/e/29418.html

Chabon, M. (2000). *The amazing adventures of kavalier and clay.* New York, NY: Random House.

Charon R. (1993). The narrative road to empathy. In H. Spiro, M. G. M. Curnen, E. Peschel, & D. St. James (Eds.), *Empathy and the practice of medicine: Beyond pills and the scalpel* (pp.147–159). New Haven, CT: Yale University Press.

Charon, R. (2001). The patient-physician relationship: Narrative medicine: A model for empathy, reflection, profession and trust. *JAMA, 286*(15), 1897–1902.

Clark, H. H. (1996). *Using language.* Cambridge, UK: Cambridge University Press.

Conklin, E. J. (1996). *Designing organizational memory: Preserving intellectual assets in a knowledge economy.* Glebe Creek, MD: CogNexus Institute. Available from: http://cognexus.org/dom.pdf [Site visited 25th September 2002]

Conle, C. (2000). Narrative inquiry: Research tool and medium for professional development. *European Journal of Teacher Education, 23*(1), 49–62.

Connelly J. (1999). Being in the present moment: Developing the capacity for mindfulness in medicine. *Academic Medicine, 74,* 420–424.

Cook, B. G., & Odon, S. L. (2013). Evidence-based practices and implementation science in special education. *Exceptional Children, 79,* 135–144.

Denning, S. (2011). *The leader's guide to storytelling: Mastering the art and discipline of business narrative.* San Francisco, CA: Jossey-Bass.

Drucker, P. (1993). *Post-Capitalist society.* Newton, MA: Butterworth Heinemann.

Edmonstone, J. (2011). *Action learning in health care—a practical handbook.* London, UK: Radcliffe.

Edvinsson, L., & Malone, M. (1997). *Intellectual capital: Realizing your company's true value by finding its hidden brainpower.* New York, NY: Harper Business.

Elwyn, G., & Gwyn, R. (1999). Stories we hear and stories we tell: Analyzing talk in clinical practice. *British Medical Journal, 318*(7177), 186–188.

Ephron, N. (2006). *I feel bad about my neck and other thoughts on being a woman.* New York, NY: Vintage Books.

Estes, C. P. (1995). *Women who run with the wolves.* New York, NY: Ballantine Books.

Freyd, J. (1993). Five hunches about perceptual processes and dynamic representations. In D. Meyer & S. Kornblum (Eds.), *Attention and performance XIV: Synergies in experimental psychology, artificial intelligence and cognitive neuroscience.* Cambridge, MA: MIT Press.

Gabbay, J., & le May, A. (2011). *Practice-based evidence for healthcare: Clinical mindlines.* New York, NY: Routledge.

Glasziou, P. (2005). Evidence based medicine: Does it make a difference? *British Medical Journal, 330*(7482), 92–94.

Goffee, R., & Jones, G. (2000). Why should anyone be led by you? *Harvard Business Review,* pp. 62–70.

Graham, I. D., Logan, J., Harrison, M. B., Straus, S. E., Tetroe, J., Caswell, W., & Robinson, N. (2006). Lost in knowledge translation: Time for a map? *Journal of Continuing Education in the Health Professions, 26,* 13–24.

Grimshaw, J. M., Eccles, M. P., Lavis, J. N., Hill, S. J., & Squires, J. E. (2012). Knowledge translation of research findings. *Implementation Science, 7,* 50.

Green L.W. (2008). Making research relevant: If it is an evidence-based practice, where's the practice-based evidence? *Family Practice, 14,* 20–24.

Gupta, J. N. D., & Sharma, S. K. (2004). *Creating knowledge based organizations.* Boston, MA: Idea Group.

Haidt, J. (2006). *The happiness hypothesis.* New York, NY: Basic Books.

Hildreth, P., & Kimble, C. (2002). The duality of knowledge. *Information Research, 8* (1). Paper no. 142. Available from http://InformationR.n et/ir/8-1/paper142.html

Hildreth, P., Wright, P., & Kimble, C. (1999). Knowledge management: Are we missing something? In *Proceedings of the 4th UKAIS Conference* (pp. 347–356). London, UK: McGraw Hill.

Hinckley, J. J. (2008). *Narrative-based practice in speech-language pathology.* San Diego: CA: Plural.

Holland, A., Cohen-Schneider, R. Kagan, A. et al. (2016, November). *The moral implications for conversational and personal narratives in aphasia treatment: Implications and applications.* Presentation at ASHA Conference, Philadelphia, PA.

Hunter, K. M., Charon, R., Coulehan, J. L. (1995). The study of literature in medical education. *Academic Medicine: Journal of the Association of American Medical Colleges, 70*(9), 787–794.

Hurwitz, B. (2000). Narrative and the practice of medicine. *The Lancet, 356,* 2086–2089.

Kazdin, A. E., & Kendall, P. C. (1998). Current progress and future plans for developing effective treatments: Comments and perspectives. *Journal of Clinical Child Psychology, 27,* 217–226.

Labov, W. (1997). Some further steps in narrative analysis. *Journal of Narrative and Life History, 7,* 395-415.

Laine, C., & Davidoff, F. (1996). Patient-centered medicine: A professional evolution. *Journal of American Medical Association. 275:* 152-156.

Lakoff, G. (2004). *Don't think of an elephant: Know your values and frame the debate.* White River Junction, VT: Chelsea Green.

Law, M. (2000). Strategies for implementing evidence-based practice in early intervention. *Infants and Young Children, 13,* 32–40.

Law, M., & Baum, C. (1998). Evidence-based practice occupational therapy. *Canadian Journal of Occupational Therapy, 65,* 131–135.

Lee, J. (2000). Knowledge management: The intellectual revolution. *IIE Solutions, 32*(10), 34–37.

Lesser, E. (1999). *The new American spirituality.* New York, NY: Random House.

Levenstein, J. H. (1984). The patient-centered general practice consultation. *South African Family Practice, 5,* 276–282.

Lewin, K. (1946). Action research and minority problems. *Journal of Social Issues 2*(4), 34–46. Retrieved from http://onlinelibrary.wiley.com/doi/10.1111/j.1540-4560.1946.tb02295.x/abstract

Leonard, D., & Sensiper, S. (1998). The role of tacit knowledge in group innovation. *California Management Review, 40*(3), 112–132.

Montgomery, K. (2006). *How doctors think: Clinical judgment and the practice of medicine.* New York, NY: Oxford University Press.

Moore, B. J., & Montgomery, J. K. (2008). *Making a difference for America's children: Speech-language pathologists in public schools.* Eau Claire, WI: Thinking Publications.

Morris, D. M. (1998). *Illness and culture in the postmodern age.* Berkeley, CA: University of California Press.

Morrow-Bradley, C., & Elliot, R. (1986).Utilization of psychotherapy research by practicing psychotherapists. *American Psychologist, 41,* 188–197.

National Institute on Disability and Rehabilitation Research, (2005). *Long-range plan for fiscal years 2005–2009.* Retrieved September 23, 2009, from http://www.ed.gov/legislation/FedRegister/other/2006-1/021506d.pdf

Nelson, K., Moskowitz, D., & Steiner, H. (2008). Narration and vividness as measures of event specificity in autobiographical memory. *Discourse Processes, 45,* 195–209.

Nonaka, I. (1991) The knowledge creating company. *Harvard Business Review, 69,* 96–104.

Nonaka, I. (1994). A dynamic theory of organizational knowledge creation. *Organizational Science, 5*(1), 14–37.

Nonako, I., & Hirotaka, T. (1995). *The knowledge creating company: How Japanese companies create the dynamics of innovation.* Oxford, UK: Oxford University Press.

Novack, D. H., Suchman, A. L., Clark, W., Epstein, R. M., Najberg, E., & Kaplan, C. (1997). Calibrating the physician: Personal awareness and effective patient care. Working Group on Promoting Physician Personal Awareness, American Academy on Physician and Patient. *JAMA, 278,* 502–509.

O'Dell, C., & Grayson, C. J. (1998). *If only we knew what we know: The transfer of internal knowledge and best practice.* New York, NY: The Free Press.

Ormrod, J. E. (1999). *Human learning* (3rd ed.). Englewood Cliffs, NJ: Prentice Hall.

Orr, J. (1997) *Talking about machines: An ethnography of a modern job.* Ithaca, NY: Cornell University Press.

Papir-Bernstein, W. (2012). The artistry of practice-based evidence (PBE): One practitioner's path—Part I. In R. Goldfarb (Ed.), *Translational speech-language pathology and audiology.* San Diego, CA: Plural.

Pascarella, P. (1997, October). Harnessing knowledge. *Management Review,* pp. 37–40.

Polkinghorne, D. E. (1988). *Narrative knowing and the human sciences.* Albany, NY: State University of New York Press.

Polyani, M. (1958). *Personal knowledge.* Chicago, IL: University of Chicago Press.

Quinn, J. B., Anderson, T., & Finkelstein, S. (1996). Managing professional intellect: Making the most of the best. *Harvard Business Review,* pp. 71–80.

Rogers, E. (2003). *Diffusion of innovations* (5th ed.). New York, NY: Simon and Shuster.

Rycroft-Malone, J. (2004). The PARIHS framework: A framework for guiding the implementation of evidence-based practice. *Journal of Nursing Care Quality, 19,* 297–304.

Rycroft-Malone, J., Kitson, A., Harvey, G., McCormack, B., Seers, K., Titchen, A., & Estabrooks, C. (2002). Ingredients for change: Revisiting a conceptual framework. *Quality and Safety in Health Care, 11,* 174–180.

Sahai, S. (1998, August). *Indigenous knowledge is technology: It confers rights on community.* Paper presented at the Conference on Gender and Technology in Asia, Bangkok, Thailand.

Sbordone, R. J. (1996). Ecological validity: Some critical issues for the neuropsychologist. In R. J. Sbordone & C. J. Long (Eds.), *Ecological validity of testing* (pp. 15–41). Delray Beach, FL: GR Press/St. Lucie Press.

Seely Brown, J., & Duguid, P. (1998). Organizing knowledge. *California Management Review, 40*(3), 90–111.

Sensky, T. (2002). Knowledge management. *Advances in Psychiatric Treatment, 8*(5), 387–395.

Sharma, H., & Grover, D. (2004). Knowledge management: A human perspective. In Y. Moon, A. Osman-Gani, K. Shinil, G. Roth, & H. Oh (Eds.), *Human resource development in Asia: Harmony and partnership:* Edited Proceedings of the 3rd Conference of the Asian AHRD Chapter, pp. 50–57). Seoul, Korea: Academy of Human Resource Development.

Shedroff, N. (2000). Information interaction design: A unified field theory of design. In R. Jacobson (Ed.), *Information design.* Cambridge, MA: First MIT Press.

Shlain, L. (1998). *The alphabet versus the goddess: The conflict between word and image.* New York, NY: Viking Press.

Silver, N. (2012). *The Signal and the noise: Why so many predictions fail—but some don't.* New York, NY: Penguin Press.

Smith, E. A. (2001). The role of tacit and explicit knowledge in the workplace. *Journal of Knowledge Management 5*(4), 311–321.

Smith, B. H. (1981). Narrative versions, narrative theories. In W. J. T. Mitchell (Ed.), *On narrative* (p. 228). Chicago, IL: University of Chicago Press.

Stetler, C. B. (2001). Updating the Stetler model of research utilization to facilitate evidence-based practice. *Nursing Outlook, 49,* 272–278.

Stewart, M., Brown, J. B., Weston, W. W., Mc-Whinney, I. R., McWilliam, C. L., & Freeman, T. R.. (1995). *Patient centered medicine: Transforming the clinical method.* Thousand Oaks, CA: Sage.

Sudsawad, P. (2005). A conceptual framework to increase usability of outcome research for evidence-based practice. *American Journal of Occupational Therapy, 59,* 351–356.

Sudsawad, P. (2007). *Knowledge translation: Introduction to models, strategies, and measures.* Austin, TX: Southwest Educational Development Laboratory, National Center for the Dissemination of Disability Research.

Swan, J., Newell, S., Scarborough, H., & Hislop, D. (1999). Knowledge management, innovation networks and networking. *Journal of Knowledge Management, 3(4),* 262–275.

Swenson, M. M., & Sims, S. L. (2000). Toward a narrative-centered curriculum for nurse practitioners. *Journal of Nursing Education, 39,* 109–115.

Szulanski, G. (1994). *Intra-firm transfer of best practices project.* Houston, TX: American Productivity and Quality Center.

Tobin, D. R. (1997). *The Knowledge-enabled organization.* New York, NY: AMACOM.

Trungpa, C. (2004). *The collected works of Chogyam Trungpa* (Vol. 8). Boston, MA: Shambhala.

U.S. Department of Health and Human Services. (2013). *Dissemination and implementation research in health (R01).* Retrieved May 24, 2013, from http://grants.nih.gov/grants/guide/pa-files/PAR-10-038.html

von Krogh, G. (1998). Care in knowledge creation. *California Management Review, 40*(3), 133–153

Wah, L. (,999). Making knowledge stick. *Management Review.* pp. 24–29.

Wagner, R. K., & Sternberg, R. J. (1987). Tacit knowledge in managerial success. *Journal of Business and Psychology,* 303–312.

Wilson, J. (2007). *The performance of practice: Enhancing the repertoire of therapy with children and families.* London, UK: Karnac Books.

Winckler, M. (2000). *The case of Dr. Sachs* (L. Asher, Trans.). New York, NY: Seven Stories Press.

Winfrey, O. (2014). *What I know for sure.* New York, NY: Hearst Communications.

Wolf, M. M. (1978). Social validity: A case for subjective measurement or how applied behavior analysis is finding heart. *Journal of Applied Behavioral Analysis, 11,* 203–214.

World Health Organization. (2005). *Bridging the "know-do" gap: Meeting on knowledge translation in global health.* Retrieved September 25, 2006, from http://www.who.int/kms/WHO_EIP_KMS_2006_2.pdf

Wurman, R. S. (1996). *Information architects.* Zurich, Switzerland: Graphic Press.

CHAPTER 3

Obtainment and Orientation of Wisdom

1. WHAT IS WISDOM?

It Evolves From Knowledge Acquisition

In the world of knowledge management and information design, wisdom is the ultimate level of understanding that evolves from knowledge acquisition (Papir-Bernstein, 2012a). We achieve this state of wisdom when we see enough patterns in our knowledge base that we can synthesize and then use the information in novel ways. Through wisdom and the ability to discern patterns, we are able to take our eyes off the rear-view mirror of our past experiences and predict the future (Aldo de Moor, 2006; Wurman, 2001).

Patterns can be discerned within and throughout all subject matter: goals, communications, information, tasks, and concepts (Aldo de Moor, 2006). Once we have gathered enough patterns and linked them together, we are able to make inferences for interpreting and predicting new uses for the patterns. We see what is missing, and wisdom enables us to create something new (Papir-Bernstein, 2012a; Shedroff, 2000).

Wisdom of Practice

There is a newly acknowledged type of pedagogical scholarship in our field referred to as *wisdom of practice*, largely based upon professional experiences. Such experiences may include personal accounts of change resulting from the implementation of new instructional practices or policies and personal narratives (Papir-Bernstein, 2012b; Weimer, 2011). Our ability to self-reflect, evaluate and interpret knowledge leads to personal growth and the acquisition of wisdom. Wisdom, in this sense, implies a larger vision, and the ability to connect holistically that vision with the well-being of the larger community (Allee, 1997; Papir-Bernstein, 2012b).

The definition of wisdom can be a bit elusive, however, philosophers through the ages have considered the attainment of wisdom to be the goal of human existence (Bruce, 2011a). In earlier chapters, we have discussed how wisdom is different from knowledge in the sense that knowledge is more easily codified and thus passed down from person to person and generation to generation. The acquisition of technical knowledge has little to do with a person's character (Bruce, 2011b). Such is not the case with the acquisition of wisdom. If knowledge comes from *without*, wisdom comes from *within*. Wisdom comes from the mindful application of our daily learning's to our daily actions. You might say that professional wisdom is the ability to apply theory to practice, and model it for others. It becomes a way of life for those professionals who have it.

Wisdom is based upon tacit knowledge, largely internalized and often unconscious (Peterson & Seligman, 2004). Tacit knowledge, which is difficult to quantify, is thought of as *know-how*, as opposed to *know-what* (the facts), *know-why* (the science), or *know-who* (the networking) (Papir-Bernstein, 2012a). Wisdom relates to personal goals and values, is context-specific, and derives from skills acquired throughout life's experience. It allows us to balance priorities, such as the needs of the individual with the demands of bureaucracy. The wise are able to see things from others point of view. Wisdom cannot be directly taught, but it can be illustrated through actions, demonstrated through metaphor, and modeled.

2. SPIRITUALITY

The Conjunction of Spirituality and Health Care

Spirituality is more than simply a buzzword of the times. Today, the term relates to universality and inclusivity rather than religiosity (Spitzform, 2015). It implies more than compassion, mindfulness, and engagement. Medical practitioners and health care providers are infusing elements of spirituality into their clinical routines, as a complement to their professional practice, collaborations, and a support to themselves and their patients and clients (Silverman, 2003).

Spirituality refers to connections we all share, and enhances our ability to be maximally effective and fully present with our hearts as well as with our eyes and ears. Just recently, the term "interspirituality" was introduced to the field of clinical practice in psychology, as akin to and as important as multicultural skills or fluency in languages (Spitzform, 2015).

This section of the book is about the dimension of life that we refer to as spiritual and its place in our field of communication disorders. The conjunction of spirituality and health care is historical, intellectual, and practical because both intersect around human concern and the critical interest we have in health and healing (Cobb, Puchalski, & Rumbold, 2012). The examination of spirituality helps us understand the human capacity for sustaining health, and how we respond to those things that disrupt our health and communicative abilities. It keeps us connected to the *humanity* of those we serve, and informs the maintenance of living traditions of practice and wisdom (Cobb, Puchalski, & Rumbold, 2012).

Today, we sometimes see spirituality on the agenda of journals, conferences, and online continuing education course brochures. However, research in the field that involves spiritual components and care is still in its infancy. Nevertheless, we as practitioners need opportunities to learn about spirituality and develop our skills and capacities to attend to the spirituality of our clients as well as that of our own (Cobb et al., 2012; Hermans, 1988). As stated by Cobb, Puchalski, & Rumbold (2012), "the engagement of spirituality with healthcare can thus be seen as a core strategy for humanizing health care through its focus on inner meaning, approaches to suffering (and loss), and compassionate practice" (p. viii).

Our feelings about the word "spiritual" will influence how we are able to integrate it with our work (Lesser, 1999). Is it mysterious and unexplained? Is it something anti-scientific or anti-intellectual? Is it connected to religion, or antireligion? Is it about the occult? Is it scary and irrational? Spirituality is for many people a way of engaging with the purpose and meaning of human existence. As such, it provides a perspective and orientation to the world, a way of cultivating the mind, thinking about the soul, and a general way of life (Cobb, Puchalski, & Rumbold, 2012). The scientific investigation of spirituality in relationship to health and wellness is still relatively immature, and practitioners need opportunities "to learn about spirituality and develop their skills to attend to the spirituality of patients as well as their own" (Cobb, Puchalski, & Rumbold, 2012, p. viii). We need training, intentional educational programming, inter-professional education and collaborative learning—just for starters.

Spirituality, Health, and Ancient Cultures

New Age and holistic movements associated with complementary and alternative medicine describes the state of well-being as achieved by creating a harmony with mind, body, and spirit. Historically, concepts of health have been as varied as the ancient culture from which they emanate. Ferngren (2012) and Gregory (2012) do an interesting job discussing various universal concepts through the ages and the importance of the spiritual dimension in each one. Some examples are:

- In the Hebrew Bible, health is consistently described in spiritual rather than in medical terms. The term *shalom* was a Hebrew concept that denoted a broad concept of health, and included spiritual well-being.
- In the ancient Greek culture, moral virtue was considered a balance for the elements of the soul when there was a disturbance of

equilibrium. Moderation and self-control guarded individuals against diseases of the soul. Most writers in Greek schools of philosophy used this body-soul analogy.

- From a Buddhist perspective, the Noble Path describes practices for the ideal person with a healthy mind to have wisdom, be moral, demonstrate mental fortitude, and understand the universality of our individual experiences.
- Members of the Taoist tradition believe we are all components of a harmonious universe, and that all aspects of our lives (including health) extend into spiritual realities where bodies and spirits are intertwined and interactive. That perspective in fact defines traditional Chinese health care.

A Humanistic Theory of Spirituality

Van Hooft proposes that the adoption of a humanist theory of spirituality be incorporated with the practice of health care, and include an understanding of the concept of *transcendence,* accepting things we cannot know (2012). Knowledge is the way we structure our world through empirical experiences, conceptual classifications, and scientific explanations. As long as we focus on what is objective, real, and measureable, we are working within the world of productivity and efficient service delivery. However—we are aware of something more, something difficult to define and impossible to measure.

Spiritual but not religious (SBNR), has become a popular acronym used to identify oneself as valuing spiritual growth as a life stance (Cranfill & Mahanna-Boden, 2012). The adaptation of a spiritual life stance sometimes occurs for us when we struggle with issues of how our lives fit with a greater scheme, or questions we have have give rise to new practices, or even when we become moved by experiences and values that reveal new meaning for our lives (Scheurich, 2003; Schulz, 2005)

Spirituality is a subjective experience that exists both within and outside of traditional systems of religion. It relates to the way in which people live their lives and understand its ultimate meaning and value. We all have a longing to see our lives in some larger context, whether the context is family, community, a club, a religious framework, our life's work, or the universe (Hardy, 1979; Hillman, 1996). We long to aspire for something that takes us beyond ourselves, beyond our egos, and gives our actions a sense to worth. Our search for meaning is a primary motivation in our lives (Frankl, 1985; Palmer, 2003).

Dimensions of Spirituality

Two central dimensions to spirituality are *meaningfulness* and *relationship* (Spillers, 2011). Meaningfulness relates to what we believe is our life's purpose and how we find meaning in life events and circumstances. Relationship includes our relationship to nature, others, a higher power, and ourselves (Pesut, 2002).

Helping our clients find meaning in experiences of change and suffering is one of the most compelling reasons to infuse elements of *spirituality and soul* within our therapeutic relationships (Spillers, 2011). A third concept of spirituality is called *communion*, which allows each being, although feeling isolated and solitary, to share a hidden wholeness and interconnection with each other (Spillers, 2011). Dimensions of meaning, self-direction, personal growth, responsibility, and advocacy all may arise from one's spiritual center (Pesut, 2002; Spillers, 2011).

This is fundamentally a spiritual perspective: we have what we need, we already are what we seek, and life is a matter of being what we are rather than trying to become something we are not. Whatever we yearn for is already within us, and our job is to uncover rather than discover. We need to release it from our inner space, rather than seek it outside of ourselves. This principle is exemplified in the *Wizard of Oz*. The tin man already had a heart, the scarecrow his brain, and the lion his courage. Dorothy and Toto had to go through much turmoil to get home, only to find out that they were home all along (Hawley, 1993).

A narrative about the waterfall and the bucket of water may be used to illustrate two types of knowledge and experience (Swinton, 2012). We see a beautiful waterfall, and are struck by its mystery, the sound of the water, the way the light dances, the rainbows, the glistening, the spray. You ask, "What is this thing called waterfall, and what is it made of?" In your attempt to break it down and analyze it, you scoop up some water into a bucket from this magnificent waterfall, and something is lost. The awe is left behind. The experience of water now is quite different. Which is more real, the crashing of the waterfall or the still water in the bucket? Science and health care tend to focus on the bucket, but is it possible to understand the fullness of the human experience by looking only at the more obvious constituent parts? Can spirituality present us with a bridge and help us answer the question, "How do we know what we know?"

Two Knowledge Systems Relevant to Health Care

It is suggested that spirituality is related to a form of knowledge that is different from but connected to scientific knowledge. Two forms of knowledge systems are relevant to health care: *nomothetic* knowledge and *idiographic* knowledge (Hermans, 1988; Swinton, 2012). We need to be reminded that the relationship between the general and the particular is a fundamental property of all scientific thought, and a classic theme as taught by Socrates.

Nomothetic knowledge is gained through the use of the scientific method, and thus must be "falsifiable, replicatable and generalizable" (Swinton, 2012, p. 99). Nomothetic approaches investigate large groups of people to find general laws of behavior through the use of quantitative experimental methods. This mode of knowing affirms the water in the bucket. We see it, we can measure it, and we understand the purpose it serves.

Our second mode of knowing is *idiographic,* and presumes that meaning can be discovered in unique and non-replicable experiences. No two people experience the same event in the same way, and these experiences that are deeply individualized are not often generalized. Idiographic approaches investigate individuals in personal detail to achieve a unique understanding of them through the use of qualitative methods and case studies. Idiographic knowledge alone cannot explain the chemical constituency of water, although it can help one understand the mystery and wonder of the waterfall (Swanton, 2003). A great deal of spirituality (both within and outside of religion) occurs within the realm of idiographic knowledge.

Spiritual Intelligence (SQ)

In the mid-1990s, Daniel Goleman synthesized research from neuroscience and psychology showing how important emotional intelligence (EI or EQ) is related to overall intelligence (1995). Zohar and Marshall talk about the third Q, spiritual intelligence, the intelligence with which we address and solve problems of meaning and value, place our actions and lives in a wider and richer context, express our creativity; sanctify everyday experience; and temper rigid rules with understanding and compassion (2001).

In her book about corporate structures, Zohar describes three distinct but interrelated functional systems of mental operation: mental, emotional, and spiritual. Healthy organizations, like healthy minds, learn to respond and adapt to external stimuli through a union of these three structures (2000). Zohar further delineates a variety of principles that underlie the development of spiritual intelligence:

1. *Self-awareness:* beliefs, values, and motivations
2. *Vision and value:* acting from principles and deep beliefs
3. *Holism:* seeing larger patterns, relationships, and connections
4. *Compassion:* having the quality of "feeling-with" and deep empathy
5. *Celebration of diversity:* valuing everyone's differences and uniqueness
6. *Ability to reframe:* standing back from a situation or problem and seeing the bigger picture or wider context
7. *Sense of vocation:* feeling called upon to serve, to give something back

Spirituality and Speech-Language Pathology

One documented area of research explores the relationship between spirituality and disability (Kahn, 1997; Palmer, 2003; Schulz, 2005; Spillers, 2007). Trauma and illness are often accompanied by a crisis in meaning when major life questions loom large on our universal horizons. As we make way through those questions, we embark on a journey of our soul and get opportunity to experience our interconnectedness with others as well as our differentiation, to experience our own pain, suffering, grief, and sense of loss, as well as to find compassion and renewal (Palmer, 2003; Spillers, 2011).

In Schulz's research about spirituality and disability (2005), she interviewed adults with childhood-onset and adult-onset disabilities. Both groups noted the importance of spirituality in relationship to understanding their disability. The adults with child-onset disabilities saw their disability as the avenue for connection to a higher power and helped them find a sense of purpose and meaning early in their lives. The adults with adult-onset disabilities experienced their disability as a call to awakening the spiritual dimension of their lives. All participants in this study viewed their disabilities as positive because it facilitated growth, resilience, self-reflection, connection, and learning. In essence, their disabilities helped shape their lives and give them greater meaning (Schulz, 2005).

Spirituality has been defined as the innate human need to find meaning in life and in experiences, as well as to connect with something larger than ourselves (Palmer, 2003; Winslow & Wehtje-Winslow, 2007). While alternative health care practices have reintroduced Western health care to the body-mind-spirit perspective for health and healing, spirituality has not yet entered the formal lexicon of speech-language pathologists (Spillers, Bongard, Deplazes, Gerard, & Narveson, 2009).

Whereas religion is about organized beliefs, practices, and rituals, spirituality is broader and considered to be more of an individualized experience (Mathisen et al., 2015). Although other disciplines have conducted research on the role of a person's spiritual experiences as it relates to both treatment of and recovery from disease and disability, we are just getting started (Handzo & Koenig, 2004; Hilsman, 1997; Perez, 2004). In fact, the clinical relevance of spiritual beliefs as they relate to client and clinician perspectives and outcomes across the lifespan has been largely neglected.

Although there is a surge of interest in spirituality in health, education, business, and ethics, there is a very limited array of literature linking spiritual dimensions and SLP clinical services (Bruce, Shields, & Molzahn,

2011; Koenig, King, & Carson, 2012; Spillers, 2011). There is increasing research with regard to spirituality, but much of it pertains to medicine and little is specific to the role of the speech-language pathologist. We do know that there is evidence indicating improved physical, emotional, and mental health outcomes when a holistic and client-centered approach to treatment includes the role of spirituality (Bruce et al. 2011; Mathisen et al., 2015). We also know that unaddressed spiritual needs can interfere with positive treatment outcomes (Perez, 2004; Spillers, 2007; Spillers et al., 2009). Perhaps it is time for us to include spirituality in our field of study and thus undertake needed research, relevant education, and professional development programs (Mathisen et al., 2015).

What Does SLP Research Tell Us?

Spillers and colleagues explored the role of spirituality in professional practice (2009). In a series of questionnaires, they investigated students, clients, and practitioners regarding the inclusion of spirituality with treatment models and curricula. Over 70% of students and adult clients felt it appropriate for SLPs to address spirituality.

Mathisen and colleagues conducted a review via a database search of spirituality cross-referenced across a range of SLP practice areas, and only 15 published articles were identified. The publications focused on three broad themes: holistic practice, patient-centered care, and cultural and linguistic diversity (2015). *Holistic practices and patient-centered care* is enhanced through the SLP's development of empathy, compassion, and rapport, as reflected with the clients' core beliefs. In turn, the client's core beliefs (including aspects of gratitude and spirituality) influence their own behaviors and expectations regarding SLP outcomes (Carey-Sargeant, Carey, Mathisen, & Webb 2012; Mathisen et al., 2015; Spillers, 2011). Spiritual resources and beliefs also provide a means to help clients cope with grief, loss, and decision-making that can improve quality of life (Mathisen, 2010; Mathisen et al., 2015).

With regard to issues related to *cultural and linguistic diversity* (CALD), literature indicates that there are explicit or implicit linkages between indigenous and tribal cultures, spirituality, and speech and language outcomes. Spiritual beliefs and community rituals impact community members' perceptions of communication disorders, as well as implementation of language-learning routines within activities of daily living (Jonk & Enns, 2009). For many indigenous people, "health" implies social, emotional, spiritual, and cultural well-being within a community framework that forms a basis of their traditional life. Their transcendental beliefs, rituals, and mythologies are sacred to their identity, bond individuals to each other, and to their land, and confirm community, wholeness, and a state of general well-being (Eckermann et al., 2010; Mathisen et al., 2015; Mol, 1976).

Spirituality in Clinical Education

All health professionals, including SLPs, must remain sensitive to the beliefs and needs of the individuals being treated, regardless of age or cultural background. Our philosophical and spiritual world view are part of what makes us so different from each other, and contribute to our dynamic systems of forming judgments, values, and preferences. We must be familiar with our own beliefs, and "adopt strategies that focus on the well-being of the client and are in keeping with a patient-centered, holistic approach to clinical decision-making and ethical reasoning" (Mathisen et al., 2015, p. 2313). It is important to keep in mind that both the

World Health Organization's International Classification of Functioning (ICF) for adult clients, and the International Classification of Functioning-Child and Youth (ICF-CY) for pediatric clients include religious/spiritual classifiers (Threats, 2010; WHO, 2001).

It has been suggested that our clients travel two parallel journeys in their treatment programs. Spillers describes a physical journey, as distinguished from a metaphysical journey (2011). The client's *physical journey* consists of their movement through traditional assessments, treatment approaches, and rehabilitation programs. Their *metaphysical journey* is based on their feelings about their physical voyage, such as imperfection, isolation, fear, anxiety, and loneliness (Bruce et al., 2011; Spillers, 2011). Both need acknowledgment within our clinical treatment approach.

Why is it important to include spirituality in SLP practice and clinical education? Mathisen and colleagues cite several reasons worth considering (2015).

- There is increasing evidence linking improved outcomes in health and wellness with attention to spirituality.
- In Western culture, there is a return to the mind-body-spirit paradigm, and a separation of such may conflict with natural healing processes and health outcomes.
- It reinforces the belief that people function as whole complex systems, and are not to be viewed as an impaired body part or a disability.
- It ensures client-centered practice that is meaningful to the client, ethical, and respectful of culture and diversity.
- It reinforces the importance of inclusive and family-centered practice because it considers family issues and cultural traditions.
- It encourages self-awareness, mindfulness, and realistic expectations related to beliefs and practices that may inhibit or advance therapy.

- It encourages the SLP to develop reflective practices and clinical philosophies that highlight their own systems of beliefs and values.

Including Spirituality in Clinical Practice

Palmer (2003) explains that while we have become quite competent in our abilities to create opportunities for intellect and emotions, not so is the case with inviting "the soul" to the clinical table. Why do so few practitioners include spirituality in their clinical practice? That question was asked of occupational therapists and speech therapy students, and five main reasons emerged (Mathisen, 2010; Spillers, 2011): insufficient academic preparation; lack of time or opportunity; thought to be outside scope of practice; difficulty with quantifying and measuring data; and, difficulty contemplating their own spirituality, much less approaching the topic with clients. Students, in particular, were uncertain about the difference between religion and spirituality, the meaning of patient-centered and holistic care, and the importance of "whole person" perspectives and inter-relatedness of the physical, mental, and spiritual components of wellness (Mathisen, 2010; Spillers, 2011).

If we do consider a patient-centered holistic approach central to SLP services, and if we consider spirituality as part of that care continuum, how do we build spirituality into speech-language pathology? The following strategies (as well as cautions) have been recommended by Carey-Sargeant and colleagues (2012; Koenig et al., 2012; Mathison et al., 2015):

- Be aware of and sensitive to client's spiritual beliefs, but do not pressure them to share narratives about spiritual history or preferences.

- Further your understanding of your client's cultural and spiritual needs and issues.
- Become spiritually literate, and reflect upon your own beliefs and values.
- Respect and value the belief system of your client, but do not provide spiritual counsel.
- Encourage the inclusion of spirituality in scopes of practice, university curriculum, and continuing education.

The consideration and inclusion of spiritual belief systems within the field of SLP may clearly be in the best interests of the client, family, community, and the professionals who serve such. Increasing literature in health and wellness provides evidence that spirituality can be a helpful resource, a coping mechanism, and a resilience tool that people use to navigate through a disability, communication disorder, or life change related to the aging process. The abundance of literature calling for more holistic care, patient-centered approaches, family friendly therapy, and treatment for clients who are from culturally diverse backgrounds implores us to consider our positions on spirituality (Mathison et al., 2015).

3. THE HEART AND SOUL OF OUR WORK

What Do We Mean By Heart and Soul?

When we talk about "heart and soul," many images and phrases come to mind: the divine spark, spirit, inner teacher, true self, identity, individuation, or simply finding oneself. The acknowledgment of *heart and soul* and the importance of integrating them both with our work are topics discussed by Palmer, especially as they relate to education. His works are not rooted in empirical research, but rather reflective pieces that evolved out of his decades of exploring, working with, and writing about educators and the spiritual dimensions of their work (Palmer, 1998; 2003).

Our heart and soul connections pit us against bureaucratic conventions, and fight those biases that move us to believe most power resides on the outside of ourselves in what he calls *the visible world*. With life's experience, we learn that the inward and invisible human spirit can have at least equal impact on our individual and collective lives, and that the powers of the human heart and soul can only be grown from within (Palmer, 2003). Our greatest gift is not pedagogical technique and professional content mastery, but mastery of our own inner life. Although higher education can grow people's minds with theories and facts, and train them with skills, it cannot grow larger hearts and souls (Palmer, 2003).

Academics of the Heart

Rendon, in her model of research and education called "Academics of the Heart," talks about the importance of connecting the inner and outer natures of knowledge. To do this, she turns to the ancient wisdom and timeless philosophy of the Maya and Aztec cultures (2000a). One principle core to the indigenous people of Mexico and Central America is *the unity of existence*, or the understanding of how new knowledge fits into an ever changing and expanding system of the world. They believed that all is connected through *principles of opposition*, and that "science" is inseparable from "the divine." This same principle of *connectedness* is found in cultural/religious beliefs and traditions of the contemporary world, including Christianity, Judaism, Islam, Buddhism, Hinduism, and Confucianism (Freidel, Schele & Parker, 1993; Rendon, 2000b; Spilsbury & Bryner, 1992).

The Aztecs integrated "heart" in the search for individual growth, and referred to "flor y canto" (flower and song) as an education of the heart. *Flor y canto* was a necessary component for the creation of anything artistic such as music, literature, philosophy, and architecture. It also led them to their philosophical model of development for mathematical and scientific knowledge (Rendon, 2000a). This ancient wisdom was in place in many other cultures of the world long before Descartes and other postmodern theories of knowledge (Leon-Portilla, 1963).

Intelligence of the Heart and Soul

Consciousness and ideas are part of what the ancients called intelligence of the heart and soul, the natural relation between nature within us and the same nature outside of us (Schwaller de Lubicz, 1985). Just as the mind digests ideas and produces intelligence, the soul feeds on life, digests it, and creates wisdom and character out of our world of experiences (Moore, 1992). According to Moore, the soul needs a clearly and carefully worked out scheme of values and a sense of relatedness to the whole. It also thrives on the spirit of family, arising from traditions and values that have been part of the family for generations.

Although we are showered with information, we tend to lose our sense of intuitive wisdom. As part of our modernist syndrome, we tend to literalize everything our mind touches. This is in contrast to ancient philosophers that taught the world is a cosmic animal, or a unified organism with its own living body and soul. Although we may feel a spiritual longing for a cosmic vision that only community and relatedness can bring, we tend to react with our literal hardware within our minds instead of with sensitivity of the heart (Moore, 1992). It is because we conceive education to be about skills and information, and not about depth of feeling and imagination, that we tend to write soul out of the formula.

Integrating Heart and Soul Into Research

Rendon's model Academics of the Heart suggests the incorporation of three research elements to facilitate the design, analysis, and discussion of scientific research (2000b). The first is to *view research as a relationship-centered process.* This is not a new model to the health care and educational community, and suggests that providers must enter into relationships with clients, communities, and colleagues (as opposed to keeping distance) as part of the research process. It demands balance of the subjective with objective. It honors both the science in our brain and the wisdom in our heart and spirit. We learn to rely on personal experiences, lessons from the field, and stories demonstrating both heart and spirit. Studies in this area can benefit from the blending of scientific methodologies with personal reflections and diverse ways of knowing (Freidel, Schele, & Parker, 1993; Rendon, 2000a).

The second research element is to *honor diverse ways of knowing.* We can learn from the sacred traditions of our ancestors, experiences of diverse cultures from all over the world, quantitative and qualitative research, personal experiences and even dreams—anything that invites a higher and deeper wisdom with a variety of perspectives (Broomfield, 1997). The third is to *engage in self-reflection, contemplation, and introspective practices.* Understanding ourselves is a first step in understanding the external world and its practices. Reflective training "changes the way we are and opens us to hidden wisdom and higher grades of significance in transpersonal traditions, in the world, and in ourselves" (Walsh, 1998, p. 23). Researchers, at some point in their academic careers, must ask themselves why they do what they do and if their research truly makes a difference.

4. THE VALUE OF INTUITION

What Is Intuition?

Intuitions are ideas or solutions that pop into our conscious mind without our awareness of any precipitating mental process (Haidt & Joseph, 2004; Haidt, 2013). You suddenly know, and can't explain why. Intuition and creative mental imaging all have their place when we try to develop an alternative ways of thinking that is not as directed or controlled. Scientists talk about "lightening flashes" or "paradigm shifts" that bring into view a previously unseen solution (Belveridge, 1950; Stillwagon & Bruce, 2011).

Social psychologists explain that intuitions arise because the mind is constructed as two distinct processing systems. One is intuitive, automatic, and without much conscious effort or awareness. This processing system relies on processing shortcuts or *heuristics*, decisions that are often "good enough" for the immediate goal, which are ultimately integrated with learned knowledge and facts about the social world (Ariely, 2008; Kiss, 2006). The second processing system involves slower processing that occurs deliberately and fully within conscious awareness (Haidt & Joseph, 2004).

Intuition as Related to Ethics, Morals, and Virtues

Haidt and Joseph were interested in investigating intuition, and specifically intuitions connected with ideas of morality and values, or what they refer to as *moral intuitions* (2004). In a meta-analysis, they studied and analyzed works compiled by social psychologists to locate a common core of universal moral values. It seems that in all of the human cultures studied, the following core values triggered positive (approval) or negative (disapproval) reactions: suffering/compassion, reciprocity/fairness, and hierarchy/respect. Those flashes of approval or disapproval we feel are intuitive, and we are sometimes left to struggle with our other processing system (the one that reasons rather than reacts) to explain the judgment produced by our intuitive system (Haidt & Joseph, 2004).

We are fascinated with strange, divergent, and diverse cultures. When daily lives of these cultures are studied, certain elements related to morality and ethics arise in nearly all of them. Some examples are loyalty, respect for authority and hierarchy, reciprocity and fairness, and acknowledgment of regulations and laws (Ariely, 2008; Haidt & Joseph, 2004).

Another category of thought and study related to intuition is in the area of *virtue theory*. John Dewey conceived virtues as social skills fashioned by dynamic patterns of perception, emotion, judgment, and action (Churchland, 1998; Swanton, 2003). Virtues are closely connected to the intuitive system as "they are embodied in the very structure of the self, not merely as one of the activities of the self" (Haidt & Joseph, 2004, p. 61).

Aristotle defined virtues by reference to universal features of how human beings adapt to their environments through appraisal of behavior and conduct (Nussbaum & Sen, 1993). He supposed that as we develop virtues, we acquire a second nature as a refinement of our basic nature (Gardner, 2005). The foundation begins in childhood and continues throughout our life through examples of *virtue in practice*. Through the process of feedback and "culling and discarding," a moral learner comes to recognize what information is important to retain and what can be discarded. Aristotle was an early forerunner of the *neural network theory of morality*, which tells us that the mind is a network that gradually gets "tuned up by experience" (Churchland, 1998; Clark & Friedman, 1997). Through that lens, moral maturity then is a sort of attunement and sensitivity to the world of individual virtues, and enables us to reason in a productive and constructive manner about personal or professional situations that are challenging (Haidt & Joseph, 2004).

Intuition Is Like Instinct

Intuition allows us to sense possibilities that may be inherent in a situation but have not yet been realized or actualized (Vaughan, 1979). Most of us rely on our intuitive capacities, and whether or not we are aware of those capacities, they are common to everyday functioning. Intuition is like instinct, and is used with the smallest components of everyday lives—the instantaneous impressions and conclusions that spontaneously arise when we meet someone or something new, or have to make decisions under conditions of stress (Gladwell, 2005). Intuition has been called many things: insight, practical wisdom, creative cognition, knowing of the third kind, or suspended attention. Jung was one of the first psychologists to theorize that intuition was a cognitive construct, and one of four fundamental mental processes: thinking, feeling, sensation, and intuition (Smith, 2012).

It is like trading in our binoculars for microscopes. Gladwell refers to the ability of our unconscious to find patterns in situations and behavior based on very narrow slices of experience known as *thin-slicing* (2005). It is the power of our adaptive unconscious, although we tend to be innately suspicious of this kind of rapid cognition. We grew up hearing all the expressions: haste makes waste, look before you leap, don't judge a book by its cover. Yet, our lives are composed of both fleeting moments that demand instant decisions, in addition to the broader strokes that demand conscious and deliberate thinking.

Using Intuitions to Make Decisions

The debate over how we make judgments and decisions has a long history, beginning with philosophers and writers and continuing with social and cognitive psychologists. Let's describe the debate as having two camps: intuitive and rational. Intuition and conscious rational thinking can work in concert as the two channels through which our minds make sense of the world. The word *intuition* comes from the Latin *intuir*, which means "knowledge from within" (Pigliucci, 2012).

Until recently, self-respecting scientists who feared they would be accused of being New Agers rather than serious scientists avoided studies about intuition. However, cognitive scientists now study and regard intuition as a set of nonconscious cognitive and affective processes (Ariely, 2008). The achievement of the most productive balance between intuition and analytical thinking is crucial for making the best decisions in our personal and professional lives. Some researchers have begun to pay attention as to how we can better achieve this balance (Ariely, 2008; Sinclair & Ashkanasy, 2005).

Scholars from diverse disciplines have noted that the *availability heuristic* is a mental shortcut relying on examples that quickly come to a person's mind when evaluating a topic, concept, or decision. The easier it is to recall the consequences of something, the greater those consequences are perceived to be (Schwarz et al., 1991). This may help explain why when students and practitioners remember certain information quickly; they consider that information to be more important.

We all use our everyday intuitive abilities in combination with memory, ability to recognize familiar patterns, and learned expertise to make decisions. Kahnemann tells us we have two types of thinking, fast and slow (2011). *Fast thinking* is governed by intuition and the more automatic mental activities of perception and memory. *Slow thinking* is more deliberate, rational, and effortful.

Clinical Intuition

Intuition is a component of *the art of therapy*, which utilizes our insightful ability to think on our feet and respond to the unique components of each client and every clinical session. Clinical intuition has been defined as an unconscious decision-making process (Fogle, 2008). It is rapid and extremely subtle and does not follow cause and effect type of logic. It happens based upon the entire context of the clinical situation, and is a function of personal dynamics and interactions (Flasher & Fogle, 2012). Clinically informed intuition is different from simply following one's impulses. Our intuition can be trusted so we act on clinical hunches, and later (when there is time) we think about it deliberately and reflect on it critically (Rubin, 1984).

Clinical intuition is a tool that integrates mind, heart, emotions, and spirit as part of our decision-making process. It reaches into the depths of experience to *understand* the meaning of what someone is going through, rather than to *explain* the symptoms or behaviors (Swanton, 2003). It is sometimes referred to as our "inner knowing," or that "voice in our head. Some of us are more naturally attuned to our intuitive powers through our practices of mindfulness, meditation, introspection, or self-reflection.

5. LEARNING TO FLOURISH AND ENHANCE PROFESSIONAL HAPPINESS

Intentional and Essential Activity

Happiness depends on what you are doing, and nobody else. Fulfillment is a byproduct of what researchers call "intentional activity" —proactive choices we make as we interact with our world in order to feel competent and connect with others (Robinson, 2011). First, we need to initiate participation with those activities. It's not enough that something great happens—the desire to be proactively involved with making it happen will drive feeling happy and fulfilled. It takes initiative to increase positive mood and resist the inertial pull of sedentary lifestyle and sameness

The activities that offer the best chance to increase happiness are ones that fit your affinities and values and that are engaging. Research shows that the odds of improving happiness are greater the more inherently pleasing the experience is, the better the fit with your personality, and the more the opportunity for personal growth (Robinson, 2011). When evolutionary psychologist Bloom talks about happiness, he explains how many significant human pleasures are universal because they accompany other traits that help us survive and reproduce (Bloom, 2010). For example, one such source of pleasure is a side effect of our inborn "essentialism" which enables us to understand that all things have an underlying reality or true nature that is often hidden, but really defines their essence. For our ancestors, this allowed them to categorize which plants and animals were harmful and which ones were helpful. For us now, perhaps it brings us back to our essential beliefs—the ones that steered us before we developed the reasons (Lyubomirsky, 2013).

Aristotelian's Concept of Flourishing

Aristotle and other fellow ancient Greek philosophers shared their insights about a most critical fundamental concept that *life is a project*, and our pressing purpose is to ask ourselves and discover how we are going to pursue it (Pigliucci, 2012). In order to accomplish this, Aristotle described the process of engaging in a quest for what he termed *eudemonia*, a Greek word that literally means "having a good demon" and that is often translated as "happiness," or "flourishing." We achieve eudemonia by engaging in virtuous behavior, virtuous activities, and virtuous work. The sense of that expression is not simply feeling good, but accomplishing things and taking pleasure and pride in those accomplishments (Martinich & Sosa, 2012).

Aristotle says it simply: a flourishing human being belongs to a community whose goal is to bring about the flourishing of its members ([Aristotle, Sanders translator] 1981; Oppy, 2012). A flourishing person has moral and intellectual virtues, genuine friendships, possesses theoretical and practical wisdom, and acts with courage, sincerity, and justice. Most ancient conceptions of human flourishing are similar and include mental, physical, and spiritual aspects of health care as well as self-care (Oppy, 2012).

How Do We Flourish?

Gendler's research focuses on resilience and flourishing, and the fundamental ancient insights as related to the language of the soul. Flourishing occurs when there is spiritual well-being (the Greeks called this *eudaimonea),* along with practical wisdom (which the Greeks called *phronesis*). Gendler takes that insight and break it down in to component parts in the five ancient secrets, found in the ideas of all of the five thinkers: *Socrates* (develop appropriate self-knowledge), *Plato* (cultivate internal harmony), *Aristotle* (foster virtue and change through habit), *Cicero* (pursue and appreciate true friendship), and *Epictetus* (self-reliance and recognition of what is and is not within your control) (Gendler, 2010, 2013). More regarding this is discussed in the next section of this chapter.

Happiness depends more on how we handle what happens, and less on what actually happens. Our happiness is determined by how we perceive, and interpret what happens, and then integrate it into what we already believe is true. The one variable that plays a great influence over our perceptions is our commitment. In other words, are we committed to half empty or half full? Are we committed to seeing the best in people or the worst? When we commit to something, and we turn our attention to it, it grows (Kubler-Ross & Kessler, 2000). Like a suitcase that we keep filling up with things we don't need. In addition, this baggage, as it is often called, is heavy to carry around, and slows our progress toward happiness. Happiness is our natural state, and we need to get back there.

Happiness Studies

Happiness studies are booming in the social sciences and include first-person experiences and reflections as part of the quantitative and qualitative scientific rigor (Gutting, 2011). According to Seligman, well-being theory has five elements: positive emotion, engagement, meaning, positive relationships, and accomplishment (2011). *Positive emotion* and *engagement* can only be assessed subjectively, and both are pursued for their own sake. Engagement relates to new learning, and interests. Strengths and virtues are supports for engagement and positive relationships. *Meaning* is attained through belonging to and serving something that you believe is bigger than the self. *Accomplishment*, or achievement, can also be pursued for its own sake. *Positive relationships* are all about other people, and our pursuit of personal attachments.

Happiness has been described as involving four variables (Gutting, 2011).

1. *Freedom from suffering* is described by the ancient Greeks as largely a matter of luck
2. Also described by the ancient Greeks is the *proper use of pleasure*, related to gratification of the physical senses as well as aesthetic sensibilities directed to art and nature.
3. Happiness of *human love* takes us into the world of morals, ethics, and values.
4. *Fulfilling work* is described in ancient literature as everyone taking up some task that contributes to the community's welfare.

A.R.T.: Happiness

Upon my retirement for my speech supervisory position, I was taken out to lunch by the practitioners under my supervision. We went to a Chinese restaurant, and my fortune read as follows: "Happiness is comprised of three things—meaningful work, mutual love, and hope for the future . . . "

---

6. GUIDING PRINCIPLES, RECURRING THEMES, ENDURING TRUTHS AND THEIR RELATIONSHIP TO OUR ATTITUDES, PHILOSOPHY, AND ETHICS

The Importance of Historical Perspectives

My goal in this section is not to describe any ancient philosophies in detail, or to provide a detailed narrative about the history of ideas that I will touch upon. Rather, it is to explore certain themes and their impact upon our clients, our work, and us. While there is no formula or recipe for a successful career, there are recurring interactions and experiences that have taken place over the centuries and around the world. When we recognize and understand the patterns, we can navigate through our own interactions and experiences with greater wisdom and purpose. This is a premise agreed upon by ancient sages, classic philosophers and modern psychologists (Haidt, 2006).

Judith Duchan offers a history of our field on her website, and suggests that by understanding history we build a more reflective perspective toward our clinical practice (2015). History affirms that others knew what we now know, and humbles us to realize that we perhaps need some new angles and interpretations of attitudes and practices that we may be taking for granted. That point is beautifully driven home in an article written about "the golden rule," and its impact on the work we do. The golden rule, commonly translated as, "Do unto others as you would have them do unto you." is a principle of altruism found in just about every human culture and religion (Wattles, 1996). We cover this more fully in Chapter 6 when we talk about "harmony."

Virtues of the Ancients

Ancient texts emphasize practice rather than acquisition of factual knowledge. When we read about the wisdom represented by Confucius or Buddha, it is often in the formal aphorism that is still perceived as "worldwide laws of life" (Peterson & Seligman, 2004). The Old and New Testament, Homer, and Aesop all illustrate virtuous and upstanding behaviors through the use of proverbs, maxims, fables, and role model examples (Haidt, 2006).

Oldest works of direct moral institution are the teachings of Amenemope, an Egyptian

text written around 1300 AD, a book providing "instruction about life" and a guide for well-being. The biblical "Book of Proverbs" borrowed a lot from Amenemope. One common feature of ancient texts is that they rely to a large extent on maxims and role models rather than scientific proofs and logic. The use of maxims facilitates flashes of "aha" moments, and the use of examples or role models elicits admiration and awe. Integration of moral instruction sparks the emotions (Peterson & Seligman, 2004).

In architecture school, one learns that all design endeavors express *the zeitgeist*. It is a German word that roughly means the spirit of an age, sensibility of an era, and the intellectual inclinations and biases that underlie human endeavor as flavored by a particular era (Frederick, 2007). As a result of the zeitgeist, parallel trends tend to occur in most creative enterprises such as literature, science, architecture, art, and religion. According to Hendrix (2005) some examples of intellectual trends might be:

- *Ancient's era:* tendency to accept myth-based truths
- *Classical Greek era:* tendency to value order, rationality, and democracy
- *Medieval era:* dominance of the truths or organized religion
- *The Renaissance:* embracing of science and art
- *Modern era:* tendency to favor truths revealed by the scientific method
- *Postmodern era:* truth is relative and impossible to know from only one perspective

Classic teachings are commonly seen as *eternal wisdom*, and therefore assumed to be applicable still (Venhoven, 2003). Confucianism is one of the classic Chinese schools of philosophy that deals with the question of how one should live and shed light on some *pillars of practice* that we will be discussing. It values happiness, reflection, community, rules, humanities, responsibility, and duty as very positive (Bradburn, 1969).

One of the pivotal ideas of Confucianism is the concept of "jen," a feeling of compassion and concern for the well being of others, which is discussed more fully in Chapter 5 when we talk about "character" and its relationship to our work. A second virtue that Confucius teaches us about is a positive attitude toward learning and the importance of self-cultivation, both of which are covered in Chapter 7, when professional growth is discussed (Keltner, 2009).

The Five Ancient Secrets of Classical Philosophers (Gendler, 2010, 2013)

Socrates claimed that the wise man knows that he knows nothing. One source of wisdom is *knowing what one does not know*. Self-knowledge requires humility, and we may be unaware of the sources or our emotions, our choices, and our preferences. The recognition of that brings with it an opportunity for insight about our blind spots and introspection into ourselves, and becomes the building block of all else we do in the field.

Plato's notions were translated into the *id* and *ego* in modern psychiatry, and concern the notion of *dual processing*. We have multi-parts; some parts direct us to be safe and some to take risks. Sometimes these parts are in harmony and sometimes in tension. When in tension, it takes much more energy and effort for us to control our behavior. We must cultivate the *internal harmony* that will impact our ethics, values, and help us meet the demands of the system.

Aristotle said it quite simply, "*foster change* through habit." Change can only be attained through consistent action. States of character arise out of like activities and habits. If you want to become a particular way, start acting that way. When we begin to do what

we think we "should" do, productive habits develop, and patterns of behavior initially under conscious control become automatized.

Cicero states that when we lack self-reflection, the *social support* and presence of another changes our perception of the world and we develop new patterns of perception and response. However, those supports need to be the best association, one who has already learned what we need to know, or is interested in the same learning. You learn the journey from one who has already taken it. For us, this translates into using professional resources, seeking out expertise, and enhancing peer-to-peer interactions.

Epictetus tells us that because *some things are up to us and others are not*, we should restrict our attention to what is under our control. This ultimately evolved into Reinhold Niebuhr's "The Serenity Prayer," and became the basis of step recovery programs. The key is self-knowledge, and only with that can we control ourselves and grow our self-reflective components. How does this help us? We can control our opinions, our aversions, our judgments, and our attitudes. You assume purpose and power, and others will decide your reputation.

Descartes and Western Epistemology

When Descartes wrote the *Discourse on the Method*, he might not have known that it was to become one of the most influential works in the history of modern philosophy, as well as the development of the rational sciences (Rendon, 2000; Zajonc, 1993). It was in this treatise that the intellect was separated from intuition, and two key principles were established as the basis for Western epistemology (Zajonc, 1993). Descartes and his followers believed that *intellectual training alone provides the road to understanding*; however, this is certainly not the case throughout the ancient and the modern world. Certain Eastern philosophies and traditions affirm that the mind must be given a multidimensional and contemplative training that refines "ethics, emotions, motivation, and attention" (Walsh, 1998, p. 21).

The second principle that his book affirmed, is that *reason and emotion are separate and irreconcilable* (Rendon, 2000a). This dichotomous view of reason and emotion has long been challenged. In fact, Greenspan and others assert that emotional experience is the basis of the mind's development in the areas of intelligence, academic abilities, sense of self, and morality (1997).

Despite research and the emergence of a multitude of holistic Eastern philosophies, Western allegiance to the separation of reason from emotion and of the intellect from intuition, remains steadfast (Damasio, 1994; Gaukroger, 1995). At its worst, this type of thinking perpetuates the belief that research excels over scholarship, that theory excels over practice, that quantitative data excel over qualitative data, and that numbers excel over fieldwork and personal reflections (Rendon, 2000b).

A.R.T.: Meaning For Us

As I was approaching the last chapter of this book, my friend Carol asked how things were going. When I told her, she gave me her perspective, as a social worker, about the structure of this book. It was very moving, because she mentioned so many things in this chapter—spirituality, recurring themes, heart and soul. When I told her (without having read this chapter) she had touched on much of its content—she commented that most professionals today want something that helps tie together all of the knowledge they have accumulated through coursework, independent studies, and experience. Hopefully, that has been accomplished.

What This Means For Us

We sometimes make choices from an either/or mentality: reason over faith, academic knowledge over humanity, hard knowledge over soft, mind over heart and soul, current over ancient and diverse ways of knowing. We wind up creating a competitive and conflicted atmosphere that is estranged from our nature and inner ways of knowing (Tarnas, 1998). Let us instead create a new framework that rebalances and reconfigures lost connections—let us reconnect spirit with intellect and bridge our different ways of knowing (Broomfield, 1997). Tarnas states the need to " . . . honor our humanity while incorporating high standards in our work. We need a marriage between precise inquiry and poetic intuition." (1998, p. 6)

REFLECTIVE SUMMATIVE QUESTIONS

1. How would you define wisdom and what part has it and will it continue to play in your life as a speech-language pathologist?
2. Please explain if and why or why not you consider yourself to be a spiritual person. Include your spiritual "worldview."
3. Describe a personal experience with "the waterfall and the bucket of water."
4. How would you relate three of Zohar's principles related to spiritual intelligence with the practice of speech-language pathology?
5. What speech-language pathology research or readings are you familiar with that struck a "heart, soul, or spiritual" chord?
6. What is clinical intuition and how prominent a role would it play in your professional decisions?
7. How do you "look after" yourself as a student or professional, and how have you flourished in those roles?

8. What principles, themes, and truths have impacted your studies and professional life?

REFERENCES

Aldo de Moor. (2006). Towards more effective collaboration workspaces: From collaboration technologies to patterns. Referenced from Pattberg, J., & Fluegge, M. *Towards an ontology of collaboration patterns*. Retrieved May 6, 2013, from http://subs.emis.de/LNI/Proceedings/Proceedings120/gi-proc-120-007.pdf

Allee, V. (1997). *The knowledge evolution: Expanding organizational intelligence*. Oxford, UK: Butterworth-Heinemann.

Ariely, D. (2008). *Predictable irrational: The hidden forces that shape our decisions*. New York, NY: HarperCollins.

Aristotle. (1981). *The politics* (T. A. Sinclair, Trans.). Harmondsworth, UK: Penguin

Beveridge, W. (1950). *The art of scientific investigation*. New York, NY: W. M. Norton.

Bloom, P. (2010). *How pleasure works: The new science of why we like what we like*. New York, NY: W. W. Norton.

Bradburn, N. M. (1969). *The structure of psychological well-being*. Chicago, IL: Aldine.

Broomfield, J. (1997). *Other ways of knowing*. Rochester, VT: Inner Traditions International.

Bruce, D. (2011a, July). Knowledge and wisdom, Part I. *Theosophical Society in America*. Retrieved from https://www.theosophical.org/files/resources/reflections/Reflections-2011-07.pdf

Bruce, D. (2011b, August). Knowledge and wisdom, Part II. *Theosophical Society in America*. Retrieved from https://www.theosophical.org/files/resources/reflections/Reflections-2011-08.pdf

Bruce, A., Shields, L., & Molzahn, A. (2011). Language and the (im)possibilities of articulating spirituality. *Journal of Holistic Nursing, 29*(1), 44–52.

Carey-Sargeant, C. L., Carey, L. B., Mathisen, B., & Webb, G. (2012). *Holistic practice: Speech language pathologists and spirituality [Keynote Presentation III]*. Paper presented at the Lynda R. Campbell Memorial Lecture Series: ATLAS Week Topics in Diversity, St. Louis University, Missouri.

Churchland, P. (1998). Toward a cognitive neurobiology of the moral virtues. *Topoi, 17*, 83–96.

Clark, A, May, L., & Friedman, M. (Eds.) (1997). *Mind and morals*. Cambridge, MA: MIT Press.

Cobb, M., Puchalski, C., & Rumbold, B. (Eds.). (2012). *Oxford textbook of spirituality in healthcare*. New York, NY: Oxford University Press.

Cranfill, T. & Mahanna-Boden, S. (2012). *Spirituality and healthcare: What can we do?* Atlanta, GA: ASHA Conference.

Damasio, A. R. (1994). *Descartes' error*. New York, NY: Avon Books.

Duchan, J. (2015). *History of speech-language pathology*. Retrieved from http://www.acsu.buffalo.edu/~duchan/index.html 1/18/16

Eckermann, A. K., Dowd, T., Chong, E., Nixon, L., Gray, R., & Johnson, S. (2010). *Bridging cultures in aboriginal health* (3rd ed.). Sydney, Australia: Churchill Livingstone.

Ferngren, G. (2012). Medicine and religion: A historical perspective. In M. Cobb, C. Puchalski, & B. Rumbold (Eds.), *Oxford textbook of spirituality in healthcare*. New York, NY: Oxford University Press.

Flasher, L. V., & Fogle, P. T. (2012). *Counseling skills for speech-language pathologists and audiologists*. Clifton Park, NY: Delmar Cengage Learning.

Fogle, P. T. (2008). *Foundations of communication sciences and disorders*. Clifton Park, NY: Thomas Delmar Learning.

Frankl, V. E. (1985). *Man's search for meaning*. New York, NY: Washington Square Press.

Frederick, M. (2007). *101 Things I learned in architecture school*. Cambridge, MA: MIT Press.

Freidel, D., Schele, L., & Parker, J. (1993). *Maya cosmos*. New York, NY: Quill William Morrow.

Gardiner, S. M. (Ed) (2005). *Virtue ethics, old and new*. Ithaca, NY: Cornell University Press.

Gaukroger, S. (1995). *Descartes: An intellectual biography*. New York, NY: Oxford University Press.

Gendler, T. S. (2010). *Intuition, imagination, and philosophical methodology*. New York, NY: Oxford University Press.

Gendler, T. (2013). *The five ancient secrets to modern flourishing*. Psychiatry/Yale School of Medicine. Retrieved from http://medicine.yale.edu/psychiatry/education/grand/2013/0524.aspx

Gladwell, M. (2005). *Blink: The power of thinking without thinking*. New York, NY: Little, Brown and Company.

Goleman, D. (1995). *Emotional intelligence*. New York, NY: Bantam Books.

Gregory, K. (2012). Buddhism: Perspectives for contemporary world. In M. Cobb, C. Puchalski, & B. Rumbold (Eds.), *Oxford textbook of spirituality in healthcare*. New York, NY: Oxford University Press.

Greenspan, S. I. (1997). *The growth of the mind*. Reading, MA: Perseus Books.

Gutting, G. (2011). *Thinking the impossible: French philosophy since 1960*. London, UK: Oxford University Press.

Haidt, J. (2006). *The happiness hypothesis*. New York, NY: Basic Books.

Haidt, J. (2013). *The righteous mind: Why good people are divided by politics and religion*. New York, NY: First Vintage Books.

Haidt, J., & Joseph, C. (2004, Fall). Intuitive ethics: How innately prepared intuitions generate culturally variable virtues. *American Academy of Arts and Sciences: Daedalus*, pp. 55–56.

Handzo, G., & Koenig, H. G. (2004). Spiritual care: Whose job is it anyway? *Southern Medical Journal*, *97*(12), 1242–1245.

Hardy, A. (1979). *The spiritual nature of man*. Oxford, UK: Oxford University Press.

Hawley, H. (1993). *Reawakening the spirit in work*. New York, NY: Simon & Shuster.

Hendrix, J. S. (2005). *Aesthetics & the philosophy of spirit*. New York, NY: Peter Lang.

Hermans, H. (1988). On the integration of nomothetic and idiographic research methods in the study of personal meaning. *Journal of Personality*, *56*(4), 785–812.

Hillman, J. (1996). *The soul's code*. New York, NY: Random House.

Hilsman, G. J. (1997). The place of spirituality in managed care. *Health Progress*. *78*(1), 43–46.

Jonk, L., & Enns, C. (2009). Using culturally appropriate methodology to explore Dene mothers' views on language facilitation. *Canadian Journal of Speech-Language Pathology and Audiology*, *33*(1), 33–44.

Kahn, M. (1997). *Between therapist and client. The new relationship: An integrated approach*. London, UK: Tavistock.

Kahneman, D. (2011). *Thinking fast and slow*. New York, NY: Farrar, Straus, and Giroux.

Keltner, D. (2009). *Born to be good: The science of a meaningful life*. New York, NY: W.W. Norton.

Kiss, O. (2006). Heuristic, methodology or logic of discovery: Lakatos on patterns of thinking. *Perspectives On Science*. *14*(3). 302–317.

Koenig, H., King, V., & Carson, B. (2012). *Handbook of religion and health* (2nd ed.). New York, NY: Oxford University Press.

Kubler-Ross, E., & Kessler, D. (2000). *Life lessons*. New York, NY: Scribner.

Leon-Portilla, M. (1963). *Aztec thought and culture: A study of the ancient Nahuatl mind*. (J. E. Davis, Trans.). Norman, OK: University of Oklahoma Press.

Lesser, E. (1999). *The new American spirituality*. New York, NY: Random House.

Lyubomirsky, S. (2013). *The myths of happiness*. New York, NY: The Penguin Group.

Mathisen, B. (2010). *Including spirituality in speech pathology practice: A pilot study of undergraduates* (Unpublished manuscript). The University of Newcastle, New South Wales.

Mathisen, B., Carey, L. B., Carey-Sargeant, C. L., Webb, G., Millar, C., & Krikheli, L. (2015). Religion, spirituality and speech-language pathology. *Journal of Religion and Health*, *54*(6), 2309–2323.

Martinich, A. P., & Sosa, D. (Eds.). (2012). *The philosophy of language*. London, UK: Oxford University Press.

Mol, H. (1976). *Identity and the sacred: A sketch for a new social-scientific theory of religion*. Oxford, London, UK: Blackwell.

Moore, T. (1992). *Care of the soul*. New York, NY: HarperCollins.

Nussbaum, M., & Sen, A. (Eds.). (1993). *The quality of life*. New York, NY: Oxford University Press.

Oppy, G. (2012). Philosophy. In M. Cobb, C. Puchalski, & B. Rumbold (Eds.), *Oxford textbook of spirituality in healthcare*. New York, NY: Oxford University Press.

Palmer, P. J. (1998). *The courage to teach: Exploring the inner landscape of a teacher's life.* San Francisco, CA: Jossey-Bass.

Palmer, P. J. (2003). Teaching with heart and soul: Reflections on spirituality in teacher education. *Journal of Teacher Education., 54*(5), 376–385.

Papir-Bernstein, W. (2012a). The artistry of practice-based evidence (PBE): One practitioner's path —Part I. In R. Goldfarb (Ed.), *Translational speech-language pathology and audiology* (pp. 51–57. San Diego, CA: Plural.

Papir-Bernstein, W. (2012b). The artistry of practice-based evidence (PBE): One practitioner's path—Part II. In R. Goldfarb (Ed.), *Translational speech-language pathology and audiology* (pp. 83–87). San Diego, CA: Plural.

Perez, J.C. (2004). Healing presence. *Care management Journals, 5*(1), 41–46.

Pesut, B. (2002). The development of nursing students' spirituality and spiritual care-giving. *Nurse Education Today, 22,* 128–135.

Peterson, C., & Seligman, M. (2004). *Character strengths and virtues.* New York, NY: Oxford University Press.

Pigliucci, M. (2012). *Answers for Aristotle: How science and philosophy can lead us to a more meaningful life.* New York, NY: Basic Books.

Rendón, L. (2000a). Academics of the heart: Reconnecting the scientific mind with the spirit's artistry. *Review of Higher Education, 24,* 1–13.

Rendón, L. (2000b). Academics of the heart: Maintaining body, soul and spirit. In M. Garcia (Ed.), *Microcosms of diversity: Succeeding as a faculty member of color* (pp. 141–154). Westport, CT: Greenwood Press.

Robinson, J. (2011). *Don't miss your life: Find more joy and fulfillment now.* Hoboken, NJ: John Wiley & Sons.

Rubin, J. A. (1984). *The art of art therapy.* New York, NY: Brunner/Mazel.

Scheurich, N. (2003). Reconsidering spirituality and medicine. *Academic Medicine. 78*(4), 1123–1128.

Schulz, E. K. (2005). The meaning of spirituality for individuals with disabilities. *Disability and Rehabilitation, 27*(21), 1283–1295.

Schwaller de Lubicz, R. A. (1985). *The Egyptian miracle: An introduction to the wisdom of the temple.* New York, NY: Inner Traditions.

Schwarz, N. , Strack, F., Bless, H., Klumpp, G., Rittenauer-Schatka, H., & Simons, A. (1991). Ease of retrieval as information: A look at the availability heuristic. *Journal of Personality and Social Psychology, 61,* 195–202.

Seligman, M. (2011). *Flourish: A visionary new understanding of happiness and well-being.* New York, NY: Free Press.

Shedroff, N. (2000). Information interaction design: A unified field theory of design. In R. Jacobson (Ed.), *Information design* (pp. 267–292). Cambridge; London, UK. First MIT Press.

Silverman, E. M. (2003). Shared connections: Spirituality in clinical practice. *The ASHA Leader, 8*(17), 40.

Sinclair, M., & Ashkanasy, N. (2005). Intuition: Myth or a decision-making tool? *Management Learning, 36,* 353–370.

Smith, H. (2012). *The spaces in-between: How the art of intuition informs the science of evidence based practice in psychotherapy.* Master of Social Work Clinical Research Papers. Paper 93. Retrieved from http://sophia.stkate.edu/msw_papers/93

Spillers, C. S. (2007). An existential framework for understanding the counseling needs of clients. *American Journal of Speech-Language Pathology, 16,* 191–197.

Spillers, C. S. (2011). Spiritual dimensions of the clinical relationship. In R. F. Fourie (Ed.), *Therapeutic processes for communication disorders: A guide for students and clinicians* (pp. 229–243). East Sussex, UK: Psychology Press.

Spillers, C. S., Bongard, B., Deplazes, B., Gerard, B., & Narveson, B. (2009) *Exploring the role of spirituality in professional practice.* ASHA Mini-seminar presentation, New Orleans, LA.

Spilsbury, A., & Bryner, M. (1992). *The Mayan oracle.* Santa Fe, NM: Bear and Co.

Spitzform, M. (2015). Interspiritual and clinical practice. *Spirituality in Clinical Practice, 2*(4), 285–288.

Stillwaggon, L., & Bruce, M. (2011). *Just the arguments: 100 of the most important argu-*

ments in western philosophy. New York, NY: Wiley-Blackwell.

Swanton, C. (2003). *Virtue ethics: A pluralistic view.* Oxford, UK: Oxford University Press.

Swinton, J. (2012). Healthcare spirituality: A question of knowledge. In M. Cobb, C. Puchalski, & B. Rumbold (Eds.), *Oxford textbook of spirituality in healthcare.* New York, NY: Oxford University Press.

Tarnas, R. (1998). The passion of the western mind. In H. Palmer (Ed.), *Inner knowing* (pp. 14–20). New York, NY: Jeremy P. Tarcher/Putnam.

Threats, T. (2010). The ICF and speech-language pathology: Aspiring to a fuller realization of ethical issues. *International Journal of Speech-Language Pathology, 12*(2), 87–93.

Van Hooft, S. (2012). The western humanist tradition. In M. Cobb, C. Puchalski, & B. Rumbold (Eds.), *Oxford textbook of spirituality in healthcare.* New York, NY: Oxford University Press.

Vaughan, F. E. (1979). *Awakening intuition.* Garden City, NJ: Anchor Press/Doubleday.

Venhoven, R. (2003). Hedonism and happiness. *Journal of Happiness Studies, 4,* 437–457.

Walsh, R. (1998). Hidden wisdom. In H. Palmer (Ed.), *Inner knowing* (pp. 21–23). New York, NY: Jeremy P. Tarcher/Putnam.

Wattles, J. (1996). *The golden rule.* New York, NY: Oxford University Press.

Weimer, M. A. (2011). A primer on pedagogical scholarship. *ASHA Perspectives on Issues in Higher Education, 14*(1), 5–10.

Winslow, G. R., & Wehtje-Winslow, B. J. (2007). Ethical boundaries of spiritual care. *Medical Journal of Australia, 186*(10), S63–S66.

World Health Organization (WHO). (2001). *International classification of functioning of disability and health.* Geneva, Switzerland: Author.

Wurman, S. (2001). *Information anxiety 2.* Indianapolis, IN: Que.

Zajonc, A. (1993). *Catching the light.* New York, NY: Oxford University Press.

Zohar, D. (2000). *SQ: Connecting with our spiritual intelligence.* London, UK: Bloomsbury.

Zohar, D., & Marshall, I. (2001). *Spiritual intelligence: The ultimate intelligence.* New York, NY: Bloomsbury.

PART II

Supporting Our Path:
Philosophical Pillars of Practice

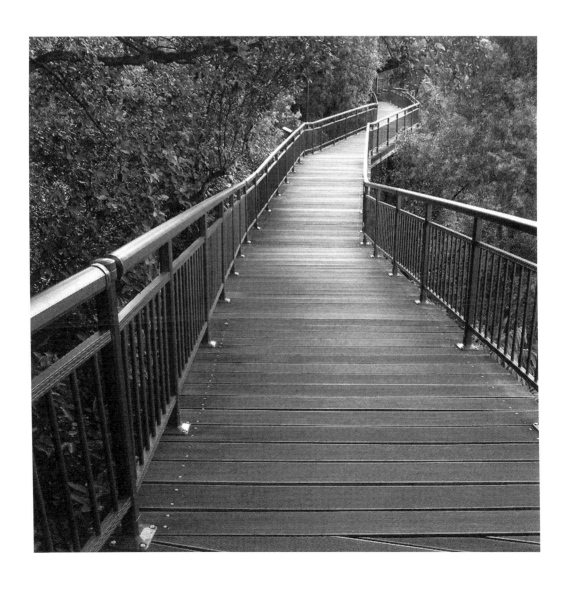

INTRODUCTION

Part II begins our discussion about supporting the practitioner's path in speech-language pathology with principles that frame our thinking and support our path: the *philosophical and therapeutic pillars of practice*. It contains five chapters presented as qualities and attitudes for the practitioner in relationship to self, clients, and emerging professional issues in the field of speech-language pathology. Much of the information introduced in Part II provides the foundation for a solid therapeutic approach and the underpinnings of *the therapeutic attitude* (Cornett & Chabon, 1988).

In some ways, the formulation of this section became one of the principle drivers for its need. Part II was born out of my interest in positive psychology, as a field whose practical application is to help individuals and organizations identify and use their strengths to increase and sustain levels of well-being. Peterman and Seligman's book describing character strengths and virtues (CSV) represents a first attempt by a research community to identify and classify the positive psychological traits of human beings (2004).

The CSV identifies six classes of *core virtues or character strengths* recognized by the vast majority of cultures, and practiced throughout recorded history (Peterman & Seligman, 2004). The CSV defined character strengths as fulfilling to the individual as well as intrinsically valuable. They are often personified by people made famous through myth, story, or song, but can be notably absent in others. At best, these virtues are nurtured by societal norms and educational institutions, and modeled throughout our professional lives (Shryack et al., 2010).

Another way of viewing the importance of Part II, is in tribute to the laws and principles by which the universe, and all within, is

governed. Ancient mystical teachings dating back over 5, 000 years from Egypt, Greece, and India all have common threads connecting these laws (Kostos, 2013). Different cultures refer to them in different ways, but I have attempted to capture some of the overriding themes that support our practices and impact the course of our treatment programs.

The *practitioner's path* is framed by the supporting principles of reflection, counsel and care, balance and harmony, growth, and detachment. It is these guiding principles, these recurring themes, and these enduring truths that will provide the supporting backbone of our practice and set the trajectory for our professional life. Part II is about the more human aspects of competency, qualities, and, traits that are difficult to teach, even more difficult to measure, and sometimes get omitted from our textbooks, training programs and continuing education. They are aspects of our practice that need to be cultivated and taken seriously because they will impact the course of our treatment.

This section of the book is about utilizing and enhancing oneself as a *tool of practice*. The acknowledgment of our beliefs, insights, perspectives, and judgments all become the underpinnings of the therapeutic process. This process is sometimes referred to as *the therapeutic use of self* as an artful tool of practice that informs the science of evidence, and enables us to sustain the personal self as well as the professional self (Kuhaneck, Spitzer, & Miller, 2010; Mosey, 1986).

Part II introduces readers to a "port of entry" as an alternative to knowledge, skills and cognitive areas of expertise: *working from the inside out* (Geller, 2002; Geller & Foley, 2009). When we work from the *inside out* as opposed to the outside in, we are focusing on the more covert, affective, internalized, and reflective processes. It reminds us that we are in a service profession driven by humanistic values, and that professionalism consists of more than cognitive expertise and technical competencies (Remen & Rabow, 2005). When we connect with those core values, as viewed through an ancient and universal lens, we draw meaning and strength against occasional assaults from our bureaucracies and framing regulations (Bornstein, 2007). I believe that this needs to be the *professional consciousness* of our new age, because when we work on getting the inside right, the outside has a greater chance of falling into place.

In his book *The Power of Now*, Tolle distinguishes between the knower and the thinker, both of whom reside inside of ourselves (2004). Part II speaks to "the knower" in you rather than "the thinker." The knower often dwells behind the thinker, much the same way that the tacit knowledge dwells behind the explicit academic knowledge. He and many other writers of spirit make reference to one teaching that comes in many forms. Consider the possibility that beneath all of the academic rhetoric and behind all the scientific theories, there are ancient truths, teachings, and philosophies that feed into our natural states of belief, trust, and expectations. These philosophical truths help us make sense of all our other learnings. As we experience these truths, "there is then a feeling of exaltation and heightened aliveness, as something within you says: yes, I know this is true" (Tolle, p. 10).

REFERENCES

Bornstein, D. (2007). *How to change the world: Social entrepreneurs and the power of new ideas.* New York, NY: Oxford University Press.

Cornett, B. S., & Chabon, S. (1988). *The clinical practice of speech-language pathology.* Columbus, OH: Merrill.

Geller, E. (2002). A reflective model of supervision in speech-language pathology: Process and practice. *Clinical Supervisor, 20*(2), 191–200.

Geller, E., & Foley, G. M. (2009). Broadening the ports of entry for speech-language pathologists: A relational and reflective model for clinical supervision. *American Journal of Speech-Language Pathology, 18*, 22–41.

Kotsos, T. (2013). *The adventure of I.* London, UK: Amarantho House.

Kuhaneck, H. M., Spitzer, S. L., & Miller, E. (2010). *Activity analysis, creativity, and playfulness in pediatric occupational therapy.* Boston, MA: Jones and Bartlett.

Mosey, A. C. (1986). *Psychosocial components of occupational therapy.* New York, NY: Raven Press.

Peterson, C., & Seligman, M. (2004). *Character strengths and virtues: A handbook and classification.* Oxford, UK: Oxford University Press.

Remen, R. N., & Rabow, M. W. (2005). The healer's art: professionalism, service and mission. *Medical Education, 39*(11), 1167–1168.

Shryack, J., Steger, M., Krueger, R., & Kallie, C. (2010). *The structure of virtue.* Atlanta, GA: Elsevier.

Tolle, E. (2004). *The power of now.* Novato, CA: New World Library.

CHAPTER 4

Reflection

1. ATTENTION AND SELF-AWARENESS

Paying Attention

Any technique that helps us see the connectedness, relationships, and patterns of things in the world becomes valuable. According to Zen legend, the fifteenth-century master Ikkyu was asked to write down a maxim of "the highest wisdom," and he wrote one word—*attention*. When he was asked if that was all there was, he wrote down two words: *attention, attention* (Horgan, 2003, p. 226).

When we learn to objectively observe, we have a higher likelihood of discovering information we will find useful. It takes practice to learn how to observe in a nonjudgmental way, but when we do it we will notice many more details about our client's nonverbal communication as well as verbal communication (Riley, 2002). Awareness and observation are intricate aspects of active listening.

Self-Awareness

Self-awareness and attending are both prerequisites for self-reflection and will enhance our clinical performance (Silverman, 2008). We need to be aware of our personal thoughts and feelings, and our own awareness allows us to be fully present with the client (Riley, 2002). Self-awareness can be defined as knowledge about your thoughts, feelings, and actions at any given moment in time (Riley, 2002). It involves something called *presence*, and is the opposite of being "on automatic."

Self-awareness helps us distinguish between our own thoughts and feeling and those of our client (Luterman, 1991). It will also help us be available to our clients, as we eliminate those distracting thoughts that interfere with our ability to attend to client nonverbal cues. Self-awareness, presence, and enhanced attention to our clients will heighten our memory of the session as well. They help us free our minds from the distractions that enter.

A strategy that can help us work toward increasing self-awareness is to transform some automatic action routine into something with greater awareness. For example, try it when peeling an orange or brushing your teeth as you focus on every action.

Attention is Reinforcing

Although clinician attention is one of the most powerful and effective reinforcers that clinicians have available in their toolbox, it has been rarely studied in our field and, therefore, not well understood. Attention is often indicated through a wide variety of visual and motor behaviors such as making eye contact, silent listening, smiling, head nod, head tilt, hand gestures, and eyebrow changes (Moore, 1979).

The reinforcing effects of clinician attention in the provision of speech and language therapy when working with children was studied back in 1979. Three conclusions were drawn as a result of the study and review of other relevant research (Moore, 1979).

- Attention may be a *strong positive reinforce* for any behavior upon which it is contingent.
- Attention may serve as a reinforcer *regardless of the intent of clinicians' verbal statements.*
- Clinician attention *effects behavior of others* in the peer group.

Self-Awareness Leads Us to Belief

Only when we increase our awareness of our own beliefs about ourselves and our clients can we distinguish their concerns and projections from our own. As we practice compassionate listening, our ability to provide compassionate care increases. Our responsibilities include the acknowledgment that we are part of the *change process* for our clients.

As we listen well to our clients, we communicate through our kindness that they are accepted and safe (Charon, 2006; Silverman, 2008; Spillers, 2007). Active listening and self-reflection are two of the most valuable tools we have. Whatever we can do to better know ourselves will assist our efforts to know and be helpful to others (Silverman, 2008). It all begins with belief.

2. BELIEF

What Are Beliefs and How Important Are They in Our Work?

Beliefs are part of our everyday lives and are manifested through our thoughts, actions, and things we talk about (Cobb, 2012; Kenny,

2007). Without the support of beliefs, everything begins to wobble. Our beliefs support our convictions and help us navigate through and engage with and shape our involvements with the world. Our beliefs are indications of what we consider to be true (Steglich-Peterson, 2006). Nobel laureate and neuroscientist Roger Sperry considered belief to be the force that, above any other, shapes the course of human affairs (1991).

The role that beliefs play in our field is not just a consideration for clients, but for practitioners as well. Personal beliefs are sometimes thought to be unimportant or irrelevant to clinical practice, but in fact are related to ethical and clinical values and our approach to establishing relationships with our clients that are open and congruent with their expectations (Cobb, 2012). Belief is the cornerstone of trust, faith, hope, conviction, and self-confidence. Belief is as much something we *are* as something we *do*. It is both a state of mind and a way of being (Hawley, 1993). Peters and Waterman introduced the importance of rebelieving —reacquiring the essential belief in oneself. That was the true message of their best-selling book, *In Search of Excellence*, which infused a shot of self-confidence to our nation (Hawley, 1993; Peters & Waterman, 1982).

Belief moves us to the path, to the place of wisdom. Beliefs provide the source of inspiration, the bedrock of dedication, and the very basis of commitment. Belief and faith are similar—both stem from deep within, not from external sources. We have all heard the expression, "blind faith," and in many ways faith is blind. However most of us, as data and documentation seeking scientists, are uncomfortable with that belief. We want proof, we want to see the evidence before we leap. We must be willing to take that "leap of faith" and begin to foster our own internal evidence, to create our own sense of inner authority (Hawley, 1993).

Expectations call upon the same deep power as faith and belief. We tend to meet our expectations, so when we expect the best, chances are we will get it. When we expect the worst, we are usually not disappointed. Expectations are closely tied to productivity, learning, and behavioral change in general. This has been shown to exist in many fields, including business, education, psychology, and speech-language pathology (Hawley, 1993; Locke & Latham, 2002; Pasupathy, & Bogschutz, 2013). Often beliefs and expectations, rather than abilities, bring in the results.

Our Library of Health and Wellness Beliefs

Part of our *library of beliefs* is commitment to knowing what sustains health, causes illness, and brings about healing. Health beliefs are used to explain why individuals do not always follow advice, why they vary in response to symptoms, and adapt or abandon treatment regimens (Janz & Becker, 1984). One model that is used to help predict patient attitudes and behaviors toward treatment is the Health Beliefs Model, a psychosocial model developed from behavioral and psychological theory. The model includes the following categories of belief that determine values, attitudes,and behaviors that might help or hinder the therapeutic process of healing or rehabilitation (Stretcher & Rosenstock, 1997):

- Vulnerability to contract a condition
- Belief in the diagnosis
- Perceived benefits or effectiveness of the treatment
- Negative consequences of treatment, such as time lost, cost, or inconvenience
- Perceived severity and potential consequences
- Perceived impact on their lives
- Self-efficacy and confidence in one's ability to change outcomes

The Existence of Aliefs

The term *alief* was coined by Tamar Gendler, a Professor of Philosophy and Cognitive Science at Yale University. Gendler (2008a) defines *alief* as "an innate or habitual propensity to respond to an apparent stimulus in a particular way" (p. 552). Often an alief is in tension with a person's explicit beliefs. For example, a person who believes in racial equality may nonetheless have aliefs that cause him or her to treat people differently when they are of different racial groups or ethnicity (Gendler, 2008b). Since the notion was introduced, it has been cited to explain such psychological phenomena as why we experience pleasure when we listen to stories, and the persistence of *positive illusions*. Positive illusions allow us to convince ourselves of something we know on another level is not true (Bloom, 2011).

An alief allows us to act differently than what we think we believe. Thinking in terms of alief differs from thinking in terms of traditional cognitive attitudes. *Alief* allows for another possibility: that you can be absolutely and rationally convinced of something, yet also alieve—and thus behave—quite differently (Gendler, 2008b). This view of the mind as a place where rational, strongly-held beliefs can coexist with aliefs suggests why behavioral change is so difficult. If beliefs are conscious responses to how we think things are, aliefs are conscious responses to how things seem (McKay & Dennett, 2009). You believe one thing is true, but act as if another is true because of your alief. In philosophy and psychology an *alief* is an automatic or habitual belief-like-attitude, particularly one that is in tension with a person's explicit beliefs (Gendler, 2008a, 2008b).

When our environment is stable and when we are attentive, our aliefs will be largely in accord with our reality-reflective beliefs and attitudes. However, when our environment is unstable, atypical or undesirable, and when we are largely inattentive to reality in certain ways, our aliefs will conflict with our beliefs and create a state of discord (Gendler, 2008b). Discord can be deliberate (daydreams) or unwelcome (phobias, abuses). We must learn how to respond to discordant aliefs, which the ancients considered the problem of harmonizing the parts of the soul, or in more modern terms can be described as the conflict between reason and the passions (Gendler, 2008a).

According to Gendler (2008a, 2008b), we all have aliefs. They are more primitive than beliefs and desires, and are neither rational nor irrational. They simply exist. Although we may be aware that we have aliefs, because they are habitual and instinctive automatic responses, they operate outside the realm of conscious thought. In order to better understand our reactions, it is important that we recognize the role they play in our overall framework of beliefs, attitudes, and knowledge systems. Only when we are aware of our aliefs, as well as our beliefs, can we hope to harmonize them and create a *reflective equilibrium* (Gendler, 2008a; McKay & Dennett, 2009).

Self-Efficacy Beliefs

Self-efficacy is derived from social cognitive theory, which explains human behavior as an interaction of cognition, emotion, behavior, and the environment (Bandura, 1997; Pasupathy & Bogschutz, 2013). We discuss self-efficacy in more detail in Chapter 7 as a component of growth. Self-efficacy is not related to knowledge and skills that an individual possesses, but to what an individual believes he or she can accomplish with the knowledge and skills possessed. Perceived self-efficacy directly relates to confidence and beliefs in one's capabilities to execute actions that are required to produce specific outcomes (Bandura, 1997).

Self-efficacy beliefs play a critical role in how we learn as we acquire knowledge and skills. Competent functioning requires harmony between self-beliefs and possessed skills and knowledge (Pajares, 1996; Schunk, 1983). The creation and use of self-beliefs is an intuitive process that influences and directs future behavior (Ormrod, 2006). For example, as students, we develop beliefs about our academic capabilities that play a large role in determining what we do with the knowledge and skills we have learned (Pintrich & De Groot, 1990).

Self-beliefs develop from four sources: interpretations of experience, the modeled actions of others, verbal feedback of others, and physiological states such as anxiety, stress, and fatigue (Bandura, 1997; Pajares, 1996; Schunk, 1983). Self-efficacy beliefs inform motivation and self-regulation in several ways. They influence our choices, our courses of action, our accomplishments, and our personal well-being (Bandura, 1997; Pajares, 1992, 1996). They will impact new learnings and changes in behavior, both personally and professionally.

Self-efficacy beliefs have been shown to be predictive of performance, because effort invested in a particular action is regulated by an individual's belief in his or her ability to perform that action (Bandura, 1982). In addition, individuals with strong self-efficacy beliefs have high motivation and strong commitment to their goals, and are, therefore, not easily discouraged by obstacles or barriers (Pasupathy & Bogschutz, 2013). They tend to be persistent, resilient, and exhibit greater staying power and less burn-out (Crowe, Deppe, & Karr, 2008).

Clinical self-efficacy, or the individual's belief in his or her clinical capabilities, is to be distinguished from treatment efficacy or outcomes. However, the strength of a clinician's self-efficacy (confidence in beliefs) can positively impact the goals chosen and achieved. Higher goals may be chosen, and outcome achievement is more likely through clinician determination and perseverance (Locke & Lathan, 2002). Understanding the importance of self-efficacy beliefs can help us enhance educational pedagogy, foster skill mastery, build clinical confidence, and facilitate more positive clinical performance and experiences (Pasupathy & Bogschutz, 2013). Self-efficacy is discussed in more detail in Chapter 7.

Our Beliefs About Our Students

Research studying the beliefs of teachers has shown that internal personal efficacy beliefs can impact external instructional outcomes through the influence of personal orientation and philosophy about the educational process (Marsh, Walker, & Debus, 1991; Woolfolk & Hoy, 1990). Teachers with a low sense of efficacy tend to hold a more *custodial rather than educational* view of student's behavior. Teachers with a high sense of efficacy create mastery rather than maintenance experiences in the classroom (Ashton & Webb, 1986).

Although we cannot accomplish tasks beyond our capabilities simply by believing that we can, our beliefs become the internal rules that help us determine the effort and perseverance required for performance success (Runne, 2012). It is helpful for us, as students and practitioners, to understand the conditions and contexts under which self-beliefs will carryover to professional learning situations. This will help us build confidence as well as competence and self-perceptions of both. Perception of competence, rather than competence itself, may more accurately predict motivation, effort, and opportunity to challenge oneself with new learnings and continuous growth.

---

3. REFLECTIVE KNOWLEDGE SYSTEMS

History of Reflective Practice

Precursors of reflective knowledge and practice can be found in ancient texts such as Buddhist teachings and the *Meditations* of Stoic philosopher Marcus Aurelius (Winter, 2003). *Reflective practice* actually has its roots in an idea from the Enlightenment, that if we venture to stand outside of ourselves, we will have a clearer understanding of who we are and what we do (Brookfield, 1995). Reflection means the incorporation of thought, consideration, and questions about what we do, what works, what doesn't, and how we can best change things around (Hubball, Collins, & Pratt, 2005). It is an active and largely internalized process that requires encouragement, support, and time. Reflective practices need to be part of the "bigger picture" of academic and institutional work environments through their training and staff development approaches.

The need for reflective practice is certainly not new, but seems to be having a revival. In fact, the concepts underlying reflective practice are quite old. Early in the 20th century, John Dewey was among the first to write about reflective practice with his exploration of experience, interaction, and reflection (Dewey, 1933). According to Dewey, when confronted with situations, we act either in routine ways or reflective ways (1933). Dewey was among the first to identify reflection as a different way of thinking that prompted purposeful inquiry and problem resolution (Sinclair, 1998). Dewey's initial work was solidified when Schön's book was published (1983). Whereas Dewey talked about the process of reflection, Schön's interest was to facilitate the development of *reflective practitioners.*

Reflective Practice Evolved from Knowledge Systems

In 1978, Barbara Carper, a professor of nursing, attempted to classify the different sources from which knowledge and beliefs in professional practice can be derived. The typology identifies five fundamental patterns of knowing and created a professional impetus for incorporating reflection as a professional practice habit (Carper, 1978).

1. *Empirical:* This is the factual knowledge from science, or other external sources, that can be empirically verified. *What knowledge informed me?*
2. *Personal:* These are the knowledge and attitudes derived from personal self-understanding and empathy, including imagining one's self in the client's position. *Why did I feel the way I did within this situation?*
3. *Ethical:* These are those attitudes and knowledge derived from an ethical framework, including an awareness of moral questions and choices. *What factors were influencing me, and did I act for the best reasons?*
4. *Aesthetic:* This is an awareness of the immediate situation, seated in immediate practical action, including awareness of the patient and their circumstances as uniquely individual, and of the combined wholeness of the situation. *What was I trying to achieve?*
5. *Reflexive:* This is connecting the immediate situation with past situations. *How could I have handled the situation better?*

A Crisis in Confidence: Technical Rationality

In 1987, Donald Schön reintroduced us to the concept of reflective practice. He described it as a critical process in refining one's artistry or craft in a particular discipline, and involves thoughtfully considering one's own experiences when applying knowledge (Schön, 1987). Schön recommended reflective practice as a way for beginners in a discipline to recognize consonance between their own individual practices and those of successful practitioners.

Schön (1983) was one of the first to discuss what he called "the crisis in confidence in professional knowledge" (p. 3) He attributes this crisis to our emphasis on *technical rationality* as resulting from the scientific method as being the dominant epistemology of practice in most professional training programs. This causes a gap between the rigor of research and the demands of real-time practice (Tremmel, 1993). Whereas technical rationality is based on the results of research usually conducted off site, reflection generates knowledge directly from experience. In a sense, the practitioner is acting as a researcher on site, and the practice becomes the laboratory (Schön, 1983; Tremmel, 1993).

Schön tells us that knowledgeable practice is shaped by more than this technical type of knowledge (1983). It is shaped by what he called "knowing-in-action," which is fueled by self-reflection or *reflection-in-action*. Feelings play a large influential factor in one's ability to interpret and respond to situations, and to reflect. The artistry of our practice is influenced and framed by the knowing that comes from doing, which eventually develops into our tacit knowledge and professional intuition. The art of implementation and improvisation are necessary neighbors to the rigor of science and research (Dilello, 2010).

Competent practitioners usually know more than they can say. Their capacity to *do the right thing* exhibits more about what they know in what they do by the way in which they do it. Their practices exemplify the difference between *knowing that* and *knowing how*. Our intuitive and sometimes spontaneous knowing is often used in the midst of action to cope with situations that are unique, uncertain, or even conflicted (Schön, 1983). Over the years, we have seen reference to the crisis in professional confidence and the decline in professional self-image calling for a greater acknowledgment of the *art of practice* (Schön, 1983).

When we reflect both in and on our practice, we may reflect on many things: appreciations that underlie a judgment; strategies and theories implicit in a pattern of behavior; feelings about a situation that led us to adopt a particular course of action; how we have framed a problem we are trying to solve; or even about our role with a larger macrosystem (Schön, 1987; Visser, 2010). Reflection-in-action involves experiment, and we become researchers in a practice context, and bring to life *practice-based evidence.*

4. REFLECTIVE PRACTICES

What Is Reflective Practice?

Although *reflective practice* conjures up a multitude of interpretations, even with the same discipline, it is generally understood as the process of learning through and from experience for the purpose of gaining new insights of one self and one's practice habits (Boud, Keogh, & Walker, 1985; Finlay, 2003). It allows us to examine assumptions about our everyday practice, and encourages self-awareness and critical evaluation of our responses to everyday, real-time situations. Reflection can mean anything from solitary introspection to the engagement of critical dialogue with others. For some, it means adopting a thought-infused and carefully crafted approach to practice, while others find reflection too self-indulgent (Smyth, 1992).

Reflective practice is the capacity to reflect on action and engage in a process of continuous learning (Schön, 1983). According to one definition, it involves a process of paying critical attention to the practical values and theories that inform everyday actions, by the examination of practice both reflectively and reflexively. This leads to developmental insight

(Bolton, 2010). A key rationale for reflective practice is that knowledge alone does not necessarily lead to learning; deliberate reflection on experiential learning is essential (Cochran-Smith & Lytle, 1999). It has been described as a self-directing learning approach taught to professionals from a variety of disciplines, applicable to all professions, and commonly used in health and teaching professions, though applicable to all professions (Boud et al., 1985; Larrivee, 2000). Reflective practices enable us to think about what, how and why we do what we do. They facilitate our ability to step out of "one size fits all" action routines.

Reflective practice can be an important tool in practice-based professional learning settings where people learn from their own professional experiences, and may be one of the most important sources of personal professional development and improvement (Johns & Burnie, 2013). A person who reflects throughout his or her practice is not just looking back on past actions and events, but is taking a conscious look at emotions, experiences, actions, and responses, and using that information to add to his or her existing knowledge base and reach a higher level of understanding (Paterson & Chapman, 2013).

Types of Reflection

Schön differentiates between two types of reflection: *reflection-in-action* and *reflection-on action* (1987, 1996). Reflection-in-action happens while working, and cites the importance of being aware of decisions as you make them. The majority of teachers and other professionals practice this level of reflection. The second level of reflection, reflection-on-action, happens after decisions and actions have occurred. It involves the cognitive processes of review, analysis, and evaluation—all of which enhance professional development (Schön, 1996).

We reflect both during and after action to improve practices. When we *reflect in action,* we heighten our awareness of our clinical decisions at the time they are happening, evaluate outcomes in real time, and make changes as they need to be made. When we *reflect on action,* we are doing so after the action has been completed. We review, analyze, evaluate, and then adapt future courses of action (Moon, 1999).

This level of reflection can be achieved by thinking back about our experiences, testing our existing beliefs, and questioning decisions and their results. This can be expressed in writing reflective journals, audio journals, professional exchanges, peer observations, action research, and keeping professional portfolios. In other words, it is a deeper level of reflection and more time-consuming, which may be the reason that reflection-in-action is more commonly reported in research than is reflection-on-action (Moon, 1999; Odeh, Kurt, & Atamturk, 2006; Postholm, 2008; Van Manen, 1995).

In both types of reflection, in-action and on-action, professionals seek to connect with their feelings as they attend to theory. Reflection-in-action was the core of *professional artistry,* as Schön described it, in contrast to the technical-rationality demanded by the rigorous application of science. Today, we would translate this dominant positivist paradigm of technical-rationality into the evidence-based practice (EBP) movement. We know from earlier chapters that EBP tends to favor quantitative studies over qualitative ones, and established testing protocols over intuitive practice (Fish & Coles, 1998). In Schön's view, professionals had to confront the dilemma of *rigor verses relevance* created by the strict adherence to technical-rationality (EPB).

One of the keys to thinking-in-action is to take a step back, a skill that novices rarely have. They feel more comfortable following established rules and procedures (often mechanically), until they develop the skill of simultaneously being able to monitor and adapt their actions. Practitioners who feel more expert in their practice are comfortable with thinking-in-action, as it calls upon intuition, creativity, and tacit knowledge (Finlay, 2008; Fish & Coles, 1998).

Levels and Skills

Reflective practice can be viewed as a synthesis of *reflection, self-awareness,* and *critical thinking* (Eby, 2000). *Reflection* can be described as tool for promoting self-awareness, social awareness, self-expression, and cooperative learning. Reflection links theory with practice. *Self-awareness* can be described as a cognitive ability to sense, think, feel, and know through intuition. We evaluate all that we acquire through self-awareness to develop understanding. *Critical thinking* is a tool for helping us identify and challenge assumptions, question context, and explore alternatives. Zeichner and Liston (1996) have differentiated between the five R's, or the five levels of reflection:

1. *Rapid reflection:* involves automatic and immediate action
2. *Repair:* involves using client cues to alter actions and revise decisions
3. *Review:* involves discussing or writing about decisions and actions
4. *Research:* involves collecting data or reading research in a systematic way
5. *Re-theorizing and reformulating:* involves examining your own practice in light of academic theories

Models of Reflective Practice

Many models of reflective practice have been proposed from differing fields of health care and education. It has been suggested they all involve three basic processes (Quinn, 1988).

The first is *retrospection*, such as thinking back about a situational experience. The second is *self-evaluation*, such as using theoretical perspectives to analyze and evaluate actions and feelings related to the experience. The last is *reorientation*, such as using the results of a self-evaluation to impact future decisions and approaches to similar experiences.

Graham Gibbs, a learning researcher, offers suggestions known as *Gibbs' reflective cycle*, which can be simplified into the following six distinct stages to assist in structuring reflection on learning experiences (Gibbs, 1988): description, feelings, evaluation, analysis, conclusions, and action plan. Christopher Johns, a professor of nursing, designed a structured model of reflection that provides practitioners with a guide to gain greater understanding of his or her practice (Johns, 2010; Johns & Bernie, 2013). Johns highlights the importance of experienced knowledge in combination with the ability of a practitioner to access, understand, and put into practice technical/empirical information that has been acquired. Reflection occurs though simultaneously "looking in" on one's thoughts and emotions and "looking out" at the situations and issues that seem significant (Johns, 2010).

Benefits of Reflective Practice

Reflective teaching and learning have been important trends in education, largely because they foster problem solving, decision-making, and critical thinking. Reflection begins with open-mindedness and assumption of responsibility, and evolves into a willingness to question our practices for the purpose of self-growth and improved outcomes for our clients (Odeh et al., 2006). The act of reflection is seen as an effective way of promoting the development of autonomous, qualified, and self-directed professionals. Engaging in reflective practice has been associated with improved quality of care, stimulating personal and professional growth and closing the gap between theory and practice (Johns & Burnie, 2013; Paterson & Chapman, 2013).

Numerous benefits to reflective practice have been identified, and include (Davies, 2012; Johns & Burnie, 2013):

- Increased learning from experiences
- Identification of personal and professional strengths and areas for improvement
- Acquisition of new knowledge and skills
- Further understanding of own beliefs, attitudes, and values
- Facilitation of self-directed learning
- Enhanced motivation for new learning
- Additional sources of feedback
- Improvements of personal and clinical confidence

Reflecting on one's teaching and provision of speech and language therapy should foster personal growth and development, lead to better understanding of how client's learn, help practitioners assess which practices are effective under specific circumstances, aid in the development of therapy adaptations, and enhance the scholarship of teaching and learning (Hubball et al., 2005; Schön, 1987). Reflective practice is an important component of our field and provides a framework of great value for enhancing effectiveness in professional practice, benefiting the practitioner as well as those whom the profession serves. It has potential to bridge theory with practice and generate theory about practice, balance science with client-centered care, link evidence-based practice with practice-based evidence, and contribute to the cultivation of ethical principles of practice (Caty, Kinsella, & Doyle, 2016).

Our contemporary workplace is a landscape that is constantly evolving, being driven by political, economical, technological, demographic, and social winds of change (Lubinski

& Hudson, 2013). We are asked to be more creative with fewer resources, learn about new technology, and work effectively with other professionals across disciplines all for the benefit of our students. Many of the new skills we need to learn are done so independently, and require an ongoing process of reflection about one's practice and changes that need to take place to help us better cope with our evolving professional landscape. As we discussed in this chapter, reflective practice is the deliberate examination of experience that results in current learning and directs future actions. As we reflect about workplace relationships, or student clinical and educational issues, that learning becomes integrated into our repertoire of practice-based evidence (Gabbay & le May, 2011).

Through reflective practices, we understand better what we do and why we do it and thus take this first step in theorizing, generating, and sharing new knowledge (Beecham, 2004). We must pay attention to the ways in which practice-based knowledge is generated and how it contributes to our clinical expertise. Only then can we begin the process of making tacit knowledge that informs professional practice explicit (Caty et al., 2016).

Limitations and Challenges to Reflective Practice

There is no doubt that reflection is essential for professional growth and more effective teaching. However, there is still some debate over how we can best teach one to become a reflective practitioner. Reflection may not be a simple procedure that can be taught, but rather a holistic orientation or attitude about teaching and learning that can be helped to acquire (Zeichner & Liston, 1996). Familiarity with the term reflective practice is no guarantee that it will be applied to professional experiences, because the theory-practice gap dictates that formal knowledge acquisition

and awareness of theories does not necessarily lead to changes in action (Harris, 1998; McAlpine & Weston, 2000).

The concept does not come without its concerns. Three areas of concern about reflective practice have been identified: ethical, professional, and pedagogic. One *ethical concern* is that reflection can have an emotional impact on the person reflecting (Quinn, 1988). Questioning assumptions can be powerful, and the constant striving for self-improvement that reflective practices engender can also lead to feelings of self-rejection or disapproval.

Professional concerns surface when reflective practice is conducted ineffectively or inappropriately and reinforces negative practice or devalues the importance of clinical reasoning. In such cases, the point is missed and its value goes unrecognized (Boud & Walker, 1998). Reflective practices are best used as a *springboard* for personal and professional growth and development of general insight, and must be modeled and adequately supported by mentors and supervisors who are comfortable with the process (Quinn, 1988).

One *pedagogic concern* is that students and practitioners must be *developmentally ready* to participate with critical reflection. They must be willing to analyze their practice experiences, reflect on significant and meaningful incidents in context, and question their assumptions—rather than simply learning for the future (Eraut, 2004). A second pedagogic concern relates to the compulsory element when reflective exercises are *required*. "Reflection" and "assessment" are often incompatible activities, as external assessment discourages genuine, honest, and critical self-examination. A number of qualitative studies from the fields of medicine, nursing, and social work showed that when students feel compelled to write, they generally write what they think the teacher wants. In addition, they write just enough to pass the requirement, and their writings are superficial, strategic, and guarded (Eraut, 2004; Hobbs, 2007; Wellard & Bethune, 1996).

In summary, the following are identified barriers to reflective practice: (Bolton, 2010; Jasper, 2003):

- lack of understanding about the reflective process,
- discomfort with confronting challenges,
- unease with self-evaluation,
- time consuming,
- confusion about which situations/experiences to reflect upon, and
- reflection may not be adequate to resolve clinical problems.

Why Is Reflective Practice So Difficult?

Reflective practice must be nurtured, and practitioners need to apply it selectively and use it with care. It is difficult to practice, and even more so to teach or model. Why is reflective practice so difficult (Finlay, 2003)? First, there is confusion about what exactly it is. It also involves a complex interaction of processes, and there is no end to what can be reflected upon. Reflective practice taps tacit and dimensions of knowledge and practice that are taken for granted and difficult to translate. Lastly, it seeks to identify qualitative elements of practice (such as professional artistry and focus on ideological dimensions) which are hard to see, and difficult to articulate and quantify. Remember that reflective practice is highly specific to both individuals and contexts. Each practitioner needs to reflect in different ways at different times, and different contexts may demand a different type of reflecting.

Strategies for Practicing More Reflectively

Reflective practice is useful for professions as they update their skills and knowledge and consider new ways to interact with their colleagues. Somerville and Keeling suggest seven simple ways that professionals can practice more reflectively (2004).

1. Seek feedback by asking for it.
2. Every day ask and answer the question, "What have I learned today?"
3. Acknowledge your strengths and those of others with whom you work.
4. Identify positive accomplishments and areas for growth.
5. View experiences objectively by removing yourself, and imagining the situation is on stage and you are in the audience.
6. Empathize by stating out loud what you imagine the other person is experiencing.
7. Keep a journal where you record your thoughts and feelings, and look for patterns.

As students and practitioners, we tend to reflect more *in action* rather than *on action*. In fact, reflecting on action was often ignored (Moon, 2004). It is best achieved by thinking back over our experiences and questioning our beliefs and decisions. There are numerous tools we can use to accomplish this: reflective journals, action research, and professional portfolios. This involves a deeper level of reflection, and is more deliberate and therefore time consuming. In conclusion, neither the awareness of theory about reflective practices nor knowledge about the importance of reflection for profession growth will mean that professionals apply reflection as part of their professional practices (Moon, 2004).

Reflective practices are used in various professions and for different reasons (Stone-Goldman, 2012; Van Deurzen & Adams, 2011). Studies about clinical effectiveness report that reflective practices enhance rapport, foster professional growth, facilitate cultural understanding, improve clinical supervision, and help us cope with loss and tragedy (Stone-Goldman, 2012).

When we reflect on our practices, we are better able to explore and learn from our reactions to others. According to Stone-Goldman (2012), our most important reflective tools are:

- *Focused attention* or mindfulness, which is the conscious direction of our attention to our experiences (Davis & Hayes, 2011)
- *Thought analysis*, which is the conscious review and ongoing probe for deeper understanding of our clinical experiences
- *Writing*, which brings ideas to light and highlights themes

Reflective writing is also called free writing, journal writing, expressive writing, and spontaneous writing (Stone-Goldman, 2010). It is a tool we use to help us find the balance between our personal self and our professional self, as they intersect within the landscape of our clinical experiences. How do we get started with reflective writing—what do we write about? Stone-Goldman suggests we can begin with one of the following: immediate emotional, mental, or physical states; recent stressful events or anticipation of future events; or stories to tell, or stories that you have been told.

Who Are Reflective Practitioners?

Reflective practitioners look back at the work they do and the work process at regular intervals, and considers how they can improve. They reflect on the work they have done. They are not happy to carry on at the current standard because they long to improve (Osterman & Kottkamp, 1993).

In one study about the use of self-reflective practices by educators, it was found that neither gender, experience, level of education or knowledge of the importance of reflection for professional growth play a role in facilitating reflective practices (Odeh et al., 2006).

Knowledge about theories does not necessarily govern our actions or our reflections about them. Reflective practice includes a thoughtful consideration and questioning of what we do, what works and what does not. The process begins with one's willingness to question his/her practice and further develops through adapting our style with the needs of our clients.

There tends to be agreement that reflection can have many positive effects, but what does it actually mean in practice? Three ideas related to practice are crucial: First, reflective practitioners examine both *the hows* and *the whats* of their work, including their beliefs and values. Second, they examine *the underlying premises* on which their work is based. Third, they integrate a *plurality of approaches* to integrate intentional critical thinking activities into their learning experiences and work habits (Hubball et al., 2005).

REFLECTIVE SUMMATIVE QUESTIONS

1. What factors and variables do you feel are most important when selecting desired outcomes for your client?
2. What skills, knowledge, and attitudes would you like to improve in order to become a better student and better clinician?
3. What aspect of student experience/clinician experience/client experience would you like to improve?
4. What do you hope to achieve for and with your clients within the context of clinical practice?
5. What types of reflective practices have you used in your training program or work setting?
6. Keep a reflective journal for one class and/or one client. Include the following types

of information: what you have tried, what you have learned, how and why you reach the conclusions you have, and ideas for change in the future.

REFERENCES

Ashton, P. T., & Webb, R. B. (1986). *Making a difference: Teachers' sense of efficacy and student achievement.* New York, NY: Longman.

Bandura, A. (1997). *Self-efficacy: The exercise of control.* New York, NY: W. H. Freeman.

Bandura, A. (1982). Self-efficacy mechanism in human agency. *American Psychologist, 37,* 122–147.

Beecham, R. (2004). Power and practice: A critique of evidence-based practice for the profession of speech-language pathology. *International Journal of Speech-Language Pathology, 6*(2), 131–133.

Bloom, P. (2011). *How pleasure works: The new science of why we like what we like.* New York, NY: W. W. Norton.

Bolton, G. (2010) *Reflective practice: writing and professional development* (3rd ed.). Los Angeles, CA: Sage.

Boud, D., Keogh, R., & Walker, D. (1985). *Reflection, turning experience into learning.* London, UK: Kogan Page.

Boud, D., & Walker, D. (1998). Promoting reflection in professional courses: The challenge of context. *Studies in Higher Education, 23*(2),191–206.

Brookfield, S. D. (1995). *Becoming critically reflective teacher.* San Francisco, CA: Jossey-Bass.

Carper, B. (1978). Fundamental patterns of knowing in nursing. *Advances in Nursing Science 1*(1). 13–24.

Caty, M., Kinsella, E. A., & Doyle, P. C. (2016). Reflective practice in speech-language pathology: Relevance for practice and education. *Canadian Journal of Speech-Language Pathology and Audiology, 40*(1), 81–91.

Charon, R. (2006). *Narrative medicine: Honoring the stories of illness.* New York, NY: Oxford University Press.

Cobb, M. (2012). Belief. In M. Cobb, C. Puchalski, & B. Rumbold, (Eds.). *Oxford textbook of spirituality in healthcare.* New York, NY: Oxford University Press.

Cochran-Smith, M., & Lytle, S. L. (1999). Relationships of knowledge and practice: Teacher learning in communities. *Review of Research Education, 24*(1), 249–305.

Crowe, E., Deppe, J., & Karr, S. (2008). State, national efforts address personnel shortages. *The ASHA Leader, 13*(4), 8.

Davies, S. (2012). Embracing reflective practice. *Education for Primary Care, 23*(1), 9–12.

Davis, D. M., & Hayes, J. A. (2011). What are the benefits of mindfulness? A practice review of psychotherapy-related research. *American Psychological Association, 48*(2), 198–208.

Dewey, J. (1933). *How we think: A restatement of the relation of reflective thinking to the educative process.* Boston. MA: Houghton Mifflin.

DiLollo, A. (2010). The crisis of confidence in professional knowledge: Implications for clinical education in speech-language pathology. *ASHA Perspectives on Administration and Supervision, 20,* 85–91.

Eby, M. A. (2000). Understanding professional development. In A. Brechin, H. Brown, & M. A. Eby (Eds.), *Critical practice in health and social care.* London, UK: Sage.

Eraut, M. (2004). Editorial: The practice of reflection. *Learning in Health and Social Care, 3*(2), 47–52.

Finlay, L. (2003) Mapping multiple routes. In L. Finlay & B. Gough (Eds.), *Reflexivity: A guide for researchers in health and social sciences.* Oxford, UK: Blackwell.

Fish, D., & Coles, C. (1998). *Developing professional judgment in health care: Learning through practice.* Oxford, UK: Butterworth-Heinemann.

Gabbay, J., & le May, A. (2011). *Practice-based evidence for healthcare: Clinical mindlines.* New York, NY: Routledge.

Gendler, T. S. (2008a). Alief in action (and reaction). *Mind and Language, 23*(5), 552–585.

Gendler, T. S. (2008b). Alief and belief. *Journal of Philosophy, 105*(10), 634–663.

Gibbs, G. (1988). *Learning by doing: A guide to teaching and learning methods.* Oxford, UK: Further Education Unit, Oxford Polytechnic.

Harris, A. (1998). Effective teaching: A review of the literature. *School Leadership and Management, 18*(2), 169–183.

Hawley, J. (1993). *Reawakening the spirit in work.* New York, NY: Simon & Shuster.

Hobbs, V. (2007). Faking it or hating it: Can reflective practice be forced? *Reflective Practice, 8*(3), 405–417.

Horgan, J. (2003). *Rational mysticism.* New York, NY: Houghton Mifflin.

Hubball, H., Collins, J., & Pratt, D. (2005). Enhancing reflective teaching practices: Implications for faculty development programs. *Canadian Journal of Higher Education, 3,* 57–81.

Janz, N., & Becker, M. (1984). The health belief model: A decade later. *Health Education Behavior, 11*(1), 1–47.

Jasper, M. (2003). *Beginning reflective practice.* Oxford, UK: Nelson Thornes.

Johns, C. (Ed.). (2010). *Guided reflection: A narrative approach to advancing professional practice.* Chichester, UK; Ames, IA: Blackwell.

Johns, C., & Burnie, S. (2013) *Becoming a reflective practitioner.* Ames, IA: Blackwell.

Kenney, A. (2007). Knowledge, belief and faith. *Philosophy, 82*(3), 381–397.

Larrivee, B. (2000). Transforming teaching practice: Becoming the critically reflective teacher. *Reflective Practice: Multidisciplinary Perspectives, 1*(3), 293–307

Locke, E. A., & Latham, G. P. (2002). Building a practical useful theory of goal setting and task motivation: A 35-year odyssey. *American Psychologist, 57*(9), 705–717.

Lubinski, R., & Hudson, M.W. (2013). Professions for the 21st century. In R. Lubinski & M. W. Hudson (Eds.), *Professional issues in speech-language pathology and audiology.* Clifton Park, NY: Delmar.

Luterman, D. M. (1991). *Counseling the communicatively disordered and their families* (2nd ed.). Austin, TX: Pro-Ed.

Marsh, H. W., Walker, R., & Debus, R. (1991). Subject-specific components of academic self-concept and self-efficacy. *Contemporary Educational Psychology, 16,* 331–345.

McAlpine, C., & Weston, C. (2000). Reflection: issues related to improving professors teaching and students learning. *Instructional Science, 28,* 363–385.

McKay, R. T., & Dennett, D. (2009). The evolution of misbelief. *Behavioral and Brain Sciences, 32,* 493–510.

Moon, J. A. (1999). *Reflection in learning and professional development: Theory and practice.* London, UK: Kogan Page.

Moon, J. A. (2004). *A handbook of reflective and experiential learning.* New York, NY: Routledge-Falmer.

Moore, J. C. (1979). An analysis of the reinforcing function of clinician attention. *Language, Speech and Hearing Services in Schools, 10,* 93–98.

Odeh, Z., Kurt, M., & Atamturk, N. (2006). *Reflective practice and its role in personal and professional growth.* Turkey: Near East University.

Ormrod, J. E. (2006). *Educational psychology: Developing learners* (5th ed.). Upper Saddle River, NJ: Pearson/Merrill Prentice Hall.

Osterman, K. F., & Kottkamp, R. B. (1993). *Reflective practice for educators.* San Diego, CA: Corwin Press

Pajares, F. (1992). Teachers' beliefs and educational research: Cleaning up a messy construct. *Review of Educational Research, 62,* 307–332.

Pajares, F. (1996). Self-efficacy beliefs in academic settings. *Review of Educational Research, 66,* 543–578.

Pasupathy, R., & Bogschulz, R. J. (2013). An investigation of graduate speech-language pathology students' SLP clinical self-efficacy. *Contemporary Issues in Communication Sciences and Disorders. 40,* 151–159.

Paterson, C., & Chapman, J. (August 2013). Enhancing skills of critical reflection to evidence learning in professional practice. *Physical Therapy in Sport, 14*(3), 133–138.

Peters, T., & Waterman, R. (1982). *In search of excellence: Lessons from America's best-run companies.* New York, NY: Harper Collins.

Pintrich, P. R., & De Groot, E. V. (1990). Motivational and self-regulated learning components of classroom academic performance. *Journal of Educational Psychology, 82,* 33–40.

Postholm, M. B. (2008). Teachers developing practice: Reflection as key activity. *Teaching and Teacher Education, 24*(7), 47–53.

Quinn, F. M. (1998). Reflection and reflective practice. In F. M. Quinn (Ed.), *Continuing pro-

fessional development in nursing. Cheltenham, UK: Stanley Thornes.

Riley, J. (2002). Counseling: An approach for speech-language pathologists. *Contemporary Issues in Communication Science and Disorders, 29,* 6–16.

Runne, C. (2012). *Self-efficacy in people with speech or language disorders: A qualitative study* (Unpublished master's thesis). University of Washington, Seattle.

Schön, D. A. (1983). *The reflective practitioner: How professionals think in action.* New York, NY: Basic Books.

Schön, D. (1987). *Educating the reflective practitioner.* San Francisco, CA: Jossey-Bass.

Schön, D.A. (1996). *Educating the reflective practitioner: Toward a new design for teaching and learning in the professions.* San Francisco, CA: Jossey-Bass.

Schunk, D. H. (1983). Developing children's self-efficacy and skills: The roles of social information and goal setting. *Contemporary Educational Psychology, 8,* 76–86.

Silverman, E. (2008). Ongoing self-reflection. *American Journal of Speech-Language Pathology, 17*(92), 92.

Sinclair, K. (1998) Reflective practice in health care. In J. Creek (Ed.), *Occupational therapy: new perspectives.* London, UK: Whurr.

Smyth, J. (1992) Teachers' work and the politics of reflection. *American Educational Research Journal, 29,* 267–300.

Somerville, D., & Keeling, J. (2004). A practical approach to promote reflective practice within nursing. *Nursing Times, 100*(12), 42–45.

Sperry, R. (1991). Search of beliefs to live by consistent with science. *Zygon: Journal of Religion and Science, 26,* 237–258.

Spillers, C. (2007). An existential framework for understanding the counseling needs of clients. *American Journal of Speech-Language Pathology, 163,* 191–197.

Steglich-Petersen, A. (2006). No norm needed: On the aim of belief. *Philosophical Quarterly, 56*(225). 499–516.

Stone-Goldman, J. (2010, April). *Personal-professional balance: Does it exist? How do we find it?* Keynote speech presented at ASHA Health Care/Business Institute, Seattle, WA.

Stone-Goldman, J. (2012, November). *Reflective practice for emotional balance in professional relationships.* Paper presented at ASHA Convention, Atlanta, GA.

Stretcher, V. J., & Rosenstock, I. M. (1997). The health belief model. In A. Baum, *Cambridge handbook of psychology, health and medicine* (pp. 113–117). Cambridge, UK: Cambridge University Press.

Tremmel, R. (1993). Zen and the art of reflective practice in teacher education. *Harvard Educational Review, 63*(4), 434–458.

Van Deurzen, E., & Adams, M. (2011). *Skills in existential counseling and psychotherapy.* London, UK: Sage.

Van Manen, M. (1995). On the epistemology of reflective practice. *Teachers and Teaching: Theory and Practice 1*(1), 33–50.

Visser, W. (2010). Schön: Design as a reflective practice. Collection, Parsons Paris School of Art and Design. *Art + Design and Psychology,* pp. 21–25.

Wellard, S., & Bethune, E. (1996). Reflective journal writing in nurse education: Whose interests does it serve? *Journal of Advanced Nursing, 24*(5), 1077–1082.

Winter, R. (2003). Buddhism and action research: Towards an appropriate model of inquiry for the caring professions. *Educational Action Research, 11*(1), 141–160.

Woolfolk, A. E., & Hoy, W. K. (1990). Prospective teachers' sense of efficacy and beliefs about control. *Journal of Educational Psychology, 82,* 81–91.

Zeichner, K. M., & Liston, D. P. (Eds.). (1996). *Reflective teaching– An introduction.* New York, NY: Routledge.

CHAPTER 5

Counsel and Care

1. ACTIVE LISTENING

Listen to Understand

One of our most valuable tools and greatest gift may be our ability to listen for the purpose of enhancing our understanding of our clients and their disorders (Luterman, 2008; Rogers, 1951; Shames, 2006). Listening to understand allows the time and space for emotional and spiritual issues to arise. It focuses on the feeling tone beneath the words and invites response to the feeling content, rather than to the surface content of the message.

Listening to understand requires speech-language pathologists to be fully present for their clients and involves an attitude of empathy, nonjudgmental, and unconditional positive regard (Flasher & Fogle, 2012; Moses, 1989; Rogers, 1951; Spillers, 2007). In the presence of such, clients often feel affirmed and accepted and therefore more willing to trust and accept help (Brammer & MacDonald, 2003; Shames, 2006).

Discover the Client's Perspective

The word "therapy" actually means *attendance*, and comes from the Greek *therapeia* (Finlay, 2015). As we listen, we must attend to what is said and what is revealed. The process of making sense of another's world begins with *their story*. Core to the very nature of a *thera-peutic relationship* is a desire to discover the client's perspective (Barrow, 2011; Clarkson, 2003). The use of closed-ended questions, grounded in time constrains, often derail client narratives, or simply cut them short. The same can be true of overdirecting interviews. In general, we need to spend more time listening for stories as part of our everyday practice routines.

Sometimes attentive listening does not feel like an important and relevant clinical activity (Charon, 2006). Yet, therapeutic conversations can provide an opportunity to allow our *professional expertise* to interact with the *experiential expertise* of our client. There are numerous benefits to really attending to the client's story and aligning with a narrative mode of thought that impact the client as well as the therapist: improved therapist job satisfaction, access to important information relevant to diagnosis and intervention, improved clinical outcomes, and improved clinical judgment and decision-making (Barrow, 2008; White & Epston, 1990).

How can we insure that we are truly hearing the story (Barrow, 2011)?

- Incorporate mindfulness
- Trust in the experiential resources of the client
- Use open-ended conversational starters
- Suspend your own beliefs about the communication issue and disability
- Reflect on your role and the role of the client

Stereophonic Listening to Client Narratives

Charon's notion of *stereophonic listening* is described as the ability to hear *both the body and the person who inhabits it* (Barrow, 2011; Charon, 2006). This ability to listen with more than one ear allows us to simultaneously focus on the communication disability, the physical impairment, the barriers, and the personality factors that impact treatment (Charon, 2006).

When we discussed narratives in Chapter 2, we suggested that by active listening we create the conditions for a client to tell their story. This allows them an opportunity to give voice to their experiences and ultimately frame them into something more meaningful for themselves (Barrow, 2011). As listeners to another's story, we are not simply receiving what we hear. We are actively cocreating the story through our utilization of probes, searching for clues, and hypothesizing (Barrow, 2011).

A *narrative approach* to counseling was developed in 1990 by White and Epston. A narrative refers to an individual's personal story and its influence on their interpretation of events and personal experiences (Woltner, DiLollo, & Apel, 2006). The concept behind narrative therapy (as discussed in Chapter 2) is that we are all storytellers, and our stories —whether told by us or by others about us— shape our behavior and sense of selves (Dimaggio, Salvatore, Azzara, & Cantania, 2003; Woltner et al., 2006). Clients sometimes come to therapy with a thinly constructed problem-saturated account of their lives. Our role is to facilitate and encourage a richer narrative that encompasses strengths and abilities (White & Epston, 1990; Woltner et al., 2006).

A key feature of narrative-based practice using stereophonic listening is the process of describing the communication behaviors as distinct from the person (Dobkin, 2015). This is called "externalizing the problem." As that distinction is experienced by the client, the intervention becomes more manageable because behaviors can be broken down into smaller bits.

Spillers reminds us that therapy can lead clients on *two simultaneous journeys* (2007). The first is the *surface journey*, through remediation of speech and language skills. We lead this journey by doing everything we are trained to do: evaluate communication behaviors, set goals with clients, facilitate new skills, and document progress. However, far below the surface, a client may *journey inward*. The speech-language pathologist accompanies and witnesses the client's work on this journey —being fully present, listening empathically and without judgment. Within the context of our therapeutic work, we can allow space and give permission for the inner journey to unfold. Clients' successful resolution of these life issues on their inner journeys will likely enhance therapeutic efforts on the outer journeys (Spillers, 2007).

The Learnable Skill

Active listening has been described as a learnable skill and key component in the development of collaborative relationships with clients, parents, and other team members. There have been three major elements identified in the process of active listening (Thistle & McNaughton, 2015; Wegger, Castle, & Emmett, 2010): the listener conveys *unconditional attention;* the listener demonstrates *awareness of speaker's intent* by paraphrasing content and feelings in the speaker's message; and the listener asks questions and *encourages additional information* based upon this exchange.

In one study that demonstrated the effectiveness of active listening training for special educators, a four-step strategy was introduced with the acronym *LAFF*: *listen*, empathize, and communicate respect; *ask* questions and ask permission to take notes; *focus* on the immediate issues; and *find* a first step (McNaughton, Hamlin, McCarthy, Head-Reeves, & Schreiner, 2008; Thistle & McNaughton, 2015).

1. *Listen, empathize, and communicate respect:* This directs us to attend concerns by making initial statements expressing understanding and empathy, without agreement, disagreement, or judgment. Respect is communicated through use of nonverbal behaviors, indicators of attentiveness, and other body language, and provides the building blocks for rapport and collaboration.

2. *Ask questions, and ask for permission to take notes:* This directs us to gather information by asking open-ended questions.

3. *Focus on the immediate issues:* This directs us to summarize concerns and check for accuracy. This provides opportunities for clarification, and also provides evidence that the practitioner has been listening.

4. *Find a first step:* This directs us to talk about the plan, what is next, and how we will followup to ensure the plan stays on track.

Rules of Active Listening

Active listening is hard work. We remain focused, not letting distractions pull our attention away. We are observing the nonverbal messages, hearing the verbal messages, and putting all the connecting threads together (Riley, 2002). We are looking for patterns, consistencies, and contradictions where words and emotions lack congruence. We listen for expressions of grief, isolation, hopelessness, and loss. What are some of the rules (Riley, 2002)?

- We do not try to solve problems or come up with answers; we simply listen, acknowledge, and support.

- We do not question accuracy of client statements.
- We do not try to convince the client of anything.
- We separate our experiences from those of the client.
- We recognize our own anxiety and discomfort, and our tendency (in response) to intellectualize and over-talk.
- We do not turn the conversation around to us.
- Hear the client's story in a cohesive way and reflect it back.

Listening Instead of Talking

Listening, instead of talking and focusing on feelings rather than facts, can be very difficult for the beginning and the experienced SLP clinician. In fact, many of the behaviors underlying client-centered counseling are contradictory to students' prior clinical experience (Kaderavek, Laux, & Mills, 2004). With client-centered counseling or therapy, we are trained to be reflective rather than to direct client behavior. Students must also learn to subordinate their own personal reactions and opinions and to focus instead on facilitating the client's personal growth. As Shames (2006) stated, "It is a very one-sided, non-mutual relationship. One person expresses, reveals, and examines while the other facilitates the process." (p. 13)

In order to develop a client-centered session, speech-language pathology students need to become comfortable using a variety of nonverbal behaviors. These include, among other things, facial expression, head nodding, body posture, and eye contact (Shipley, 1997). Both the awareness and effective use of these variables have been associated with counseling effectiveness (Burgoon, 1994). There are specific strategies to improve nonverbal communication. In terms of *body position and leaning*, we need to maintain a relaxed by slightly forward body position. A tightly closed position (arm and leg crossing) should be avoided. Eye contact is a bit more complex, as there is a variation that occurs in typical communication (shorter) versus counseling sessions (longer). Eye contact styles also have great variations based upon culture.

Our client is central to all that takes place during our sessions. We call this client-directed, active participation, or client-centered. *Deep, focused, and nonjudgmental listening* is one of greatest skills, and it allows clients to participate more fully in the therapeutic process. As our confidence increases, we are more easily able to let go of control and enable the client to teach us what they need. As we do less and say less, more learning and changes of behavior will be facilitated. That is the irony of our work (Luterman, 2011).

Deep listening by the counselor means *it's not about me*, and requires that all personal agendas be set aside (Luterman, 2010). *Being in service* to another human being reminds us that the most important clinical tool in our clinical landscape is, now and always, the clinician. Even we need periodic care and recalibration. The practice of self-care is a preventive measure for the dreaded "burnout."

Silence Is Golden

One of the most powerful techniques for maintaining a client-centered focus is for the SLP to permit and tolerate silence during the interview (Cormier & Nurius, 2003; Kaderavek, Laux & Mills, 2004; Seligman, 2004). Silence is more than just the absence of speech; silence can indicate respect, agreement, or empathic consideration of the speaker's communication (Battle, 1997). However, depending upon ethnic and cultural background, silence may be interpreted as more positive or more negative, and steeped with interpretations of tension or uncertainty.

Discomfort with silence leads many SLP students and practitioners to dread the occurrence of silence during therapy sessions (Shames, 2006). We must increase our tolerance for conversational pauses. One effective strategy for doing this is simply to mentally count to five before commenting or reflecting feelings (Kaderavek, Laux, & Mills, 2004). Positive benefits of silence include allowing the client to process information, maintaining a client-centered versus clinician-directed focus, and providing an open invitation to the client to talk. Often, with a clinician-induced silence or pause time, clients will elaborate or explore their feelings without additional clinician input (Shames, 2006).

Along with pause time, the use of additional minimal encouragers (e.g., use of "mmm-hmm," "yes," or "I see") and head nods can be explored during the clinical or therapy sessions. Minimal encouragers act as verbal reinforcement demonstrating clinician attention and approval (Hackney & Cormier, 1994). Pause time and minimal encouragers used together establish the SLP as a listener instead of a "director" during the counseling interview (Luterman, 2008).

Mindful Listening

Mindful listening has been described as when the mind and body work together to communicate for the following purposes: information processing, information seeking, evaluative listening, therapeutic listening, or empathetic or compassionate listening (Shafir, 2003). Barriers to mindful listening include past experiences, personal agendas, and a focus on outcome rather than process, whereas reassurance and paraphrasing through reflection will support listening.

Shafir proposes a LISTEN acronym to support mindful listening (2003):

- Look interested
- Involve yourself by responding

- Stay in a listening mode
- Test your understanding with reflexive comments
- Evaluate the information
- Neutralize your feelings

We can add to that:

- Speak with integrity
- Listen with empathy
- Practice with compassion (Cranfill & Mahanna-Boden, 2012).

A.R.T.: Listen

As I was writing this chapter, I walked by a Pilates studio in my neighborhood. Something caught my eye—it was a sign that simply said, "Remember that the words LISTEN and SILENT are composed of the same letters . . . "

---

2. MINDFULNESS

How Is Mindfulness Defined?

Mindfulness has moved from a largely obscure Buddhist concept to a mainstream concept in the "helping professions" that address human services . Advocates believe that every client and practitioner would benefit from incorporating mindfulness into their therapy approach (Davis & Hayes, 2011). Among its benefits are increased patience, self-control, objectivity, insight, enhanced flexibility, improved concentration, increased empathy, increased processing speech, emotional intelligence, ability to relate to others, and oneself with kindness and acceptance and decreased reactivity (Davis & Hayes, 2011).

The term "mindfulness" refers to a psychological state of awareness and mode of processing information, or a practice that promotes that awareness (Kostanski & Hassed,

2008). The derivation of the word is from the Pali word "sati," which means having awareness, attention, and remembering (Bodhi, 2000). It is associated with a moment-to-moment awareness, and a freedom that occurs when attention is unattached to any particular point of view (Germier, 2005) Mindfulness has been defined as paying attention on purpose, nonjudgmentally, and in the present moment. It is essentially composed of two ingredients: attention to one's present experience with an accepting attitude (Brown, Marquis, & Guiffrida, 2013; Paulson, Davidson, Jha, & Kabat-Zinn, 2013).

Mindfulness as Self-Observation

Mindfulness has been described as a kind of meditative process of merging moment-by-moment experience with a certain quality of attention (Kabat-Zinn, 1990). Mindfulness can be systematically cultivated by applying one's attention to one's bodily sensations, emotions, thoughts, and the surrounding environment (Bodhi, 2000; Davis & Hayes, 2011). The capacity to evoke mindfulness is considered central for increasing clinician awareness and skillful response to emotional distress expressed by clients (Bishop, Lau, Shapiro, Carlson, & Anderson, 2004). Mindfulness involves a direct observation of something as if for the first time, and is an alternative to the more common experience of observing people and events through the filter of our beliefs, assumptions, and expectations.

Broadly conceptualized, in the state of mindfulness thoughts and feelings are observed as events in the mind. Thoughts are not suppressed, but are objects for observation. These thought events are nonjudgmental, so that each thought and sensation is acknowledged and accepted as it is (Segal. Williams, & Teasdale, 2002). It is a type of *self-observation*, with no automatic or habitual patterns of reactivity. Mindfulness is sometimes perceived as a space between perception and response, and is thought to enable one to respond to situations more reflectively, as opposed to reflexively (Bishop et al., 2004). It has been describes as a process of *investigative awareness*, and involves actively observing the *ever-shifting dynamic flow* of private experience (Bishop et al., 2004). As such, it provides opportunities to gain insight into the nature of thoughts and feelings as passing events in the mind (internal stimuli) rather that valid reflections of what is happening in the outside world (external situations) (Kabat-Zinn, 1990).

Mindfulness has been described as *embodying qualities* such as patience (allowing things to unfold in time), trust (confidence), nonreactivity (calm), wisdom (self-knowledge), and compassion (empathy) (Kabat-Zinn, 1990; Reibel, Greeson, Brainard, & Rosenzweig, 2001). It has been associated with constructs that describe similar abilities, such as introspection, observing self, presence, insight, and self-observation (Bishop et al., 2004; Parasuraman, 1998). This approach has been shown to help clients face their feelings about loss and disability, and focus on altering the impact of and response to those thoughts and feelings in order to develop more appropriate remediation strategies (Bishop et al., 2004). The benefits are key to the health and well-being of the client as well as the clinician (Seikel, Holst, Hudock, Ament, & O'Donnell, 2016).

Cultivating Mindful Habits

The first step in cultivating mindfulness is the development of *presence*, the process of fully attending to each moment without distracting thoughts about the past or future. Being present involves being open and receptive to everything that is being shared in the therapeutic relationship (Siegel, 2010). Training in mechanisms of presence that support the resonance circuit are learnable skills, and sup-port the clinical connection between client and practitioner (Baldini, Parker, Nelson, & Siegel, 2014; Parker, Nelson, Epel, & Siegel, 2014). As a result of practitioners intentionally cultivating presence, they are better able to attend to themselves, their clients, and the therapeutic relationship. Mindful practices allow one to respond wisely rather than react blindly. It has been described as a type of "superpower" that is simple, but not easy (Seikel et al., 2016).

Compassion is another tool we use to sustain and enhance mindful practice, and benefits ourselves as well as our clients. Research has found that the way in which we relate to ourselves will influence how we relate to our clients. Practitioners who treat themselves with kindness and care, are less likely to be judgmental and critical of their clients (Klimecki, Leiberg, Lamm, & Singer, 2013).

Researchers from clinical psychology have proposed an operational definition of mindfulness with the following two components: *self-regulation of attention* and *orientation to experience* (Bishop et al., 2004). *Self-regulation of attention* involves sustained attention, attention switching, and the inhibition of distracters. Because it contains monitoring and control, it is sometimes described as a metacognitive skill. *Self-regulation of attention* may be described with the following summative statements (Bishop et al., 2004; Tolor & Reznikoff, 1960):

- Bring awareness to current experience
- Regulate the focus of attention
- Maintain and sustain attention, increasing vigilance over prolonged periods of time
- Focus on breath
- Switch from attending to thought to attending to breath
- Focus on breathing inhibits secondary thoughts and feelings (unrelated to current experience) that arise in the stream of consciousness

Orientation to experience is another component of mindfulness, and may be described with the following summative statements (Bishop et al., 2004; Hayes, Strosahl, & Wilsen, 1999; Parasuraman, 1998):

- Maintain an attitude of curiosity about where the mind wanders as it drifts away from the breath
- All thoughts, feelings, and sensations are subject to notice and observation
- Take a stance of acceptance and be experientially open to each moment of experience
- Abandon your agenda
- Be open and receptive to whatever occurs in the field of awareness.

The Science Behind Mindfulness

There is evidence that mindfulness helps with the development of effective emotional regulation and gains in working memory indicated by brain function (Farb, Segal, Mayberg, Bean, McKeon, et al., 2010). In addition to the affective benefits, mindfulness has been shown to enhance brain functions associated with self-insight, morality and intuition (Davidson, Kabat-Zinn, Shumacher, Rosenkranz, & Muller, 2003; Davis & Hayes, 2011).

As we look through the lens of modern neuroscience, research tells us that the human brain is in a constant state of change. New experiences promote neuroplasticity and neural integration which can impact our emotions, thoughts, and behavior (Baldini et al., 2014). Neuroplasticity, or the rewiring that occurs in the brain as a result of experience, explains how mindfulness practices (such as focused attention, visualization, or meditation) can alter the brains physical structure and functioning (Davis & Hayes, 2011; Farb et al., 2010). In essence, as we expose our clients to new and intentional experiences, we can facilitate their growth. As we sculpt the flow of energy and information within ourselves and others, our role as *neuroarchitect* becomes more apparent (Davidson & Begley, 2012; Siegel, 2012).

Mindsight refers to this process of intentionally shaping the mind's energy and information flow within our own brain, and sharing energy and information during exchanges within our relationships. Verbal communication, nonverbal exchanges, posture and eye gaze all facilitate these exchanges (Baldini et al., 2014). Mindsight is one of the building blocks of mindfulness, and incorporates elements such as *present moment awareness* (Baldini et al., 2014; Siegel, 2010). It allows for communication between people that cultivates compassionate connections and respects differences. The neural mechanisms responsible for both mindsight and the benefits of mindfulness can be described as a type of *resonance circuit*—a neural hub for encouraging *interpersonal attunement* and subsequent emotional responses (Siegel, 2010). Interpersonal attunement can be defined as resonance with another person in that moment of time (Siegel, 2010). It is this resonance that helps the client feel part of the larger *we*, an essential component of any healing, transformative, and restorative process.

Why Is Mindfulness Helpful?

A theory of mindful practice forms the basis of educational programs for practitioners from a variety of fields, and mindfulness-based interventions are increasingly more frequent in educational programs for the health professions (Connelly, 2005; Epstein, 1999). It has been proposed that mindfulness training, as well as additional counseling training, be provided to speech-language pathology graduate students and continuing education programs for practicing practitioners (Bech & Verticchio, 2014; Seikel et al., 2016). These theories and interventions state that enhancing intrapersonal and interpersonal self-awareness can improve clinician well-being and effectiveness in clinical practice.

Mindfulness has been identified in our literature as helpful to practitioners and their abilities to relate to their patients, as it enhances core qualities of empathy, openness, acceptance, patience, intention, and compassion (Gregory, 2012; Hicks & Bien, 2008). With a mindful approach, the practitioner maintains specific attitudes while focusing attention on a situation as it unfolds (Dobkin, 2015). As mindfulness involves the ability to mute inner distractions and suspend sense of self in order to be fully in the present as we actively listen, it invokes a mutual inward and outward quiet as we project a *therapeutic presence* (Charon, 2006).

Clinical Outcomes of Mindfulness

When clients feel emotionally attuned with a practitioner, they feel connected and understood. Clinical work that is informed by mindsight and reflective mindfulness practices is more likely to promote emotional well-being, comfort and safety, and thus behavioral change (Siegel, 2010, 2012). Mindful practice requires that we reflect on ourselves, our practice, and our world.

In medical research, mindfulness outcomes for physicians experiencing burnout and distress include (Krasner, Epstein, Beckman, Suchman, & Chapman, 2009):

- The capacity to lower one's own reactivity to challenging experiences;
- The ability to notice, observe, and experience bodily sensations, thoughts, and feelings even though they may be unpleasant acting with awareness and attention (not being on autopilot);
- A focus on experience, not on the labels or judgments applied to them.

- The process of being fully present and attentive in the moment during everyday activities with their patients.

For the practitioner, engaging tools for mindful interventions have been linked with the following outcomes for practitioners and their clients (Baldini et al., 2014; Christopher, Chrisman, Trotter-Mathison, Schure, and Dahlen, et al., 2011; Irving, Dobkin, & Park, 2009; Seikel et al., 2016): reduced stress and burnout; increased resilience in the face of emotional stressors; improved self-care; enhanced therapeutic relationships; increased skillful communication such as use of positive affect, pause before reacting and increased awareness of clients' non-verbal signals; and increased empathy, compassion and focus on client needs.

Tools and Practices

Two underlying themes characterize most mindfulness practices: *awareness of awareness*, and *paying attention to intention* (Siegel, 2007). One often overlooked component is to cultivate awareness of one's body while *getting out of the thinking head* (Siegel, 2012). Another integrative exercise is called the *wheel of awareness*, used as a metaphor for the mind with the center hub representing an open state of awareness. As we focus on the individual spokes of the wheel, for example on our breathing or individual senses, we learn to differentiate and then systematically integrate areas of awareness. This type of exercise encourages response flexibility, emotional regulation, empathy, insight, and intuition (Lazar et al., 2005).

Presence and compassion are "at the heart of the art of therapy," and can be learned. They are win-win for both the practitioner and the client, and form the core of mindful practices (Baldini et al., 2014, p. 225). They strengthen our therapeutic relationships, increase practitioner resilience, and provide opportunities for our clients to experience holistic and integrative clinical outcomes. The counseling process has been described as beginning with a *self-aware clinician* (Riley, 2002). Awareness of one's own distractions and prejudices is essential in order to put them aside and be fully present with the client, both emotionally and mentally. Self-awareness allows us to have a deeper understanding of our own behavior, the client's behavior, and the dynamics between the two (Bech & Verticchio, 2014).

The ability to be *fully present* with the client and to focus exclusively on the client is one of the most powerful dynamics in the counseling process (Riley, 2002). It has been referred to, in some literature about counseling, as mindfulness. *Mental clarity* is a prerequisite to effective observation of the client, and a prerequisite to mental clarity is to still the chatter of our mind. Another important function of counseling that is facilitated by the clinician's self-awareness is *active listening*. Active listening requires the clinician to be alert, focused on the client, and observant of the client's verbal and nonverbal messages. Self-awareness also allows a clinician to maintain his or her emotional stability and not personalize emotions that are being expressed (Flasher & Fogle, 2012).

Mindfulness-Based Exercises

We are reminded of the old adage that people can guide another on a road only as far as they themselves have ventured, surely applies to the application of mindfulness practices within our therapy approaches (Davis & Hayes, 2011). The integration of such practices with our clients necessitates engaging in such practices ourselves. A good place to begin is to understand and reflect upon the following four *dispositions of mindfulness* as an ongoing component of our clinical relationships (Seikel et al., 2016):

1. *Kindness:* wishing well to others
2. *Compassion:* the desire to alleviate the suffering of others
3. *Joy:* simple and nonjudgmental desire for the success of others
4. *Equanimity:* believing that some outcomes are beyond our control

The following are examples of mindfulness-based exercises (Davis & Hayes, 2011): *Track internal responses* to client, and what makes you feel more or less empathetic toward the client. *Visualize* an image, color, or memory that elicits feeling friendly (compassion) toward yourself. Pay attention to your internal experience in the presence of different clients. Notice how *feelings shift* from moment to moment. One final exercise is called *let go of judgments* and the desire to say something, and practice fully listening to clients. Track when attention wanders and practice returning back to present moment.

Future research is needed in the following areas (Davis & Hayes, 2011): to uncover more about the potential benefits that long term mindful practices have on the changing brain; performance-based measures of mindfulness, other than self-reported questionnaires; developmental stages of mindfulness; and data reporting mindfulness curriculum and continuing education in our field.

3. COUNSELING

The Importance of Counseling for Speech-Language Pathologists

As early as the 1950s, Charles Van Riper and Wendell Johnson talked about the importance of the relationship between the client and clinician. However, in the 1950s and 1960s, the field and our role were largely defined by somewhat narrow technical terminology in order to establish its scientific credibility (Luterman, 2001; Rollin, 2000).

We are well equipped to deal with the professional content called for when we take case histories, perform diagnostics, and implement remediation approaches. However, there are emotional, communicative and counseling factors we must consider as well when working with clients and caregivers. We need to be more than simply *competent in our area of expertise* (Kendall, 2000). We have learned that possessing solid technical skills is no longer enough, and that learning about the process skills is what comprises more of the art of therapeutic intervention. It has been suggested that lack of training and experience in the area of counseling creates feelings of discomfort about using techniques related to affect counseling, as opposed to information-based counseling (Phillips & Mendel, 2008; Schum, 1986).

The importance of counseling as part of our professional repertoire of services cannot be overstated (Kendall, 2000). It reinforces the *person first* concept, that is, we treat the person first—not the disorder. Each client exists as separate and apart from their disability, and yet must be able to make choices about how to incorporate the disability and challenges in with his or her life decisions (Kottler, 2002). That is where we come in. Nothing replaces our need for human interaction. We work with clients and caregivers who are grieving for either something they lost, or something they will never have. Grief has no boundaries: not age, not culture, not disability (Luterman, 2011). Grief is normal, and when our clients are emotionally upset "grief work" may be called for.

We do not want to ignore the *emotional plane* of our work. Emotional upset interferes with a client's ability to process information and sometimes calls for our ability to listen and validate their feelings. Emotional growth does not easily lend itself to objective measurement; however, affect needs to be valued as solidly as content (Luterman, 2011). Most stages of the communication rehabilitation process call for the use of some counseling techniques. Counseling is part of our job description and our clinical responsibilities (Bradshaw & Gregory, 2014). At times, we purposefully avoid addressing emotional issues with our clients, and use factual discussions about intervention or humor to deflect emotional reactions (Bradshaw & Gregory, 2014). We do this to help us get through difficult social interactions as well as feelings related to emotional intimacy (Simmons-Mackie & Damico, 2011).

How Is Counseling Defined?

The term counsel may be defined as advice, interchange of opinion, recommendation or instruction regarding the judgment or conduct of another (Phillips & Mendel, 2008). Counseling skills are especially important because practitioners must be aware of how the disability affects the client and family from a psychosocial and emotional point of view. Counseling skills help us increase effectiveness of treatment and assist our clients in dealing with the emotional impact of the situation that brought them to our service (Schum, 1986). Bradshaw and Gregory tell us that counseling is largely a listening process. As clinicians, we must recognize our own emotions, as well as the emotions of the clients. When we listen to our clients, we acknowledge and empower them (2014).

Counseling has been described as a process that helps us explore and clarify our thoughts and feelings about life's challenges and accompanying decisions (Kendall, 2000; Rollin, 1987). Those who write about the importance of using counseling techniques in speech-language pathology, do so by adapting information from the *behavioral, humanistic, and existentialist models* used in the fields of psychology and social work (Kendall, 2000; Luterman, 1991). The goal of counseling is to empower our clients to make decisions and *take ownership* for their behaviors during the therapeutic process. No meaningful change can take place without ownership of responsibility (Luterman, 2011).

Counseling is a process that empowers clients to make informed decisions concerning their own welfare and assume ownership (Luterman, 2008). It is described as both a science and an art. The science enables our technical understanding of therapies and skills, which the art gives us the understanding of when and how to use them (Cranfill & Mahanna-Boden, 2012; Nystul, 2006). Our use of active listening, facial expressions, body language, posture, and tone of voice give our clients strong messages about our acceptance and feelings about the person, and will thus impact our interactions (Nystul, 2006).

Our Training and Scope of Practice

The ASHA scope of practices in speech-language pathology and audiology include counseling as one of the roles and responsibilities. Counseling/interpersonal skills influence significant aspects of the clinician/client/family triad (Atkins, 2007). Counseling has been described as a scholarly discipline, an applied science, a social science, and a clinical process, which makes it an applied science (Crowe, 1997). This aspect of our profession has been called an art and a science. It involves the clinician's personal characteristics and helping skills as an art as well as applying the scientific process of observing, presupposing, inferring, hypothesizing, testing, and theorizing as

a science. The *science* of counseling is related to understanding psychological and therapies and skills, whereas the *art* of is related to understanding how and when to use these therapies and skills (Nystul, 2006).

It has been reported that speech-language pathology students receive little training in counseling during their graduate education. There is no question that counseling skills are essential in establishing and maintaining a strong relationship with the client, and in assisting clients and their families in coping with concerns and reactions to communication disabilities (Phillips & Mendel, 2008; Shrum, 1986).

A literature review in 1986 reported that 40% of accredited communication sciences and disorders programs offered counseling courses within their departments (McCarthy, Culpepper, & Lucks). In 1994, a similar study was conducted with little change (Culpepper & McCarthy).

Over 80% of students indicated a need for more counseling coursework and practicum (Kaderavek, Laux & Mills, 2004; Luterman, 2008). In addition, there are limited studies in our field that report research related to counseling issues. Many clients we see, or their family members, may have emotional and psychological overlay resulting from ramifications of their communication disorders. Learning to deal with clients' affective responses can be challenging, but each one provides learning opportunities.

Eighty percent of the respondents reported completing no coursework pertaining to counseling while in graduate school, although more than 90% did see it within their role (Phillips & Mendel, 2008). It is not surprising that students and clinicians feel largely unprepared to offer counseling to their clients, if they do not feel adequately prepared to do so. Yet we know that through counseling, clients feel more empowered to make decisions regarding their independence and are better able to cope with their disability (Luterman, 2001; Phillips & Mendel, 2008; Schum, 1986). When prepared, clinicians can help their clients reduce feelings of frustration, anger, guilt, and anxiety relating to adjustments to their communication disability (Rollin, 2000).

The number of graduate programs that offer counseling courses or coursework to emerging SLPs is still lower than we would like to see. In addition to receiving little or no counseling training in graduate programs, practicing SLPs have not been exposed to a substantial increase of continuing education activities in this area (Atkins, 2007; Rollin, 2000). Not only does this potentially impact clinician comfort, knowledge, and confidence, it impacts client outcomes (Kaderavek et al., 2004).

According to ASHA (2007), counseling clients and their family members is within the speech-language pathologists' and audiologists' scope of practice if it is related to the communication disorder. Many clinicians experience uncertainty concerning the boundaries of counseling (Shipley, 1997). Professionals need to be able to differentiate between parents who want counseling for themselves and those who want to discuss their children. If the concerns are not focused on the client or the communication disorder, we should refer clients and/or family members who need help beyond the field to other specialized professionals who are more qualified to help them with their particular concerns (Haynes & Pindzola, 2014).

Counseling is one of the most important ways that we have to help our clients achieve lifelong goals (Holland & Nelson, 2013) Although counseling is a broad term, and many counseling models do exist, one counseling approach often talked about in our field as our most fitting approach is personal adjustment counseling (Holland & Nelson, 2013; Kendall, 2000; Phillips & Mendel, 2008). The communication skills needed include

the ability to talk less, listen more, and listen actively. The professional needs to differentiate between content and affective components of the client's message, and then respond appropriately (English et al., 2007).

What Is Our Role as Counselor?

We continue to have problems identifying how we as professionals should engage with counseling activities, what should be the goals of such activities, and where are the boundaries between our responsibility and that of other professionals (Toner & Shadden, 2002). According to Shipley, there are three different terms that may help us understand perspectives and responsibilities: counseling, guidance, and psychotherapy (1997). Counseling relates primarily to personal adjustment rather than changes of personality. *Guidance* refers to the process in which suggestions and information are used to positively influence another person's thoughts and behavior. *Psychotherapy* is seen as the job of professionals who are trained to deal with individuals with chronic and serious life problems. As described here, both counseling and guidance would be roles we can be comfortable performing (Luterman, 2008; Shipley, 1997).

Successful counseling depends upon the clinician's understanding of the client, as well as the dynamics of counseling. The following are *rules of the counseling exchange* to guide the process (Toner & Shadden, 2002):

1. Know what is considered "normal"
2. Learn as much as possible about the client
3. Provide sufficient time for conversational exchange
4. Create a therapeutic partnership
5. Develop and maintain trust
6. Adjust your communication style to the client and caregivers

7. Accommodate styles of learning
8. Adapt to changing needs and expressed concerns

The Counseling Relationship

The goals of any type of counseling approach or program have commonalities across the professions: to help clients facilitate the discovery of alternative possibilities and options a sense of control and independence, and new perspectives and confidence about adjusting to and caring for themselves (Riley, 2002). One of the most important dynamics for counseling is the clinician's communication of *care for* the client. Caring may be describes as having empathy and concern for the well-being of another (Riley, 2002). It is not a technique, but rather a state of being. It is expressed throughout the clinical process in everything we do.

The counseling relationship places a specific and unique set of demands on us. We have to give ourselves permission to offer emotional support, and sometimes that opportunity is present and necessary even before we offer clinical information (Luterman, 2006). As we enter the realm of feelings, our role includes (Crandall, 1997; Flahive & White; 1982; Luterman, 2006):

- Deep, selfless listening
- Putting aside your personal agenda
- Recognizing the wisdom that resides within the client
- Suspending judgments.

Dealing With Content and Feelings

We have an obligation to provide both information (teach) and emotional support (coun-sel) to our clients, and must learn to recognize when one is needed over the other (Luterman, 2006; Stone, 1992). When parents ask us about the work we are doing with their children, it may seem as if they are asking for information. However, what they may need is to express their feeling of loss, fear, or anger regarding their child's disability.

Some counseling skills are easier to learn than others. While gathering information and giving interviews generally focus on *facts*, counseling sessions frequently concern clients' *feelings*. In order to help clients work through attitudes and feelings, students must develop a client-centered focus in contrast to a clinician-directed focus (Shames, 2006). This process includes learning to tolerate silence during the client/clinician interaction. Silence is a clinical tool that helps reflect client emotions and clarifies clients' self-perceptions.

Another variable connected to client-centered therapy is the type of response we offer: *content-related or feeling-related*. When paraphrasing content, we often rephrase the words said by the client. *Content responses* are the more frequently used response by clinicians. Content responses have the positive benefit of encouraging clients to elaborate on specific informational aspects (Shames, 2006), but can make the session fairly predictable. As a result, these types of responses may not encourage the client to elaborate on his or her emotional reaction to the event (Luterman, 2008).

In contrast, *affect/feeling-related responses* relate to the client's emotional expressions. Clients may minimize or hide their emotional reaction to their communication disorder. They may also feel that if they express feelings, they might be rejected by the practitioner (Shames, 2006). Luterman (2008) stated that the beginning clinicians too might feel that emotion-related responses are risky. However, the use of feeling-related comments is one of the most significant illustrations of empathic listening (Luterman, 2008; Rogers, 1951) and is influential in building a supportive clinical environment.

Verbal Exchanges

It is important to consider the differences between *paraphrasing* and *summarizing*. When paraphrasing content or feelings, the SLP attempts to closely and immediately mirror the client's utterances (content) or immediately capture the underlying emotion (feelings) after it is expressed (Kaderavek et al., 2004). When summarizing, however, the SLP condenses the content or feelings expressed over a longer period of time (Shames, 2006). Summaries are most useful to conclude an interview or a therapy session and allow the SLP to confirm clinical impressions. Very often, the client will respond to a summary statement by confirming or denying aspects of the message or feelings expressed. The goal of summarization is to express the "big picture" in as few words as possible (Shames, 2006).

Another clinical variable with client-centered therapy the students were introduced to the issue of *open versus closed questions* and the importance of supporting a client's discussion of feelings. We are to be reminded that because silence increases a client's responses, questions were to be considered a secondary rather than a primary interviewing behavior. Open or open-ended questions allow the client or family member to respond in a number of different ways, whereas closed questions typically require a specific response (Cormier & Nurius, 2003; Kaderavek et al., 2004; Seligman, 2004). Open-ended responses will be facilitated by the use of "tell me why" and "how" questions.

It is helpful to be able to identify the different question types and to discuss the relative merits of each kind of question. Whereas closed questions help the SLP secure information and are very time efficient, open questions encourage client talk, communicate SLP interest, and reveal the client's knowledge, feelings, and perspective (Shipley, 1997). Clinicians might be tempted to use too many closed questions because of a low tolerance for silence or in an attempt to "look professional." Overall, we need to reflect on the facilitative use of open-ended questions in creating a client-centered focus (Kaderavek et al., 2004).

Counseling Models Used in Speech-Language Pathology

We adapt and use a number of counseling models, including the behavioral model, the humanistic model, and the existential model. The *behavioral model* evolves from the behavioral principle that human behavior can be shaped by the environment (Skinner, 1953). These models provide frameworks that are highly structured, contain specific task breakdowns (task analysis and shaping of behaviors), and with measurement and reinforcement of each step. They are easy to teach because the methodology is so specific. Although these types of models are often used within our *therapy approaches to change behaviors*, they do not help us cope with our broader role as it impacts dealing with clients' feelings about loss of independence and self-esteem (Kendall, 2000).

The *humanistic model* addresses the underlying feelings that accompany a communication disorder, and was introduced by Carl Rogers (1951). It is also referred to as the self-theory model, which places the client in the center of and in relationship with the larger environment. Therapy outcomes are influenced by the client's perception of his communication difficulty with respect to his overall reality of the "larger environmental picture." According to this model, one of our roles is to develop an *attitude of unconditional regard* and acceptance of the client and his disability (Kendall, 2000; Luterman, 2008). A second role is that of *empathetic listener*, which involves close listening and careful restructuring of information.

Carl Rogers, founder of *person/client-centered therapy*, would say that we guide our clients in the process of becoming *self-actualized individuals* (1951, 1961). The practitioner creates a supportive environment with unconditional acceptance and respect for the client, and through this environment and feedback, the client finds resolution and answers that were always there. We help them discover or *rediscover the congruence* between reality and perception, and progress toward self-actualization as they replace faulty assumptions with perceptions that are closer to reality (Riley, 2002; Rogers, 1961).

According to Carl Rogers, the most important factor in successful therapy is the *relational climate* created by the clinician's attitude (1951, 1961). He specified that there were three interrelated core conditions that impacted the climate and the interactions within (Cooper & Hoeldampf, 2010; Rogers, 1980):

1. *Clinician congruence:* communication of transparency, self-disclosure, and authenticity
2. *Unconditional positive regard:* acceptance of the client with no disapproval, and a willingness to listen without judgment or advice
3. *Empathy:* understanding and appreciation of the client's perspective

A third model applied to communication disorders is *existentialism*, which relies on themes of existence such as freedom, loneliness, and grief (Kendall, 2000). *Freedom* is discussed more fully in Chapter 8 as a component of detachment. It refers to allowing the client and family to assume a larger responsibility, as we slowly fade out of the therapeutic picture. Freedom is a vital component of any therapeutic relationship, and is demanding of both client and practitioner. We discuss this model more fully in the section that follows.

Existential Models of Counseling

Existential and grieving models from psychology literature provide insight for us when working with our clients on loss resolution. Our field has often "borrowed" from psychology, because emotional issues sometimes accompany communication disorders. It has been suggested that this type of inner work constitutes a spiritual journey that may parallel the journey through the therapeutic process, and when we attend to these issues, we can enhance outcomes of treatment (Spillers, 2007). Some of these models and therapies include client-centered therapy (Rogers, 1961), cognitive therapy (Beck, 1995; Ellis, 1977), and models of grieving (Kubler-Ross, 1969).

We have also looked toward existential psychology, because it frames individual experiences with communication disorders in a more universal context of the spiritual implications of human experience (Flasher & Fogle, 2004; Spillers, 2007). Grief is a normal human response to loss, and we have learned that loss permeates disability (Flasher & Fogle, 2012). It is through the experience of grieving that we are able to separate from the loss and make some sense out of it (Moses, 1989; Spillers, 2007). An existential framework can offer one vantage point from which to understand a client's inner, spiritual struggles with loss resolution.

Existentialism emphasizes individual freedom, responsibility, loneliness, and meaning (Spillers, 2007; Wyatt, 2003). According to the existentialist viewpoint, events in life bring us face to face with those universal and cosmic realities that permeate the human condition (Yalom, 1980). How we embrace these challenges and find meaning in our lives becomes part of our inner work, our spiritual journeys. Although many external resources can provide support along the way (such as family, friends and religion), the journey itself is the sole work of the individual (Myss, 1997).

A communication disorder, or any type of disability, can open the door to a spiritual awakening by raising some fundamental questions of human existence: Why am I the way that I am? What is the true purpose of my life and how am I going to live it? These deeper emotional and spiritual questions sometimes surface in assessment and treatment sessions with clients and may have a bearing on their long-term rehabilitation (Spillers, 2007). Although not all clients undertake such a journey during their experience of speech and language therapy, it is important to be prepared for the possibility. For some clients, resolution of these emotional and spiritual issues may be necessary in order to face and sustain the behavioral changes that their communication disorder necessitates.

Themes: Personal Change, Grief, and Loneliness

Personal change is a lonely business, and demands responsibility. Responsibility is a critical issue in any type of personal change, specifically responsibility to one's self, which includes actively participating in one's own habilitation and living up to one's full potential. In an existential framework, the client owns the communication disorder, and has the freedom to change it and choose her or his attitude toward it (Spillers, 2007; Yalom, 1980). We, as speech-language pathologists, can teach new communication behaviors and encourage clients to achieve the change, but we cannot make the changes for their clients. Although this seems like an intuitive statement, its

power is sometimes overlooked by a clinician's genuine desire to help clients improve.

Loneliness is universal and has always been part of the human condition. The onset of a communication disorder can precipitate an experience in existential aloneness by impelling individuals to acknowledge their emotional loneliness and their desire to belong (O'Donohue, 1999). A communication disorder can disrupt a person's most salient means of connecting with others—oral communication (Spillers, 2007). Our connections to others enhance our sense of belonging. When clients feel their emotional loneliness acutely, their longing to belong may intensify. This need for belonging and reconnecting sometimes emerges within the therapy process. The speech-language pathologist may be the first person in clients' lives who understands their experiences with their impairments and who treats them with acceptance, support and unconditional positive regard (Shipley, 1997).

While it may be true that a communication disorder can precipitate a potential loss of belonging, the disorder can also invoke loneliness through the necessary process of change (Luterman, 2008; Yalom, 1980). By definition, change requires us to give up the familiar and the known in exchange for something unfamiliar and unknown. The unknown often breeds anxiety, some of which stems from our existential aloneness, because we face our changes alone. As we stated earlier, others can lend help and support; however, they cannot do the work for us. The client is the only one who can make the needed changes (Spillers, 2007). As we support this life-altering process of change, we must be willing to restrain from solving clients' problems and be willing to witness the emotions that often accompany our work.

Each one of us bears the responsibility of finding meaning in our lives and constructing a truthful and valid way of living (Yalom, 1980). We can process that meaning on a cosmic or existential level and on an implicit or experiential level (Reker & Chamberlain, 2000). Cosmic meaning refers to the big picture—how we understand events in our lives in relationship with the universe. For many people, religious and spiritual beliefs provide a template for deriving cosmic meaning. Implicit meaning refers to how we may process a particular experience with reference to our life. For example, what does it mean to have a communication disorder, and how does this impact my life? This implicit meaning often emerges over time and does not present itself immediately in the situational circumstances (Young-Eisendrath, 1996).

It is not unusual for a person with a disability to experience a sense of grief, which allows them to reflect on loss and make sense of it (Spillers, 2011). Grief, when experienced through a disability, represents a struggle to confront a type of symbolic death and loss of a sense of "normalcy," or dream of such for the future (Luterman, 2011). Parents also experience this when they have a child born with a disability. They need to confront the loss of the "perfect" child before they can embrace the uniqueness and value of they child they have.

Part of the grief process is confronting change, and both change and grief are lonely places to live. They require us to let go of the safe and familiar, for the foreign and unfamiliar. They also reflect back to us the fact that we are different, isolated, and disconnected from the rest of the world. Grief is often associated with emotions such as denial, depression, fear, and anger—however, let us not focus on the emotions and miss the opportunities for spirit and soul work that grief facilitates.

Finding meaning in life (cosmic) and in our experiences (implicit) allows us to shift our attention away from our personal circumstances and focus on fulfilling that meaning (Blair, 2004). Attending to meaning can open us to transcendence and growth. Our attention to existential elements and grieving states can give us, as students and practitioners, an additional lens through which to view some of the emotional experiences and needs of clients. When the process through speech and language therapy evokes a hidden spiritual journey, speech-language pathologists need to draw upon their reservoir of counseling skills.

A.R.T.: Emotional Support

I can so clearly remember the first couple years of my work, when my supervisor told me I had to be careful about two things: I should not touch my students anywhere, and I should *stay away from offering emotional support* because I was not a psychotherapist. Fortunately, it was difficult for me *not* to do either. Years later, as a supervisor myself, I understood the concerns, but it was now a different era and our role was broadened out a bit more thanks to ASHA and an evolving scope of practice.

REFLECTIVE SUMMATIVE QUESTIONS

1. Think of a recent conversation you had with a child or adult that didn't go the way you expected it to. Identify at least one active listening strategy that you might have improved upon.

2. Record yourself when you are conversing with another person. What are your most prevalent nonverbal communicators, and how do they impact the responses of the other person?

3. Practice mindful observing when you are outside and walking around. Pay attention to your thoughts, emotions, and bodily sensations. Consciously alternate your experiences by focusing first on these internal stimuli and then on the

external situations, or what is happening in the outside world.

4. Do you consider yourself a focused and nonjudgmental listener, and how can you increase your ability to do so?

5. How do you really feel about your upcoming role as counselor for your clients? What can you do to increase your comfort and confidence?

REFERENCES

American Speech-Language-Hearing Association. (2007). *Scope of practice in speech-language pathology.* Rockville, MD: Author.

Atkins, C. P. (2007). Graduate clinicians on counseling: Self-perceptions and awareness of boundaries. *Contemporary Issues in Communication Science and Disorders, 34,* 4–11.

Baldini, L. L., Parker, S. C., Nelson, B. W., & Siegel, D. J. (2014). The clinician as neuroarchitect: The importance of mindfulness and presence in clinical practice. *Clinical Social Work Journal, 42*(3), 218–227.

Barrow, R. (2008). Listening to the voice of living life with aphasia: Annie's story. *International Journal of Language and Communication Disorders, 43,* 30–46.

Barrow, R. (2011). Shaping practice: The benefits of really attending to the person's story. In R. J. Fourie (Ed.), *Therapeutic processes for communication disorders: A guide for clinicians and students.* (pp. 21–34). New York, NY: Psychology Press.

Battle, D. (1997). Multicultural considerations in counseling communicatively disordered persons and their families. In T. Crowe (Ed.), *Applications of counseling in speech-language pathology and audiology* (pp. 118–144). Baltimore, MD: Williams & Wilkins.

Beck, A. (1995). *Cognitive therapy: Basics and beyond.* New York, NY: Guilford Press.

Beck, A. R., & Verticchio, H. (2014). Counseling and mindfulness practice with graduate students in communication sciences and disorders.

Contemporary Issues in Communication Science and Disorders, 41, 133–148.

Bishop, S., Lau, M. Shapiro, S., Carlson, L., Anderson, N. D., Carmody, J., . . . Devins, G. (2004). Mindfulness: A proposed operational definition. *Clinical Psychology: Science And Practice, 11,* 230–241.

Blair, R. G. (2004). Helping older adolescents search for meaning in depression. *Journal of Mental Health Counseling, 26,* 333–347.

Bodhi, B. (2000). *A comprehensive manual of Adhidhamma.* Seattle, WA: BPS Pariyatti.

Bradshaw, J & Gregory, K. (2014). The other side of CCCs: Communication, counseling and clinicians. *The ASHA Leader, 19,* 3–4.

Brammer, L. M., & MacDonald, G. (2003). *The helping relationship: Process and skills* (8th ed.). Boston, MA: Allyn & Bacon.

Brown, A. P., Marquis, A., & Guiffrida, D. A. (2013). Mindfulness-based interventions in counseling. *Journal of Counseling and Development, 91,* 96–104.

Burgoon, J. K. (1994). Nonverbal signals. In M. L. Knapp & G. R. Miller (Eds.), *Handbook of interpersonal communication* (2nd ed., pp. 229–285). Thousand Oaks, CA: Sage.

Charon, R. (2006). *Narrative medicine: Honoring the stories of illness.* New York, NY: Oxford University Press.

Christopher, J. C., Chrisman, J. A., Trotter-Mathison, M. J., Schure, M. B., Dahler, P., & Christopher, S. B. (2011). Perceptions of the long-term influence of mindfulness training on counselors and psychotherapists: A qualitative inquiry. *Journal of Humanistic Psychology. 51*(3), 318–349.

Clarkson, P. (2003*). The therapeutic relationship.* London, UK: Whurr.

Connelly, J. E. (2005). Narrative possibilities: Using mindfulness in clinical practice. *Perspectives in Biological Medicine, 48*(1), 84–94.

Cooper, M., Watson, J. C., & Hoeldampf, D. (2010*). Person-centered and experiential therapies work: A review of the research on counseling, psychotherapy and related practices.* Ross-on-Wye, UK: PCCS Books.

Cormier, S., & Nurius, P. S. (2003). *Interviewing and change strategies for helpers: Fundamental skills and cognitive behavioral interventions* (5th ed.). Pacific Grove, CA: Brooks/Cole.

Crandall, C. (1997). An update on counseling instruction in audiological programs. *Journal of the Academy of Rehabilitative Audiology, 30,* 1–10.

Cranfill, T., & Mahanna-Boden, S. (2012). *Spirituality and healthcare: What can we do?* Atlanta, GA, ASHA Conference.

Crowe, T. A. (1997). Counseling: Definition, history, and rationale. In T. A. Crowe (Ed.), *Applications of counseling in speech- language pathology and audiology* (pp. 3–29). Baltimore, MD: Williams & Wilkins.

Culpepper, B., & McCarthy, P. (1994). Counseling and training offered by ESB-accredited programs. *ASHA, 36,* 55–58.

Davidson, R. J., & Begley, S. (2012). *The emotional life of your brain: How its unique patterns affect the way you think, feel and live—and how you can change them.* New York, NY: Penguin.

Davidson, R. J., Kabat-Zinn, J., Schumacher, J., Rosenkranz, M., Muller, D., Santorelli, S. F., . . . Sheridan, J. F. (2003). Alterations in brain and immune function produced by mindfulness meditation. *Psychosomatic Medicine, 66,* 149–152.

Davis, D. M., & Hayes, J. A. (2011). What are the benefits of mindfulness: A practice review of psychotherapy-related research. *Psychotherapy. 48*(2), 198–208.

Dimaggio, G., Salvatore, G., Azzara, C., Catania, D. (2003). Rewriting self-narratives: The therapeutic process. *Journal of Constructivist Psychology, 16,* 155–181.

Dobkin, P. L. (Ed.). (2015). *Mindful medical practice: clinical narratives and therapeutic insights.* New York, NY: Springer.

Ellis, A. (1977). The basic clinical theory of rational-emotive therapy. In A. Ellis & R. Gruger (Eds.), *Handbook of rational-emotive therapy.* New York, NY: Springer.

English, K., Naeve-Velguth, S., Rall, E., Uyehara-Isono, J., & Pittman, A. (2007). Development of an instrument to evaluate audiologic counseling skills. *Journal of American Academy of Audiology, 18,* 675–687.

Epstein R. M. (1999). Mindful practice. *JAMA. 282*(9), 833–839.

Farb, N., Segal, Z, Mayberg, H., Bean, J., McKeon, D., Fatima, Z., & Anderson, A. K. (2007). Attending to the present: Mindfulness meditation reveals distinct neural modes of self-reference. *Social Cognitive and Affective Neuroscience, 2,* 313–322.

Finlay, L. (2015). *Relational integrative psychotherapy: Engaging process and theory in practice.* Chichester, UK: Wiley.

Flahive, M., & White, S. (1982). Audiologists and counseling. *Journal of the Academy of Rehabilitative Audiology, 10,* 275–287.

Flasher, L. V., & Fogle, P. T. (2012). *Counseling skills for speech-language pathologists and audiologists* (2nd ed.). Clifton Park, NY: Delmar Cengage Learning.

Germer, C. K. (2005). Mindfulness: What is it? What does it matter? In C. K. Germer, R. D. Siegel, & P. R. Fulton (Eds.), *Mindfulness and psychotherapy* (pp. 3–27). New York, NY: Guilford Press.

Gregory, K. (2012). Buddhism: Perspectives for the contemporary world. In M. Cobb, C. Puchalski, & B. Rumbold (Eds) *Oxford textbook of spirituality in healthcare.* New York, NY: Oxford University Press.

Hackney, H., & Cormier, S. (1994). *Counseling strategies and interventions* (4th ed.). Boston, MA: Allyn & Bacon.

Hayes, S. C., Strosahl, K., & Wilson, K. G. (1999). *Acceptance and commitment therapy: An experiential approach to behavior change.* New York, NY: Guilford Press.

Haynes, W. O., & Pindzola, R. H. (2014). *Diagnosis and evaluation in speech pathology.* London, UK: Pearson.

Hicks, S. F., & Bien, T. (Eds.). (2008). *Mindfulness and the therapeutic relationship.* New York, NY: Guilford Press.

Holland, A. L., Nelson, R. L. (2013). *Counseling in communication disorders: A wellness perspective.* San Diego, CA: Plural.

Irving, J. A., Dobkin, P. L., & Park, J. (2009). Cultivating mindfulness in health care professionals: A review of empirical studies of mindfulness-based stress reduction (MBSR). *Complementary Therapies in Clinical Practice. 15*(2), 61–66.

Kabat-Zinn, J. (1990). *Full catastrophe living: Using the wisdom of your mind to face stress, pain and illness.* New York, NY: Dell.

Kaderavek, J.N., Laux, J. M., & Mills, N. H. (Fall, 2004). A counseling training module for students in speech-language pathology training programs. *Contemporary Issues in Communication Science and Disorders, 31,* 508–518.

Kendall, D. L. (2000). Counseling in communication disorders. *Contemporary Issues in Communication Science and Disorders, 27,* 96–103.

Klimecki, O. M., Leiberg, S., Lamm, C., & Singer, T. (2013). Functional neural plasticity and associated changes in positive affect after compassion training. *Cerebral Cortex, 23*(7), 1552–1561.

Kostanski, M., & Hassed, C. (2008). Mindfulness as a concept and a process. *Australian Psychologist, 43,* 15–21.

Kottler, J. A. (2002). *Theories in counseling and therapy: An experiential approach.* Boston, MA: Allyn & Bacon.

Krasner, M. S., Epstein, R. M., Bechman, H., Suchman, A. L., Chapman, B., Mooney, C. J., & Quill, T. (2009). Association of an educational program in mindful communication with burnout, empathy, and attitudes among primary care physicians. *JAMA, 302*(12), 1284–1293.

Kubler-Ross, E. (1969). *On death and dying.* New York, NY: Macmillan.

Lazar, S. W., Kerr, C. E., Wasserman, R. H., Gray, J. R., Greve, D. N., Treadway, M. T., . . . McGarvey, M. (2005). Meditation experience is associated with increased cortical thickness. *NeuroReport, 16*(17), 1893.

Luterman, D. (2006, March). The counseling relationship. *The ASHA Leader, 8,* 8–33.

Luterman, D. M. (2008). *Counseling persons with communication disorders and their families.* Austin, TX: Pro-Ed.

Luterman, D. (2011). Ruminations of an old man: A 50-year perspective on clinical practice. In R. J. Fourie (Ed.), *Therapeutic processes for communication disorders: A guide for clinicians and students.* New York, NY: Psychology Press.

McCarthy, P., Culpepper, N., & Lucks, L. (1986). Variability in counseling experiences and training programs among ESB-accrediated programs. *ASHA, 28,* 49–52.

McNaughton, D., Hamlin, D., McCarthy, J., Head-Reeves, D., & Schreiner, M. (2008). Learning to listen: Teaching an active listening strategy to pre-service education professionals. *Topics in Early Childhood Special Education, 27,* 223–231.

Moses, K. (1989). *Fundamentals of grieving: Relating to parents of the disabled.* Evanston, IL: Resource Networks.

Myss, C. (1997). *Why people don't heal and how they can.* New York, NY: Three Rivers Press.

Nystul, M. (2006). *Introduction to counseling: An art and science perspective.* Boston, MA: Allyn & Bacon.

O'Donohue, J. (1999). *Eternal echoes.* New York, NY: HarperCollins.

Parasuraman, R. (1998). *The attentive brain.* Cambridge, MA: MIT Press.

Parker, S. C, Nelson, B. W., Epel E., & Siegel, D. J. (2014). The science of presence: A central mediator of the interpersonal benefits of mindfulness. In K. W. Brown, J. D. Creswell, & R. M. Ryan (Eds.), *Handbook of mindfulness: Theory and research.* New York, NY: Guilford Press.

Paulson, S., Davidson, R., Jha, A., & Kabat-Zinn, J. (2013). Becoming conscious: The science of mindfulness. *Annals of the NY Academy of Sciences, 1303,* 87–104.

Phillips, D. T., & Mendel, L. L. (2008). Counseling training in communication disorders: A survey of clinical fellows. *Contemporary Issues in Communication Science and Disorders, 35,* 44–53.

Reibel, D. K., Greeson, J. M., Brainard, G. C., & Rosenzweig, S. (2001). Mindfulness-based stress reduction and health related quality of life in a heterogeneous patient population. *General Hospital Psychiatry, 23,* 183–192.

Reker, G., & Chamberlain, K. (Eds.). (2000). *Introduction: Exploring existential meaning* (pp. 1–4). Thousand Oaks, CA: Sage.

Riley, J. (2002). Counseling: An approach for speech-language pathologists. *Contemporary Issues in Communication Science and Disorders, 29,* 6–16.

Rogers, C. (1951). *Client-centered therapy.* Boston, MA: Houghton Mifflin.

Rogers, C. (1961). *On becoming a person.* Boston, MA: Houghton Mifflin.

Rogers, C. (1980). *A way of being*. Boston, MA: Houghton Mifflin.

Rollin, W. J. (1987). *The psychology of communication disorders in individuals and their families*. Englewood Cliffs, NJ: Prentice-Hall.

Rollin, W. J. (2000). *Counseling individuals with communication disorders: Psychodynamic and family aspects*. Boston, MA: Butterworth-Heinemann.

Schum, R. L. (1986). Counseling in speech and hearing practice. *National Student Speech and Hearing Association, 9*, 1–77.

Segal, Z. V., Williams, J. M. G., & Teasdale, J. D. (2002). *Mindfulness-based cognitive therapy for depression: A new approach for preventing relapse*. New York, NY: Guilford Press.

Seikel, T., Holst, J. Hudock, D., Ament, R., O'Donnell, J., Guryan, B., . . . Hatzenbuehler, L. (2016). *The mindful practitioner: Incorporating mindfulness into classroom, supervision and clinic*. Presented at ASHA Conference, Philadelphia, PA.

Seligman, L. (2004). *Techniques and conceptual skills for mental health professionals*. Upper Saddle River, NJ: Prentice-Hall.

Shafir, R. Z. (2003). *The Zen of Listening: Mindful communication in the age of distraction*. Wheaton, IL: Quest Books.

Shames, G. H. (2006). *Counseling the communicatively disabled and their families: A manual for clinicians*. Boston, MA: Allyn & Bacon.

Shipley, K. G. (1997). *Interviewing and counseling in communication disorders: Principles and procedures* (2nd ed.). Boston, MA: Allyn & Bacon.

Siegel, D. J. (2007). *The mindful brain: Reflection and attunement in the cultivation of well-being*. New York, NY: W.W. Norton.

Siegel, D. J. (2010). *The mindful therapist: A clinician's guide to mindsight and neural integration*. New York, NY: W.W. Norton.

Siegel, D. J. (2012). *Pocket guide to interpersonal neurobiology: An integrative handbook of the mind*. New York, NY: W.W. Norton.

Simmons-Mackie, N., & Damico, J. S. (2011). Counseling and aphasia treatment. *Topics in Language Disorders, 31*(4), 336–351.

Skinner, B. T. (1953). *Science and human behavior*. New York, NY: Macmillan.

Spillers, C. S. (2007). An existential framework for understanding the counseling needs of clients. *American Journal of Speech-Language Pathology, 16*, 191–197.

Spillers, C. (2011). Spiritual dimensions of the clinical relationship. In R. F. Fourie (Ed.), *Therapeutic processes for communication disorders: A guide for students and clinicians* (pp. 229–243). East Sussex, UK: Psychology Press.

Stone, J. R. (1992). Resolving relationship problems in communication disorders treatment: A systems approach. *Language, Speech, and Hearing Services in Schools, 23*, 300–307.

Thistle, J. J., & McNaughton, D. (2015). Teaching active listening skills to pre-service speech-language pathologists: A first step in supporting collaboration with parents of young children who require AAC. *Language, Speech, and Hearing Services in Schools, 46*, 44–55.

Tolor, A., & Reznikoff, M. (1960). A new approach to insight: A preliminary report. *Journal of Nervous and Mental Disease, 130*, 286–296.

Toner, M. A., & Shadden, B. B. (Spring, 2002). Counseling challenges: Working with older clients and caregivers. *Contemporary Issues in Communication Sciences and Disorders, 29*, 68–78.

Weger, H., Castle, G. R., & Emmett, M. C. (2010). Active listening in peer interviews: The influence of message paraphrasing on perceptions of listening skill. *International Journal of Listening, 24*, 34–49.

White, M., & Epston, D. (1990). *Narrative means to therapeutic ends*. New York, NY: W.W. Norton.

Woltner, J., DiLollo, A., & Apel, K. (2006). A narrative therapy approach to counseling: A model for working with adolescents and adults with language-literacy deficits. *Language, Speech, and Hearing Services in Schools, 37*, 168–177.

Wyatt, C. S. (2003). *Existentialism: A primer*. Retrieved February 15, 2013, from http://www.tameri.com/csw/exist/

Yalom, I. (1980). *Existential psychotherapy*. New York, NY: Basic Books.

Young-Eisendrath, P. (1996). *The gifts of suffering*. New York, NY: Addison-Wesley.

CHAPTER 6

Balance and Harmony

1. PERSPECTIVES, FRAMES, AND LENSES

A.R.T.: Outside the Circle

As a supervisor, I would wind up visiting schools for students with physical disabilities during "mealtime," as both breakfast and lunch were instructional programs that took up a good portion of the day. Breakfast had been finished, and the students being seen by the speech practitioner were now working on mealtime strategies to enhance their choice-making and requesting abilities, as well as peer/ social communication strategies. The four students were sitting in their wheelchairs, and they were lined up opposite and all were facing the practitioner. I asked the practitioner to step "outside the circle" with me, and tell me what she saw. She saw no opportunity for the peer interaction because none of the students were facing each other, and immediately made the necessary directional adjustments. As a supervisor, I was usually able to spot things they could not, simply because I was standing "outside the circle," giving me a much more global perspective.

Perspectivism

The philosophical construct that all ideas take place from particular viewpoints and interpre-

tations is called perspectivism, and was coined by German philosopher Friedrich Nietzsche (Hayman, 1980). Although there are many different conceptual schemes through which the perception of truth and value can be assumed, no one vantage point is considered more or less true. The greatest truth is created by integrating and weaving together as many different perspectives as one can gather (Mautner, 2005).

A good sense of perspective enables us to have a clear and focused worldview of events, people, and choices. It helps us lead a life of purpose and direction. Our philosophical perspective will stay with us and direct our lives (Hornfischer & Hornfischer, 1997). If we have ever heard the expression "walking in someone else's shoes," we understand a bit about perspectives and point of view.

We have a tendency to link what we encounter in the present to past experiences; however this sometimes narrows our views and causes us to generalize and narrow our perspectives. We all make sense of the world by comparing, generalizing, and categorizing things we experience. Perspective helps us make sense of what we see, much the same way that theories help us make sense of science (Dervin, 1998).

Conceptual Frames of Reference

Conceptual frames are ways that we organize our experiences, and they structure our perceptions and actions within our culture and society. A frame is a set of concepts and perspectives that organize experiences and guide the actions of individuals (Goffman, 1974). To hold the frame of a subject is to choose one particular set of meanings over another. Frames originate as a result of both our nature, and those experiences that nurture us along the way. A frame, much like a picture frame, holds together the picture or content of life's experiences. Frames are the mental structures that allow us to understand reality—and sometimes to create what we take to be reality. Social institutions and situations are shaped by mental structures (frames), which then determine how we behave in those institutions and situations (Goffman, 1974). Our frameworks direct our perspectives one way or another, with the danger that we may miss opportunities to understand experiences in different ways.

Frames of reference all come down to points of view. The notion of framing simply means to focus on a set of ideas within a particular perspective to arrive at an interpretation. We all have ways of observing, interpreting and acting in the world based upon what we believe to be true—that is our frame of reference. Our frames have limitations, simply because we have and limitations and gaps in our perceptions, knowledge, experience, processing abilities, and ability to accurately report (Fairhurst & Sarr 1996). We do, however, use frames to make sense of situations (Kolko, 2011).

Although frames can be subjective and biased and thus manifest with constraints, framing is one of the most useful strategies we have for attempting to make sense of complex problems and conditions. Frames give us opportunity to make them explicit, put them aside, shift our perspective, reflect upon alternatives, and embrace a new frame (Kolko, 2011). That process of reframing involves an artistry of pattern seeking, and a desire to integrate information from a variety of perspectives (Kolko, 2011). Each time we reframe from a new perspective, we are implementing empathetic cognitive strategies (Fairhurst & Starr, 1996).

Sense-Making

It is only through our short-term perspectives and frames that the long-term sense-making occurs. Sense-making is an internal, personal, and ongoing cyclical process of acquisition, reflection, and action that we automatically use to integrate our experiences into our understanding of the world around us (Kolko, 2010).

Dervin's description of sense-making helps us understand the complexity of our frames and perspectives. He describes the human as:

> . . . a body-mind-heart-spirit living in a time-space, moving from a past, in a present, to a future, anchored in material conditions; yet at the same time with an assumed capacity to sense make abstractions, dreams, memories, plans, ambitions, fantasies, stories, pretenses that can both transcend time-space and last beyond specific moments in time-space (Dervin, 1998. p. 38).

A.R.T.: Rainbone

I had a cartoon hanging on my refrigerator for years. There was a dog, lying on a sofa in a psychiatrist's office, obviously in the midst of psychotherapy. Being a dog lover who was dating a psychiatrist at the time, that in and of itself gave me the giggles at 3:00 AM. However, the best part was written in the dialogue bubble. The psychiatrist said something like this to the dog, "Now, I want you to think of something happy." The dog thought of a rainbow, and in his *mind cartoon,* it showed a picture of a rainbow, but with the word "rainbone." From that day on, everything I said to my dog had the word "bone" on the end. It taught me much about perspective and its place in clinical interactions.

Reframing

A frame is a schema of beliefs and values that we use when inferring meaning. When we reframe, or change part of the frame, the meaning that is inferred may also change. To reframe, try the following actions (Watzlawick, Weakland & Fisch, 1974):

- Step back from what is being said and done, consider the frame or lens through which this reality (perspective) has been created.
- Consider alternative lenses and look at it another way
- Challenge the beliefs or attributes of the frame
- Stand in the frame and describe what you see
- Select aspects of the frame to ignore, so that the frame assumes less importance.

Reframing allows us to change our emotional state, and that of others. For example, you can reframe a *problem into an opportunity* or *unkindness into a lack of understanding* (Hale, 1998). Reframing has been described as a gentle process, through which we change the conceptual or emotional setting and viewpoint in relation to how a situation is experienced (Watzlawick et al., 1974). It is used in most fields where persuasion is important. In politics, enemies are reframed as friends to rally support. In sales, reframing transforms an objection into a reason to buy. In education, reframing helps people understand what they did not understand the first time it was presented (Phillips, 1999). Shifting our gaze has been known to open up new ways of thinking about the world. In her essay about certainty and uncertainty, Nelson reminds us that Copernicus looked at the same scientific evidence that had been looked at for thousands of years, but only when he shifted his perspective from the earth to the sun, and questioned the movement, was he able to show us our solar system (2011; Rothchild, 2006).

How Frames and Reframes Work

We tend to frame situations based upon our perceived interests. It is usually not possible to convince someone that their frame is incorrect by giving them more information, because that information will be processed into the existing frame. So basically, more data won't ever change frames, and we need to engage people at the level of their assumptions. A frame gives meaning to information with its own logic. Most frames are tacit; they are inside of us and usually very difficult to change. We are not aware of the way we frame situations, or of the way other people are framing the same situation. The way to solve this difficulty is to try to make the frames explicit (McDowell, Canepa, & Ferriera, 2007).

The most effective tool that we have for changing the effectiveness of our resources is reframing. We have all been in a situation where the best we can do is what we are already doing. Sometimes, the best way to change is not to work harder, or organize better, or have more resources—but to rethink what we are doing. Reframing is very useful for accomplishing the following (Schon & Rein, 1994):

- analyzing and specifying a problem
- setting new parameters or limits
- exploring alternative dimensions
- making tacit assumptions explicit
- transforming personal perspective
- discovering alternative dimensions
- removing preconceived barriers

Assumptions and Lenses

Reflective practice, which was discussed in the previous chapter, has been defined as a process of inquiry in which practitioners try to discover and research the assumptions that frame how they work (Brookfield, 1998). When we practice this, we become more aware of the power dynamics that infuse all practice settings. It also helps us detect *hegemonic* assumptions—assumptions that we sometimes think are in our own best interests, but which actually often work against us in the longer term (Brookfield, 1995).

Assumptions are interesting, in as much as we are rarely able to view them with one lens. It is like turning our head to catch a glimpse of the back of our neck, but of course our body turns at the same time and we are left with the same view. In a sense, we are trapped within our perceptual frameworks, much like prisoners, unable to stand outside of ourselves and see how some of our deepest values and beliefs distort and constrain our ways of thinking (Brookfield, 1998). We use our interpretive filters and assumptions to shape our awareness and ultimate actions, and those actions then serve to confirm the truth of these same interpretive filters and assumptions. What a cycle . . . and it is no wonder that becoming aware of our assumptions is so daunting a task.

Three Lenses

Brookfield suggests that assumptions can more adequately be researched by seeing practice through three complementary lenses: the lens of our own autobiographies as learners of reflective practice, the lens of our students' eyes, and the lens of our colleagues' experiences (1995, 1998). These three lenses will reflect back to us very different pictures of who we are and how we work. The first lens is through *our autobiographies as learners, or self-reviews.* When we visit our autobiographies as learners, this distances us from ourselves and puts us in the role of "other." It involves an experience that touches our emotions in a substantive way. In this way, we begin to see our practice from the point of view of what our students experience. Investigating our autobiographies as teachers is a logical first reflective step and

provides one of the most important sources of insight into practice that we have (Brookfield, 1998). Personal experience is sometimes dismissed as subjective and impressionistic. The fact that we recognize aspects of our own individual experiences in the stories that others tell pays tribute to the importance of narratives and sharing tacit knowledge. We may think that our practice is based upon theory and science, but we find that the foundation of how we work has been laid in our autobiography as learner. Our autobiographies help explain those parts of our practice to which we feel strongly committed, but are unable to find it supported in a particular theory, model, or approach. They also help explain our preferences and motivations (Jalongo & Isenberg, 1995).

Our second lens is through *our students' eyes, or student review.* Seeing ourselves from our students' perspectives can lead to many surprises. We may be reassured or quite startled with the feedback we receive, and we need to be prepared to listen to what they have to say. This lens helps us understand the diversity of meanings people read into our words and actions: those incidental comments that were heard as criticisms, those gentle suggestions that were heard as commands, and the joke that was heard as an insult. One of the biggest difficulties with this lens is the reluctance of our students and their caregivers to be honest with us. They have probably learned that honest commentary can backfire. Without this lens, we will not have an appreciation of how students are experiencing their communication-learning journey.

Our third lens is through *our colleagues' experiences, or peer review.* Our colleagues serve as mirrors, reflecting back to us the image of our actions. When we foster critical conversations about our work with trusted colleagues, we may receive useful insights. Patterns will become apparent that can be helpful to us in exploring alternatives and opening up new ways of seeing and thinking about our practice. One of the biggest difficulties with this lens is the implicit "shroud of silence" that sometimes silences commentary. Feedback is essential, and we must request it.

A.R.T.: Don't Stand in the Desert

In the late 1980s, I participated in a human potential training movement called Lifespring (Hanley, 1990). Although it was somewhat controversial because of its New Age affiliation, I learned much about perspectives, perceptions, lenses, and context. One of the most helpful Lifespring-isms that stayed with me all of these years is the following: *If you want to grow orchids, don't stand in the desert.* That helped me understand the importance of context, and how easy it is to self-sabotage our own efforts by simply standing in or viewing from a perspective that is incompatible with what we are trying to accomplish.

---

2. PERSONAL AND PROFESSIONAL LIVES

Work-Life Balance

We have heard a lot of chatter about the importance of work-life balance. Consider this possibility: there is no such thing as work-life balance. However, we keep trying to live up to that impossible standard until we lose ourselves in the struggle. Why does this happen? It has been called "the sacrifice syndrome," a condition that is more than burnout (Mckee, Boyatzis, & Johnston, 2008). It's a way of life. Maybe it's familiar: we snap at people, make bad decisions, rarely smile, and move at the speed of light.

The sacrifice syndrome doesn't strike out of the blue. It starts with an insidious form of chronic, intense stress. We call it "power stress," a brutal brand of stress that often accompanies the types of diverse and ongoing responsibilities that come with our work (Mckee et al., 2008). We know about the results of stress: it triggers the release of powerful substances like epinephrine, norepinephrine, and corticosteroids. Blood pressure goes up and large muscles prepare for movement or battle. The immune system is compromised and the brain shuts down nonessential neural circuits, so we don't take in as much information (Segerstrom & Miller, 2004). We become less creative, anxious, nervous, or even depressed. The answer lies here: there really is no way to balance all that we do, until and unless we balance ourselves. McKee proposes an antidote: create a cycle of sacrifice and renewal with mindfulness, hope, and compassion (Mckee et al., 2008). We will talk a bit more about this in the next chapters focusing on *growth and self-care.*

Creating Significance and Meaning

As we mature, we get busy learning things that are not simply the acquisition of information and skills. We learn how to deal with life, with work, with family. We become wiser, and when faced with thoughts about our mortality, begin to ponder the importance of leading a life with meaning (Brooks, 2015; Gardner, 1981). Gardner describes meaning as something we build into our life from affections, loyalties, and humanistic experiences. We piece them together in a unique pattern that only we can make, and this creates the beginnings of a meaningful life (1981). We experience our life with meaning when we have found a way of serving others that leads to feelings of significance (Brooks, 2015). Although there is no practical manual or hierarchy of values that lead to meaning, there is an individual moral compass that lets us know when we are heading in the right direction.

The Merits of Reflective Writing

When work experiences intersect with personal concerns, stressors, and emotional reactions, opportunities are created for imbalanced thoughts and actions (Stone-Goldman, 2011). Stone-Goldman talks about the merits of reflective writing, as one tool for helping us reach a renewed sense of emotional calm and clarity (2011).

We all face situations that challenge our inner homeostasis and threaten our sense of balance, which is where the phrase "personal-professional intersection" comes in as a helpful strategy (Stone-Goldman, 2011, p. 24). Regardless of how separate we try to keep them on the service, there are times that they simply do interact (Katz & Johnson, 2006). Our life stories are very much alive within each of us, and sometimes, when lying dormant *story threads* weave their way into our work and trigger unexpected emotions (Stone-Goldman, 2011). The importance of using writing as a tool for personal wellness and professional growth is not a new concept. Writing has been shown to support a number of positive outcomes across a variety of professions as it (Stone-Goldman, 2010a, 2011):

- Bridges the theoretical with the practical
- Deepens creativity
- Reduces anxiety
- Facilitates reflective practices
- Brings emotional content to the surface
- Opens us to new ways of thinking

Stone-Goldman proposes the following procedure to begin developing reflective writing as "a tool for understanding the personal-professional intersection and restoring balance" (2011, p. 25). The first step is to *decide on the content* or topic for your writing. There are three categories that can help you choose: immediate states of perception (mind, body, or emotions), a recent or upcoming event, and past situations that had a large impact on you. Then, make a topics list, using a brainstorming technique. Write down everything that comes to mind. Third, begin to write, using the writing prompts and cues on Stone-Goldman's webpage (Stone-Goldman, 2010b). When your internal critical voice shows up, just keep writing. Finally, read what you have written and reflect on it with a more conscious perspective. Nothing it right or wrong. Look for stories and themes, and make note of what catches your attention.

A.R.T.: Detailed Records

A good majority of the professionals working under my supervision were conscientious, talented, dedicated, and very hard working. One of those practitioners, M., had occasion to work with a student who was being transferred to another school program. The student's new speech practitioner, who happened to be in my office one day, made a point of stopping in to see me and told me the following. She said that when she received the speech therapy records from the sending school, she had never seen anything written in such detail and found it surprising that anyone could find the time to do such detailed work on paper. This got me curious, so the next time I visited M. in her school, I browsed through her speech record folders, and I too was surprised with the details. As she and I began to talk, she confessed to me that her husband was getting a bit frustrated with her excessive work at home. By the end of our dialogue, M. promised to devote less time at home to her record keeping.

3. SCIENCE AND PRACTICE

Art, Philosophy, Spirit, and Science

Our work is not dissimilar to art and design. Art has no external constrains. It is the artist that imposes the constraints through use of materials, telling of a story, or creating a specific aesthetic. Designers always work with constraints—the design project requirements and the client come with specific demands to stay within certain rules.

It has been suggested that education in general needs to be an interactive combination of the Taoist (or Daoist) philosophical principles of yin (earth) and yang (heaven), and this can be accomplished through a dynamic interplay between the "mystical intuition and scientific analysis" (Nagel, 1994, p. 2). Intuition must be balanced with reason. We have many ways of knowing, and we need to embrace them all (Barnes, 1978; Costa & Kallick, 2008).

This idea that philosophy and science can be combined to give us the best possible knowledge about the world and how to act within it is an old one. The concept can be encapsulated by *scientia*, a Latin word that means "knowledge" in the broader sense and encompasses both the sciences and the humanities (Pigliucci, 2012). Pigliucci points out that Aristotle and other fellow ancient Greek philosophers not only give us broad insight into the content of their science, but their philosophical positions as well. In his role as psychologist, Aristotle explained that it is often difficult to balance or align our rational assessment of what is right to do, with our emotional inclination of what gives us pleasure—which usually comes to us more easily. The Greeks would say that happiness can only be achieved when it connects to the goal of improving oneself or affect the world in a positive way.

Scottish philosopher David Hume introduced us to the central idea that the conjunction of science and philosophy has much to offer in making our lives significantly better (Pigliucci, 2010). Using his thinking, if we acknowledge that science (dealing with matters of fact) is not enough, we also need philosophy (dealing with matters of value). However, our philosophy can and should be informed by the best science available because scientific knowledge can guide us, and help us revise our philosophical intuitions. Philosophy, then, can guide the general direction in which science goes.

Only recently in human history has a clear distinction has been made between science and philosophy. Galileo and Isaac Newton, in the seventeenth and eighteenth centuries, saw themselves primarily as naturalistic philosophers, not scientists (Pigliucci, 2010). Pigliucci has attempted to suggest that they be brought back together for people working in the service of "human flourishing," and to call it "sci-phi." Both science and philosophy track progress. Science can be said to make progress in proportion to how its understanding of the world matches the way the world actually is. Philosophy also makes progress when it understands more about the meaning and implications of human concepts and how they relate to the world. The two approaches are complementary. As the philosopher Immanuel Kant (1724–1804) famously put it, "Experience without theory is blind, but theory without experience is mere intellectual play" (Pigliucci, 2012). Ken Wilber is a writer who synthesizes science with spiritual thought. In his book, *A Brief History of Everything*, he discusses the process of evolution as one that transcends, includes, incorporates and goes beyond (2000). When we travel *the path*, we include and honor the wisdom of those who came before, and we incorporate the traditions of our ancestors.

Miller (2014) discusses the collaborations that take place between artists and scientists, and how both art and science benefit as artists find their muse in science. In his first chapter he states,

> From the beginning of time, people have assumed there was an invisible world of some sort—of the spirits, the mind, or the world as explored by science. . . . The play between the visible and the invisible has always been at the heart of Western art and scientific thought. (p. 3)

As an artist, Picasso's ability to transform images was driven by both mathematics and science (Miller, 2014; Ross, 2009). He was especially impressed with the concept of x-rays, that what you saw was not necessarily, what you got. We all can see the impact that geometry had on his representational imagery, and his interest in the fourth dimension being projected on a two-dimensional plane (Wilson, 2010).

Kandinsky, too, was interested in the unseen, and desired to represent the *spiritual existence and absolute forces* behind material objects (Miller, 2014, p. 12). He expressed his art as appealing more to the soul and less to the eye, and attempted to integrate into his imagery the concepts of mass, energy, and movement as they related to Einstein's relativity theory (Edwards, 2008; Isaacson, 2007). In the 1930s art began to be influenced by the emergence of quantum physics, and artists, such as Dali, searched for imagery to capture the juxtaposition of waves verses particles. One school of thought holds firm to the argument that the emotions, passion, and intuition of artists is little different from the scientist's quest for data and logic. There have been times in our history when the two branches of processing and understanding the world have drifted apart, but in the last century (and certainly post digital age); they have

once again been reunited. This reunion is not unlike our own reunion of science with practice, and rigor with relevance (Wilber, 2000).

EBP and PBE

How can we balance EBP with PBE without compromising the validity of either one? The idea is an appealing one, as this type of framework validates the importance of integrating treatment evidence with real-world evidence derived from client experiences and family perspectives. We must not ignore empirical evidence simply because it does not support our clinical experiences. On the other hand, we can collect observational evidence about effectiveness of our treatment approaches as it relates to treatment outcomes. The PBE studies, although not meant to replace research evidence, do provide another source of information to advance clinical practice (Kamhi, 2011). It may take many forms including personal experience, reflective practice, and evaluation of practice, and practice-based research (Payne & Barker, 2010).

The principles of EBP can help us achieve confidence in our ability to make clinical decisions. In its most narrow interpretation, EBP is viewed as the static implementation of an intervention that has been scientifically proven to be valid (Justice, 2008). The more common interpretation is as a process, whereby practitioners gather and integrate information from a variety of sources, evaluate different approaches, update their knowledge, provide justification for clinical decisions, review client progress, and question their beliefs and assumptions (Dollaghan, 2007; Kamhi, 2011).

In Chapter 1, we discussed the EBP triad as an approach that includes the integration of high-quality research evidence with clinical expertise and client/caregiver values and preferences. Although these principles are often depicted as the three points on a triangle, the weight or clinical significance of each point changes depending on perspective. For example, universities and clinical training institutions will identify research-based evidence as the best evidence to guide clinical decisions; practitioners working in schools will cite the importance of clinical expertise and student/caregiver values when making decisions about assessment and intervention approaches (Kamhi, 2011; Papir-Bernstein, 2012a).

As we progress in our attempts to affirm the value of different forms of evidence and knowledge, clinical experience is sometimes referred to as a branch of practice-based evidence or PBE (Horn & Gassaway, 2007; Kamhi, 2011). PBE provides the bridge, connecting scientific effectiveness with what practitioners are already doing (Kamhi, 2011). PBE is defined as the ability to use our clinical skills and past experience to identify each client's unique health variables, personal values, and expectations (Sackett, Rosenberg, Gray, Haynes, & Richardson, 1996).

Remember the Blue Highways

One of the best explanations about the importance of practice-based arenas is stated by Westfall, Mold, and Fagnan (2007), who refer to the *blue highway*, and the need to increase the use of practice-based research and evidence to better serve the people living on those highways. Donald Schon talks about the varied topography of professional practice consisting of the high ground and the swamp. On the high grounds, manageable problems lend themselves to neat solutions through evidence and research. In the swampy lowlands, problems are messy but of greatest human concern (Schon, 2001).

In the field of medicine, the blue highway, or swamp, is where most of the health care is delivered, and a far cry from the medical centers and universities where research is funded and takes place. In the field of education, blue highway or practice-based evidence takes place in the schools. It is within the "blue highway" of practice-based educational programs, where most of our children learn (Westfall, Mold, & Fagnan, 2007). On these blue highways, the learning context becomes the laboratory (Papir-Bernstein, 2012b). When the school setting is viewed as analogous to a scientific laboratory, the scientist-practitioner model is enacted (Stricker & Trierweiler, 2006). It has been suggested that most fields of practice in medicine and social sciences have a *bimodal approach* to training and practice, with science on one end and practice on the other (Stricker & Trierweiler, 2006).

Science and Practice are Partners

As we discussed in earlier chapters, clinical practice can and does inform research (the science), much the same way that research informs clinical practice. Research and practice are partners, and the relationship is not a unidirectional process (Apel, 2011). In fact, practitioners have been using the scientific method in clinical practice as standard fare: they observe a behavior, develop a hypothesis, and observe results to determine if the hypothesis was proven through a change in behavior (Apel, 2011; Bachus, 1957). We, too, are problem-solving scientists. The difference is that our laboratory is the classroom (if working with students), and our research may be completed in one or two therapy sessions.

Although there are areas of incompatibility between theory and practice that encourage and support a divergence in training and continuing education, there are many more reasons supporting synergy and convergence of principles pertaining to both science and practice (Stricker, 1992). An illustration of this synergy can considered from Flexner's classic book about medical education:

> The intellectual attitude of the two are—or should be—identical: Neither investigator nor practitioner should be blinded by prejudices or jump at conclusions; both should observe, reflect, conclude, try, and, watching results, continuously reapply the same method until the problem in hand has been solved or abandoned. (Flexner, 1925, p. 4)

Stricker and Trierweiler, in their research about clinical psychology, suggest that although the activities of science and practice are different in their orientation to problems, the attitude of science can benefit practitioners and the attitude of practitioners can benefit the science (2006; Kanfer, 1990). Science, in its traditional form, seeks answers that are public and general. Practice, in its traditional form, is private and personal more than public. Practice is also considered local, whereas science is general and universal. For the scientist, universal laws are established, and individual differences are at best, of secondary interest (Sticker & Trierweiler, 2006).

Our field of speech-language pathology embraces both science and practice, and has applauded and validated the importance of the scientist's universal quest for generalized knowledge, as well as the practitioner's local quest for applications specific to their individual clients (Sticker & Trierweiler, 2006). It is our scientific attitude that enables us to interpret, translate, and apply the evidence to our practice—thus creating the context for the development of the therapeutic and professional attitudes. By doing this, we become scientist-practitioners, and build bridges between the research and practice communities. As we learned in Chapter 1, application and translation between science and practice is a complex process, and it continues to be complex as we progress to dissemination and

implementation. This is further discussed in Part IV of the book.

Certainty and Uncertainty

The clinician is skilled in *local thinking* and problem solving, as opposed to universal or general problem solving. Local knowledge is specific to a particular group or cultural subgroup, context dependent, and unique to the ever-changing nature of events and relationships (Stricker & Trierweiler, 2006). In addition, the unique qualities of behavior and experiences emerge depending on perception and interpretation (Baron & Misovich, 1993). All of this impacts local knowledge, and as practitioners, our level of awareness and ability to reflect from within our scientific attitude is critical to the synergy.

However, we, as practitioners, are sometimes reluctant to express or admit uncertainty or to question our clinical practices. It breaks our confidence, and brings up fears that our clients too will loose confidence in our ability to remediate. Clinicians are reluctant to admit uncertainty to their peers, or their supervisors, for fear they will be perceived as not knowing their craft (Apel, 2011; Kamhi, 2011).

Clinical decision-making skills are developed when we are open to studying and implementing new ideas that may be different from the status quo. This process begins with *uncertainty*, which is a vital component in science and clinical practice (Apel, 2011). We must be open to and establish comfort with uncertainty, as it presents itself in our work. The appearance of uncertainty is a good thing. Uncertainty flags a question about a clinical practice, and creates an opportunity or reason to make a change. It is the first step in growth. Apel reminds us that progress only occurs when we question theories, explain phenomenon differently, or discover alternative means for achieving outcomes (2011).

In our world, perspectives give shape to our paradigms and philosophies about clinical practice. Both scientists and practitioners must use uncertainty to generate insightful and focused question (Nelson, 2011). The questions clinicians ask will be answered by obtaining multiple perspectives of key stakeholders, and will inform decisions regarding assessment areas and intervention targets. The "theory of uncertainty orientation" helps us understand basic differences in our approaches to problem solving (Hudson & Sorrentino, 1999). We all fall somewhere on the continuum. A person who is uncertainty-oriented will strive to achieve clarity, whereas a person who operates more on the opposite end will strive to maintain clarity (Nelson, 2011). Understanding this about oneself is the first step to incorporating the attitudes and values of our clients as a critical part of the clinical decision-making process. There is no question that uncertainty challenges comfort zones and willingness to change.

Accountability and Verification

As practitioners, we have two different levels of accountability or practice verification. One is local and internal, and the other is global or external (Apel, 2011; Stricker & Trierweiler, 2006). In the world of research, *external verification* happens through peer review and scientific discovery. In the world of practice, it happens through insurance agencies and school boards. Client outcomes and improvements in performance on state tests are expected to occur. If client improvement does not occur, practitioners are expected to change their practices (Apel, 2011). External verification serves as a type of accountability, and is a major driver in health care and education.

There is, however, another type of accountability that is at least equally as important: the personal monitoring of our professional practices. This is known as *internal verification*, or client-based (Apel, 2011; Stricker & Trierweiler, 2006). As we are responsive to the specific needs of our clients, we are following one of the basic tenets of evidence-based practice (EBP)—sensitivity to the needs, preferences and values of our clients and their caregivers (ASHA, 2005).

4. CLINICAL INTERACTIONS

Meaningful Relationships

Ancient systems of healing approach wellness as related to a state of balance and harmonious relationships. Illness and disease are viewed as the result of physical or relational disharmony rather than specific disease (Galland, 1997). How do we cultivate meaningful relationships with our clients, and how are these relationships perceived by our clients and their caregivers? Research has explored the balance of power within therapeutic relationships when working with children and adults. By understanding how our clients experience and describe their relationships with us, we are better able to reflect on *the how* of therapy, rather than just *the what* (Fourie, 2009).

During my career, I have worked within various settings and in a variety of roles. One of my key observations concerns relationships, and how they have a major impact in directing and determining outcomes of therapy. Clients, whether children or adults, ultimately want to accomplish two things: please themselves and please you. Motivation, commitment, and enjoyment will all determine how well therapy progresses (Fourie, 2011).

The Therapeutic Equator

Therapy has been defined as a collaborative and co-constructed sequence of events in which both the client and clinician work together to effect change (Simmons-Mackie & Damico, 2011). Clinical encounters have been described as having an actual *plot structure* within a clinical time frame (Mattingly & Fleming, 1994). The plot informs actions within the therapy sessions. The unfolding story, or clinical narrative, will be influenced by broad elements such as cultures, expectations, and institutional directives.

We need to be cautious about over-helping, instilling helplessness, and creating client dependence. This balance has been called *a tightrope*, or a *therapeutic equator of supportive help*, and reminds us to be responsible *to* rather than responsible *for* our client (Ciccia, 2011; Luterman, 2003). One strategy to insure that your clients remain engaged in their treatment is to ask them to note the differences in their performance from session to session. The *clinical interactions*, or social exchanges and the relationship between client and clinician, is the essence of a *therapeutic event* (Simmons-Mackie & Damico, 2011). The client's behavior influences the clinician as much as the clinician's behavior influences the client (Brookshire, Nicholas, Krueger, & Redmond, 1978). Although subtle aspects of the clinical interaction can affect the therapeutic relationship in a positive or negative way that interactive aspect of therapy is rarely described in evidence-based research reviews (Horton & Byng, 2000).

Although the definition of therapy may be a bit elusive, we certainly know what it is not. *Therapy is not* a unidirectional process of *what the clinician does to* the client, and it is not the sequence of picture card activities or naming tasks while ignoring the expertise and experiences of the participants. At best, the process of therapy facilitates the mutual arrival at a place of shared narrative that accommodates the worlds of all participants (Hinckley, 2008; Simmons-Mackie & Damico, 2011).

Balancing Our Talk

Counseling is viewed as a communication exchange. We need to be aware of and make adjustments in our style of speaking to our clients, depending upon client age and many other factors (Toner & Shadden, 2002). We may be unconsciously changing our style of speaking based upon our perspectives and feelings about age or disability. When we talk, if we sound either too caring or too controlling, we may be perceived as "talking down" in the communication exchange. The following communication styles are examples of *talking down* (Ryan et al., 1995):

- *Baby talk:* may be perceived as both caring and controlling, especially with older populations. It often contains diminutives, endearments, and cute phrases.
- *Overly personal talk:* may be perceived as high in caring and contains sometimes-inappropriate reference to person, clothing, or activities with lots of praise.
- *Directive talk:* may be perceived as very controlling, and contains lots of inference about what should and should not be done. Tone may be interpreted as cold or angry, and imply that the client is not being compliant.
- *Superficial talk:* is usually neither caring nor controlling, but may be perceived as if the presence of the client has little to do with what the practitioner is saying. Sometimes, there is a disconnect between the emotions and the content of the expression.

Analyzing Clinical Interactions

If we look for common therapeutic factors that exist that may account for treatment outcomes, there seem to be four categories of potential influence: the client, the clinician, the structure of the session, and the beliefs. Most of the qualitative research from the last 25 years indicates that clinicians are most prominent in listings of common factors, which means that individual clinicians affect therapy outcomes (Ebert & Kohnert, 2008; Grencavage & Norcross, 1990).

The importance of the clinician-client relationship cannot be overstated, and is sometimes referred to as *therapeutic alliance*. (This is rewieved more fully in Chapter 16.) In one study, two prominent groups of clinician factors studied were *behaviors* and *traits*, and the two of these factors that earned the highest rating were *rapport* and *communication with the client* (Ebert & Kohnert, 2008). Studies like these help us answer the question, "What makes speech-language treatment work?"

As we think about *clinical interactions*, we must acknowledge that communication exchanges between clients and clinicians contain multiple layers of linguistic, personal, social, and cultural aspects within each narrative. Interactions can be analyzed from a multitude of perspectives (Simmons-Mackie & Damico, 2011):

- Local aspects: what is happening at the time of the exchange
- Content aspects: what is being discussed
- Ethnographic aspects: how culture is informed within an interaction
- Narrative aspects: what is meaningful to each stakeholder (client, clinician, family)
- Conversational aspects: how language is used to create relationships

We have made a complex commitment that demands ongoing balance, as we exist as a scientific profession, an educational profession, and a helping profession. Our education tends to be more discipline-specific, and knowledge that is relational, reflective, and

experiential can easily get overlooked (Caty, Kinsella, & Doyle, 2016; Hinckley, 2010). At our best, we blend different types of knowledge that help us balance the demands of science with the care of the client.

Reflective Accountability

Reflective practice does not free us from the need to worry about professional accountability within our relationships. However, accountability may look a bit different when we are operating within the context of *reflective practitioner*, and our conversational exchanges take on, literally, a more reflective tone. Here are some examples from the perspective of a practitioner (P), and a reflective practitioner (RP) (Schon, 1983, 1987):

- (P) is presumed to know, and will claim so, regardless of uncertainty. (RP) is presumed to know, however, acknowledges that they are not the only member of the relationship to have relevant and important knowledge. They also acknowledge that uncertainties exist and provide learning opportunities for both parties.
- (P) keeps distance from the client, and holds on to the role of expert. Uses warmth and empathy as a strategy, which often comes across as something like an artificial sweetener. (RP) seeks out connections to the client's thoughts and feelings, and allows client's respect for knowledge to naturally emerge within situational contexts.

Balancing Jargon

The knowledge base of our profession comes from a variety of disciplines including, medicine, psychology, education, linguistics, physical therapy, nursing, and social work. Is it no wonder that we have an abundance of technical terminology and "professional-ese"? Although our technical vocabulary is important for helping us define precisely what we are talking about, one of our roles is to clarify information for our clients and caregivers (Bowen, 1998).

Teachers, too, can feel alienated with our overuse of technical jargon. Our inappropriate use of technical and incomprehensible jargon can facilitate feelings of anxiety and confusion, negative reactions, feelings of denial, embarrassment, distraction, or simply a lack of processing (Bowen, 1998). On the other hand, we need to be equally careful about over-simplifications and watered-down explanations, which can change the essence of information as well as get interpreted as patronizing value judgments about the client's capacity to understand.

Goals, Tasks, and Bonds

Therapy has been described as a process that includes three primary and essential components: goals, tasks, and bonds. Goals relate to expected outcomes, tasks to activities and materials, and bonds to the relationship between clinician, client, and caregivers (Bordin, 1979; Fourie, Crowley, & Oliviera, 2011). However, goals and bonds are interconnected, as the bonds of therapy provide the context for achievement of outcomes. First, the bond has been shown to be a consistent predictor of positive outcomes. A second predictor is how much the client is able or willing to contribute to the therapeutic interaction (Fourie et al., 2011; Wampold, 2001).

Clinical or therapeutic relationships have been studied in most health care professions that value client-centered approaches. Components of this relationship, although not easy to define and differentiate, generally refer to the emotional bond present between the clinician

and the client (Ackerman & Hilsenroth, 2003; Fourie et al., 2011). The therapeutic bond is an active collaboration and a necessary context for the delivery of therapy (Wampold, 2001).

Interactional Processes

Different aspects of therapeutic relationships in speech-language therapy have been studied, and include what clinician's feel about their client's behaviors and what clients feel about clinicians (Fourie et al., 2011). In general, therapists value client's behaviors such as motivation and compliance, whereas clients value empathy, careful and accepted listening, and honesty (Fourie, 2009). It has also been pointed out that client engagement in the therapeutic process can be restricted under certain circumstances. When the role of the clinician emphasizes the "expert" status, the result can create a disempowering asymmetry and dependence for the client (O'Malley, 2010). Unbalanced interactional processes can be created when clinicians control turns, request information that is known, control interpretation, and evaluate performance (Simmons-Mackie & Damico, 2011).

It has been suggested that the therapeutic relationship may have an even larger impact in therapy with children, simply because they do not initiate the treatment (Bickman et al., 2004). In addition, there is indication that emotional wellbeing in children is tied to their ability to communicate, and that an affectionate and caring relationship is a prerequisite for any type of therapeutic treatment program (Danger & Landreth, 2005; Freud, 1965). Therefore, any improvements in the emotional domain could well have a positive influence on communication.

In addition to the affective domain, another factor essential for positive engagement for children is a sense of safety. Safety allows children to feel empowered, and creates the context for the backdrop of fun to be experienced with materials and activities (Green, Crenshaw, & Kolos, 2010). Children are able to identify activities and qualities in the therapeutic environment that they value, and include being offered something to drink or eat, being made to feel comfortable, and providing them with toys (Fourie et al., 2011).

The Child's Voice

Children as young as 4 have provided perspective about their likes and dislikes during therapeutic interactions, and children's voices about preferences have begun appearing more in the literature of our field. Children with communication difficulties have reported the following insights (Bordin, 1979; Fourie et al., 2011; Markham, Laar, Gibbard, & Dean, 2009; Owen, Hayett, & Roulstone, 2004):

- They have difficulty making and retaining friends
- They are aware they have communication problems
- They perceive speech therapy as an opportunity for learning, but did not necessarily understand the purpose of speech therapy or the role of the speech-language pathologist.

Fourie and colleagues conducted a study that explored the therapeutic relationship between the practitioners and children aged 5 to 12 years (2011). The study was qualitative, and used interpretive phenomenological analysis of structured interview questions which focused on the child's experiences and life-worlds. As was discussed in Chapter 5, *Life-world* concepts refer to subjective experiences, often taken-for-granted, that constitute human social reality (Husserl, 1970).

Six descriptive themes evolved: play and fun, power dynamics, trust, routines and rituals, role confusion, and physical characteristics

of the practitioner. The following results of the study should be noted (Fourie et al., 2011):

1. *Source of fun:* Whereas children valued the play, fun, games, and rewards associated with the interaction, it is important to note that the play was usually initiated and regulated by the adult (which impacted the power dynamics).
2. *Power dynamics and trust:* Power differentials are evidenced thorough *opportunities for choice making*. When the adult is in control of dialogue and activities, the naturalness and spontaneity in meaningful communicative exchanges is limited. When the power differential is less obvious and children feel the practitioner is a confidant and someone they can trust, positive outcomes are more easily facilitated.
3. *Routines and rituals:* Predictability, opening and closing routines, and consistency all *reduce anticipatory anxiety*.
4. *Role confusion:* Although some children understood the role as distinct from teachers and medical practitioners, others described the role as just another adult in charge.

This is an important study for helping us understand the life-worlds of children as they experience the service we provide. *Play and fun* become important and valid tools through which to not only achieve outcomes, but to build bonds and relationships (Fourie, 2009, 2011). Although some of us may prefer clients who are appropriate and compliant, those values may conflict with the life-worlds of children (Stech, Curtiss, Troesch, & Binnie, 1973). *Child's play* is the innate driver for self-regulation, social, emotional, and cognitive development (Longtin & Gerber, 2008).

Most activities are initiated and driven by the adult, and that type of interaction leads to unnatural sequences of communication that can be best described as a *teaching manner* (Simmons-Mackie & Damico, 2011). However, when choices are offered to children, this sense of empowerment may counter their sense of vulnerability as a result of having a communication disorder (Ferguson & Armstrong, 2004). *When children trust* their clinician and feel safe, they are more willing to cooperate and take risks in therapy. Without taking risks, children will have limited participation in therapy activities and production tasks for fear of mistakes. Trust facilitates improved outcomes as well as generalization and transfer of learning (Weiss, 2004). Finally, both children and their caregivers need to *agree on the purpose and function* of treatment, and understand the explicit role of the clinician. Treatment goals and objectives need to be negotiated and agreed upon (Fourie et al., 2011; Paul & Haugh, 2008).

5. EMOTIONAL BALANCE

Our Emotional Core

Anything we learn that contributes to our ability to lead happy lives is useful in our work. Any learning that provides us with internal information is also providing us the ability to strengthen our emotional core (Haidt, 2006). Our *executive functions* allow us to think about and regulate our own thoughts and feelings, whereas *theory of mind* is the understanding that other people have their own feelings and motivations that are different from ours (Goleman, 2013).

We can lose our sense of emotional balance through a variety of external events or internal reactions to events. We manage our balance through greater self-awareness and the assumption of responsibility for our emotional and psychological experiences. Our reflective practices, as discussed in an earlier chapter, provide some of the tools to maintain emotional balance. Our goal is to establish a state of mental organization and emotional calm when faced with challenging or even painful interactions. We need to avoid cognitive distortions or automatic, stress-based reactions (Burns, 1989).

Levels of Emotions

We have three levels of emotions (Damasio, 1999; Tom, 2009). The "big six" primary or *universal emotions* are happiness, sadness, fear, anger, surprise, and disgust. The secondary or *social emotions* are ones such as embarrassment, jealousy, guilt, and pride. The *background emotions* are ones such as well-being, calm, anxiety, and tension.

There are other emotions such as *awe, gratitude, disgust, and elevation* that have been tied to a sense of overall well-being, including the cosmic or spiritual sides of us. Research has been conducted linking our emotions to our spiritual life, and describing them as *sources of spiritual information*. One of those emotions is *awe*. We respond to situations filled with enormous beauty and complexity of meaning and design with awe. The contexts may range from divinity to nature, music, and art. Responses have been described as a type of transport out of oneself into a higher reality (Haidt & Joseph, 2004).

Another emotion, *gratitude*, may have evolved in its initial stages to help humans engage in trade and long-term reciprocal alliances. It ultimately developed into a type of cosmic gratitude, or appreciation for the simple gift of life and for all the good things in it. And still others, *disgust and elevation*, are triggered as " . . . people show greater of lesser degrees of divinity in their actions" (Haidt, 2006, p, 424). They help us make our way in the complicated world of social relationships by providing us with spiritual clues about what is noble and virtuous in ourselves and others.

Haidt describes *disgust* as the most underappreciated emotion. It was shaped by evolution and originated as a food selection strategy, allowing us to reject food that had been contaminated with various sources of bacterial and parasitic infections. Somewhere along the evolutionary line, disgust became a social emotion triggered not only by negative response to physical things, but to social violations such as cruelty and racism (Haidt, 2006). Ultimately, the emotion of disgust may be providing us with moral information about values we consider important that have been violated, carrying with it a type of deep wisdom (Kass, 1997).

Both anthropological and psychological sources refer to social space being ordered in terms of a vertical dimension. This is in agreement with the Hindu notion of reincarnation occurring at differing vertical levels, depending on one's actions in life (karma). *Social disgust* has been described as the emotional reaction when witnessing others moving down the vertical plane, thus exhibiting their lower and baser natures (Haidt, 2006; Rozin, Haidt, & McCauley, 2000).

Elevation, on the other hand, contributes to our moral education by elevating our sentiments and providing physical feelings (a feeling of dilation or openness in the chest) with the same power that any real episode might (Haidt, 2013). We experience it as a warm and open feeling of being uplifted, and this emotion underlies human spiritual development and growth. We feel inspired by and study the lives of people who elevate others. Haidt contends that both disgust and moral elevation provide us with the spiritual clues that feed our emotions and lead us toward who and what is "good" in this world (Haidt, 2013).

Congruence

Rogers describes *congruence* as a state of balance or homeostasis between thoughts, emotions, and reality, between internal awareness and external experience (Rogers, 1961). We need to be able to recognize and accept the state of balance as well, as the state of imbalance, even before we fully understand the reasons we feel off-kilter. Congruence includes the ability to be open to uncertainty (as discussed earlier in this chapter) without being overwhelmed by fear of the unknown (Riley, 2002).

Why is emotional balance important? There are three primary reasons relative to our work with clients (Geller & Foley, 2009; Luterman, 2008; Stone-Goldman, 2012):

1. At the core of our work is the concept of *relationship*.
2. Emotions are a component of our relationships.
3. Communication is affected in a powerful way by our emotional balance.

Empathy

As students, we are certainly familiar with the term *rapport*, and understand its importance in any type of therapeutic relationship. Empathy is the component of rapport that positively impacts treatment outcomes (Moore, 2006; Rhoades, 2001). Medical research tells us that even when patients had not reached treatment goals, empathy rates high on patient satisfaction surveys (Buie, 1981; Clark, 2005, Kiesler, 1979). It has been proposed that whereas the cultivation of empathy is an important component of rapport, practitioner and client personality variables may impact empathic compatibility (Kiesler, 1979; Squire, 1990).

Empathy is defined as the capacity to understand or feel what another is experiencing from their frame of reference (Bellet & Maloney, 1991). Put another way, it is the capacity to place oneself in another's position and assume their perspective. Empathy is different from sympathy or pity—"feeling sorry" for someone leading to the desire to fix someone's problems because they are unable to help themselves (Snyder & Lopez, 2009). Barriers to empathy include work stress, perceived time constrains, tension between client and practitioners, and the belief that emotional needs are unimportant (Erdman, 2013)

Empathy can be divided into two major components: affective empathy and cognitive empathy. *Affective empathy or emotional empathy* is the capacity to respond to another's emotional state with an appropriate emotion. We join the other person in feeling along with him or her, and sometimes actually resonate with their feelings. *Cognitive empathy* is the capacity to understand and assume the perspective of another's mental state, and at the same time manage our own emotions while we take stock of theirs (Goleman, 2013; Shamay-Tsoory, Aharon-Peretz, & Perry, 2009).

Empathic Attunement

Although empathy and attunement are the most effective elements of a therapeutic relationship, they are elusive and difficult to describe (Cooper, 2008). They are very much connected, and involve a sense of connectedness, focused attention, synchronicity, immersion, and relational sense-making (Finlay, 2015). Because they are so connected and sometimes difficult to distinguish, Finlay combines them as *empathic attunement* (2015). Goleman refers to this as *empathic concern*, which leads us to care about the person and mobilize us to help if need be (2013). There are multi-layered areas of use for empathic attunement:

- Affective: relates to client affect and feelings
- Cognitive: relates to client perspective and thinking
- Rhythmic: relates to client's style of thinking and communication

Empathy is more easily convey by non-linguistic channels of communication. Research indicates that non-verbal language cues such as body posture and facial expressions convey more meaning than verbal language components (Ekman, 1993; Mehrabian, 1972). Mehrabian provides the following ratios to explain how messages are interpreted based upon non-verbal and verbal language (Moore, 2006): 93% by non-verbal cues; 55% facial expressions and 38% vocal tone; 7% words. This research supports the premise that non-linguistic language cues are critical components in communicating emotions such as anger, fear, sadness, and disgust.

Physicians have begun to make this connection and now offer courses to enhance communication through the establishment of empathetic connections. Empathy can be taught through reflective writing, role-playing, and mindfulness (Erdman, 2013). How can we facilitate empathy and enhance attunement in our professional relationships? Here are some basic suggestions (Moore, 2006; Shafir, 2000):

1. Do not interrupt when the client is speaking.
2. Actively listen.
3. Put yourself in the client's position.
4. Talk openly.
5. Ask open-ended questions.
6. Validate your client's knowledge and experiences

REFLECTIVE SUMMATIVE QUESTIONS

1. What factors related to the practitioner may positively or negatively impact therapy outcomes, given the same client and intervention program?
2. Think of a learning situation you have recently been a part of, and the instruc-

tor. Were there any particular things the instructor said or did that you found especially helpful in your learning of that new skill? What advise would you give to that instructor in the future if working with a client like yourself?

3. Describe an encounter you have had with another person who expressed a very different perspective about your field.

4. Which do you think would be more difficult to accomplish—to influence somebody's frame or their opinion, and why?

5. As a scientist-practitioner, what research ideas do you have, and how would you collect data?

6. Describe an experience you have had when you "mismatched" what you were saying to the person, the context, or the desired outcome.

REFERENCES

Ackerman, S. J., & Hilsenroth, M. J. (2003). A review of therapist characteristics and techniques positively impacting the therapeutic alliance. *Clinical Psychology Review, 23*(1), 1–33.

Apel, K. (2011). Science is an attitude: A response to Kamhi. *Language, Speech, and Hearing Services in Schools, 42,* 65–68.

American Speech-Language-Hearing Association (ASHA). (2005). *Evidence-based practice in communication disorders* [Position statement]. Available from http://www.asha.org/policy

Backus, O. (1957). Group structure in group therapy. In L. E. Travis (Ed.), *Handbook of speech pathology.* New York, NY: Appleton-Century-Crofts.

Barnes, B. J. (1978). *Accountability: Taking account of human value.* Fullerton, CA: Institute for Early Childhood Education, California State University.

Baron, R. M., & Misovich, S. J. (1993). Dispositional knowing from an ecological perspective. *Personality and Social Psychology Bulletin, 19,* 541–552.

Bellet, P. S., & Maloney, M. (1991). The importance of empathy as an interviewing skill in medicine. *JAMA, 226*(13), 1831–1832

Bickman, L., deAndrade, A. R. V., Lambert, E. W., Doucette, A., Sapyta, J., & Boyd, A. S. (2004). Youth therapeutic alliance in intensive treatment settings. *Journal of Behavioural Health Services and Research, 3*(2), 134–148.

Bordin, E. S. (1979). The generalizability of the psychoanalytic concept of the working alliance. *Psychotherapy: Theory, Research, and Practice, 16*(3), 252–260.

Bowen, C. (1998). *Communicating with clients.* Retrieved March 10, 2016, from http://www.speech-language-therapy.com/

Brookfield, S. D. (1995). *Becoming a critically reflective teacher.* San Francisco, CA: Jossey-Bass.

Brookfield, S. D. (1998). Critically reflective practice. *Journal of Continuing Education in the Health Professions, 18*(4), 197–205.

Brooks, D. (2015, Jan 6). The problem with meaning. *New York Times,* Editorial, p. A23. Retrieved from https://www.nytimes.com/2015/01/06/opinion/david-brooks-the-problem-with-meaning.html

Brookshire, R. H., Nicholas, L. S., Krueger, K. M., & Redmond, K. J. (1978). The clinical interaction analysis system: A system for observational recording of aphasia treatment. *Journal of Speech and Hearing Disorders, 43,* 437–447.

Buie, D. (1981). Empathy: Its nature and limitations. *American Psychoanalytical Association, 29*(2), 281–307.

Burns, D. (1989). *The feeling good handbook: Using the new mood therapy in everyday life.* New York, NY: W. Morrow.

Caty, M., Kinsella, E. A., & Doyle, P. C. (2016). Reflective practice in speech-language pathology: Relevance for practice and education. *Canadian Journal of Speech-Language Pathology and Audiology, 40*(1), 81–91.

Ciccia, A. (2011). Pragmatic communication. In J. Kreutzer, J. DeLuca, & B. Kaplan (Eds.), *Encyclopedia of clinical neuropsychology.* New York, NY: Springer Shop.

Clark, D. (2005, October). *Clinician patient communication to enhance health outcomes.* Proceedings of the Bayer Institute for Health Care

Communication Workshop at Southwestern Vermont Medical Center, Bennington, VT.

Cooper, M. (2008). *Essential research findings in counselling and psychotherapy: The facts are friendly.* Los Angeles, CA: Sage.

Costa, A., & Kallick, B. (2008). *Learning and leading with habits of mind: 16 essential characteristics for success.* Alexandria, VA: Association for Supervision and Curriculum Development.

Damasio, A. R. (1999). *The feeling of what happens: Body and emotion in the making of consciousness.* New York, NY: Harcourt Brace.

Danger, S., & Landreth, C. (2005). Child-centered group play therapy with children with speech difficulties. *International Journal of Play Therapy, 14*(1), 81–102.

Dervin, B. (1998). Sense-making. *Journal of Knowledge Management, 2*(2), 36–46.

Dollaghan, C. (2007). *The handbook for evidence-based practice in communication disorders.* Baltimore, MD: Brookes.

Ebert, K. D., & Kohnert, K. (2008, November). *Common factors to consider in treatment research.* Presented at ASHA Convention, Chicago, IL.

Edwards, D. (2008). *Artscience: Creativity in the post-Google generation.* Cambridge, MA: Harvard University Press.

Ekman, P. (1993). Facial expression/emotion. *American Psychologist, 48*(4), 384–392.

Erdman, S. (2013, November). *Patient-centered care: Enhancing patient satisfaction and treatment outcomes in audiology.* Presented at ASHA Convention, Atlanta, GA.

Fairhurst, G., & Sarr, R (1996). *The art of framing: managing the language of leadership.* San Francisco, CA: Jossey-Bass.

Ferguson, A., & Armstrong, E. (2004). Reflections on speech-language therapists' talk: Implications for clinical practice and education. *International Journal of Language and Communication Disorders, 39*(4), 469–507.

Finlay, L. (2015). *Relational integrative psychotherapy: Engaging process and theory in practice.* Chichester, E. Sussex, UK: Wiley.

Flexner, A. (1925). *Medical education: A comparative study.* New York, NY: Macmillan.

Fourie, R. J. (2009). A qualitative study of the therapeutic relationship in speech and language therapy: Perspectives of adults with acquired communication and swallowing disorders. *International Journal of Language and Communication Disorders, 44*(6), 979–999.

Fourie, R. J. (Ed.). (2011). *Therapeutic processes for communication disorders: A guide for clinicians and students.* New York, NY: Psychology Press.

Fourie, R., Crowley, N., & Oliviera, A. (2011). A qualitative exploration of therapeutic relationships from the perspective of six children receiving speech-language therapy. *Topics in Language Disorders. 31*(4), 310–324.

Freud, A. (1965). *Normality and pathology in childhood.* New York, NY: Norton.

Galland, L. (1997). *The four pillars of healing.* New York, NY: Random House.

Gardner, J.W. (1981). *Self-renewal: The individual and the innovative society.* New York, NY: Norton.

Geller, E., & Foley, G. M. (2009). Broadening the ports of entry for speech-language pathologists: A relational and reflective model for clinical supervision. *American Journal of Speech-Language Pathology, 18*, 22–41.

Goffman, E. (1974). *Frame Analysis: An essay on the organization of experience.* Cambridge, MA: Harvard University Press.

Goleman, D. (2013). *Focus: The hidden driver of excellence.* New York, NY: Harper.

Green, E. J., Crenshaw, D. A., & Kolos, A. C. (2010). Counseling children with preverbal trauma. *International Journal of Play Therapy, 19*(2), 95–105.

Grencavage, L. M., & Norcross, J. C. (1990). Where are commonalities among therapeutic common factors? *Professional Psychology: Research and Practice, 21*, 372–378.

Haidt, J. (2006). *The happiness hypothesis: Finding modern truth in ancient wisdom.* New York, NY: Basic Books.

Haidt, J. (2013). *The righteous mind: Why good people are divided by politics and religion.* New York, NY: First Vintage Books.

Haidt, J., & Joseph, C. (2004, Fall). Intuitive ethics: How innately prepared intuitions generate virtues. *American Academy of Arts and Sciences: Daedalus*, pp. 55–56.

Hale, K. (1998) The language of cooperation: Negotiation frames. *Mediation Quarterly, 16*(2), 147–162

Hanley, J. (1990). *Lifespring.* New York, NY: Fireside.

Haugh, S., & Paul, S. (2008). The relationship, not the therapy? In S. Paul & S. Haugh (Eds.), *The therapeutic relationship: Perspectives and themes.* Herefordshire, UK: Athenaeum Press.

Hayman, R. (1980). *Nietzsche: A critical life.* New York, NY: Oxford University Press.

Hinckley, J. J. (2008). *Narrative-based practice in speech-language pathology.* San Diego, CA: Plural.

Hinckley, J. J. (2010). The tools of our trade: Ethics, outcomes, and effects of therapeutic discourse. *Seminars in Speech and Language, 31*(2), 77–79.

Hodson, G., & Sorrentino, R. M. (1999). Uncertainty orientation and the big five personality structure. *Journal of Research in Personality, 33,* 253–261.

Horn, S. D., & Gassaway, J. (2007). Practice-based evidence study design for comparative effectiveness research. *Medical Care, 45,* S50–S57.

Hornfischer, D., & Hornfischer, E. (1997). *Father knew best: Wit and wisdom from the dads of celebrities.* New York, NY: Penguin Group.

Horton, S., & Byng, S. (2000). Examining interaction in language therapy. *International Journal of Language and Communication Disorders, 35,* 355–375.

Husseri, E. (1970). *The idea of phenomenology.* The Hague, the Netherlands: Nijhoff.

Isaacson, W. (2007). *Einstein, his life and his universe.* New York, NY: Simon & Schuster.

Jalongo, M. R., & Isenberg, J. P. (1995). *Teachers' stories: From personal narrative to professional insight.* San Francisco, CA: Jossey-Bass.

Justice, L. (2008). Evidenced-based terminology. *American Journal of Speech-Language Pathology, 17,* 324–325.

Kamhi, A. G. (2011). Balancing certainty and uncertainty in clinical practice. *Language, Speech, and Hearing Services in Schools, 42,* 59–64.

Kanfer, F. H. (1990). The scientist-practitioner connection: A bridge in need of constant attention. *Professional Psychology: Research and Practice, 21,* 264–270.

Kass. L. (1997). The wisdom of repugnance. *New Republic,* 17–26. Retrieved from https://web.stanford.edu/~mvr2j/sfsu09/extra/Kass2.pdf

Katz, R., & Johnson, T. (2006). *When professionals weep: Emotional and countertransference responses in end-of-life care.* New York, NY: Routledge.

Kiesler, D. (1979). An interpersonal communication analysis of relationship in psychotherapy. *Psychiatry, 42*(4), 299–311.

Kolko, J. (2011). *Exposing the magic of design: A practitioner's guide to the methods and theory of synthesis.* New York, NY: Oxford University Press.

Longtin, S., & Gerber, S. (2008). Contemporary perspectives on facilitating language acquisition for children on the autistic spectrum: Engaging the parent and the child. *Journal of Developmental Processes, 3*(1), 38–51.

Luterman, D. (2003). Helping the helper. *SIG 4 Perspectives on Fluency and Fluency Disorders, 13,* 19–20.

Luterman, D. M. (2008). *Counseling persons with communication disorders and their families.* Austin, TX: Pro-Ed.

Markham, C., Laar, D., Gibbard, D., & Dean, T. (2009). Children with speech, language and communication needs: Their perceptions of their quality of life. *International Journal of Language and Communication, 44* (5), 748–768.

Mattingly, C., & Fleming, M. (1994). *Clinical reasoning: Forms of inquiry in a therapeutic practice.* Philadelphia, PA: F. A. Davis.

Mautner, T. (2005). *The penguin dictionary of philosophy.* New York, NY: Penguin Books.

McDowell, C., Canepa, C., & Ferriera, S. (2000). *11.965-Reflective practice: An approach for expanding your learning frontiers.* Massachusetts Institute of Technology: MIT OpenCourseWare. Retrieved from http://ocw.mit.edu

Mckee, A., Boyatzis, R., & Johnston, F. (2008). *Becoming a resonant leader.* Boston, MA: Harvard Business School Publishing.

Mehrabian, A. (1972). *Nonverbal communication.* Chicago, IL: Aldine-Atherton.

Miller, A. I. (2014). *Colliding worlds: How cutting-edge science is redefining contemporary art.* New York, NY: W.W. Norton.

Moore, L. A. (2006). Empathy: Clinician's perspective. *ASHA Leader, 11*(10), 16–35.

Nagel, G. (1994). *The Tao of teaching: The ageless wisdom of Taoism and the art of teaching.* New York, NY: The Penguin Group.

Nelson, N. W. (2011). Questions about certainty and uncertainty in clinical practice. *Language, Speech, and Hearing Services in Schools, 42,* 81–87.

O'Malley, M. P. (2010). Exploring gender and power in clinical encounters. In R. J. Fourie (Ed.), *Therapeutic processes for communication disorders.* London, UK: Psychology Press.

Owen, R., Hayett, L., & Roulstone, S. (2004). Children's views of speech-language therapy in school: Consulting children with communication difficulties. *Child Teaching and Therapy, 2*(1), 55–73.

Papir-Bernstein, W. (2012a). The artistry of practice-based evidence (PBE): One practitioner's path —Part I. In R. Goldfarb (Ed.), *Translational Speech-Language Pathology and Audiology.* San Diego, CA: Plural.

Papir-Bernstein, W. (2012b). The artistry of practice-based evidence (PBE): One practitioner's path —Part II. In R. Goldfarb (Ed.), *Translational Speech-Language Pathology and Audiology.* San Diego, CA: Plural.

Payne, A., & Barker, H. (Eds). (2010). *Advancing dietetics and nutrition.* London, UK: Elsevier.

Phillips, B. (1999). Reformulating dispute narratives through active listening, *Mediation Quarterly, 17*(2), 161–180.

Pigliucci, M. (2010). *Nonsense on stilts: How to tell science from bunk.* Chicago, IL: University of Chicago Press.

Pigliucci, M. (2012). *Answers for Aristotle.* New York, NY: Basic Books.

Rhoades, D., McFarland, K., Finch, W., & Johnson, A. (2001) Speaking and interruptions during primary care office visits. *Family Medical Journal, 33*(7), 528–532.

Riley, J. (2002, Spring). Counseling: An approach for speech-language pathologists. *Contemporary Issues in Communication Sciences and Disorders, 29,* 6–16.

Rogers, C. (1961). *On becoming a person.* Boston, MA: Houghton Mifflin.

Ross, A. (2009). *The rest is noise: Listening to the twentieth century.* New York, NY: Harper Perennial.

Rothchild, I. (2006). *Induction, deduction and the scientific method: An eclectic overview of the practice of science.* Retrieved from http://www .ssr.org/Induction.shtml

Rozin, P. Haidt, J., & McCauley, C. (2000). Disgust. In M. Lewis & J. Haviland-Jones (Eds.), *Handbook of emotions.* New York, NY: Guilford Press.

Ryan, E. G., Hummert, M. L., & Boisch, L. H. (1995). Communication predicaments of aging: Patronizing behaviors. *Journal of Language and Social Psychology, 14,* 144–166.

Sackett, D. L., Rosenberg, W. M. C., Gray, J. A. M., Haynes, R. B., & Richardson, W. S. (1996). Evidence based medicine: What is is and what it isn't. *British Medical Journal, 312,* 71–72. Retrieved from https://www.cebma .org/wp-content/uploads/Sackett-Evidence-Based-Medicine.pdf

Schon, D. A. (1983). *The reflective practitioner: How professionals think in action.* New York, NY: Basic Books.

Schon, D. A. (1987). *Educating the reflective practitioner.* San Francisco, CA: Jossey-Bass.

Schon, D. A. (2001). Crisis of professional knowledge and the pursuit of an epistemology of practice. In J. Raven & J. Stephenson (Eds.), *Competence in the learning society.* New York, NY: Peter Lang.

Schon, D. A., & Rein, M. (1994). *Frame reflection.* New York, NY: Basic Books.

Segerstrom, S. C., & G. E. Miller (2004). Psychological stress and the human immune system: 30 years of inquiry. *Psychological Bulletin, 130*(4), 601–630.

Shafir, R. (2000). *The Zen of listening: mindful communication in the age of distraction.* Wheaton, IL: Theosophical.

Shamay-Tsoory, S., Aharon-Peretz, J., & Perry, D. (2009). Two systems for empathy. *Brain, 132*(3), 617–627.

Simmons-Mackie, N., & Damico, J. (2011). Exploring clinical interaction in speech-language therapy: Narrative, discourse and relationships. In R. J. Fourie (Ed.), *Therapeutic processes for communication disorders: A guide for clinicians and students.* New York, NY: Psychology Press.

Snyder, C. R., & Lopez, S. (Eds.). (2009). *Oxford handbook of positive psychology.* Oxford, UK: Oxford University Press.

Squier, R. (1990). A model of empathic understanding and adherence to treatment regimens in practitioner-patient relationships. *Social Science Medicine, 30*(3), 325–339.

Stech, E. L., Curtiss, J. W., Troesch, P. J., & Binnie, C. (1973). Client's reinforcement of speech clinicians: A factor-analytic study. *ASHA, 15*(6), 287–289.

Stone-Goldman, J. (2010a). *Reflective-writing for personal-professional balance.* Paper presented at ASHA Health Care/Business Institute, Seattle, WA.

Stone-Goldman, J. (2010b). *Writing prompts can help you write: The what, the why, and the how.* Retrieved from http://www.thereflectivewriter.com

Stone-Goldman, J. (2011). Reflective writing for personal-professional balance. *ASHA Perspectives SIG 11*, 23–29.

Stone-Goldman, J. (2012, November). *Reflective practice for emotional balance in professional relationships.* Presented at ASHA Convention, Atlanta, GA.

Stricker, G. (1992). The relationship of research to clinical practice. *American Psychologist, 47*, 543–549.

Stricker, G., & Trierweiler, S. J. (2006). The local scientist: A bridge between science and practice.

Training and Education in Professional Psychology, 37–46.

Tom, K. (2009, November). *Yoga in voice care.* Presented at ASHA Convention, New Orleans, LA.

Toner, M. A., & Shadden, B. B. (2002, Spring). Counseling challenges: Working with older clients and caregivers. *Contemporary Issues in Communication Sciences and Disorders, 29*, 68–78.

Wampold, B. E. (2001). *The great psychotherapy debate: Model, methods, and findings.* Mahwah, NJ: Erlbaum.

Watzlawick, P., Weakland, J., & Fisch, R. (1974). *Change: Principles of problem formation and problem resolution.* New York, NY: Norton.

Weiss, A. L. (2004). The child as agent for change in therapy for phonological disorders. *Child Language Teaching and Therapy, 20*(3), 221–244.

Westfall, J., Mold, J., & Fagnan, L. (2007). Practice-based research: Blue highways on the NIH road map. *JAMA, 297*(4), 403–406. Retrieved from http://chipcontent.chip.uconn.edu/wp-content/uploads/2015/09/Westfall-et-al.-2007.pdf

Wilber, K. (2000). *A brief history of everything.* Boston, MA: Shambhala.

Wilson, S. (2010). *Art + science now: How scientific research and technological innovation are becoming key to 21st century aesthetics.* London, UK: Thames & Hudson.

CHAPTER 7

Growth

1. SELF-EFFICACY

Theories About Behavioral Change

There are numerous theories that attempt to explain why and how behaviors change, and why they do not (Pajares, 1996). Learning theories, social-cognitive theories, and one aspect of both called self-efficacy, are of special interest to us. We talked about self-efficacy in Chapter 5 as it pertains to belief, specifically, belief in our ability to learn. Self-efficacy is thought to be predictive of *motivation* and the amount of effort an individual will expend in initiating or maintaining a change in behavior (Bandura, 1997).

According to Bandura, each one of us possesses a self-system that allows a sense of control over our thoughts, feelings, motivations and actions (1986; Pajares, 1992). This system serves a self-regulatory function as we interact with our environments. It will inform and influence our beliefs as well as our behaviors and allow us, through *self-reflection*, to make adjustments so that we can accomplish and attain our goals. However, our beliefs about our capabilities are sometimes better predictors of subsequent accomplishments than are our previous experiences (Pajares, 1996). This is where the importance of self-efficacy comes into the picture. Bandura defines self-efficacy as " . . . belief in one's capabilities to organize

and execute the courses of action required to produce given attainments" (1997, p. 3).

How Self-Efficacy Influences Outcomes and Achievements

Our self-efficacy will influence our persistence with achieving a goal and determine how long we invest time and effort. Self-efficacy impacts *self-regulation* and the *choices* we make, and therefore the learning opportunities we interact with. It enhances our memory by enhancing persistence (Berry, 1987). We tend to undertake tasks when self-efficacy is high, and avoid them when it is low. When we are operating at our optimum level of self-efficacy, we will neither be getting discouraged by overestimating our abilities nor being uninvolved with challenges and opportunities for growth (Csikszentmihalyi, 1990, 2014). Self-efficacy affects us and our *world views* in the following ways (Bandura, 1977; Runne, 2012; Schunk, 1983):

- *When it is low:* we believe tasks are more difficult than they actually are, our behavior is more often unpredictable, we blame ourselves for failure, and we see our lives outside of our control.
- *When it is high:* we consider a wider alternative of action options, we deal more efficiently with obstacles and barriers, we credit ourselves for success, we believe we are in control of our lives, and we believe that our decisions and actions shape our lives.

Self-Efficacy, Confidence, and Self-Esteem

Self-efficacy is sometimes linked to self-confidence and self-esteem or other self-concept judgments. Those of us who have the necessary skills but lack confidence, are less likely to engage in those tasks in which those skills are required, or may quickly give up when challenged (Pajares, 1992). It has been argued, however, that self-concept judgments are based on social comparisons and suffer from "frame of reference effects" when we compare our performance with those of others. Self-efficacy judgments are based on a personal ability to accomplish a specific task, and *frame of reference effects* do not play a prominent role (Marsh, Walker, & Debus, , 1991).

The stronger our self-efficacy, the more likely we are to select challenging tasks, persist at accomplishing them, and perform them successfully (Bandura, 1977). Research links self-efficacy to issues of well-being, confidence, drive, and optimism. As people evaluate their lives, they are more likely to regret challenges not confronted as a result of self-doubt rather than actions taken as a result of overconfidence and optimism (Bandura, 1997; Pajares, 1996). This is important for us to know about ourselves as well as our clients.

Factors Influencing Self-Efficacy

According to Bandura, the five primary sources of self-efficacy are success with challenges, perception of task difficulty, expenditure of effort, self-monitoring, and modeling (Hanks & Headley, 2015). There are four factors that may influence self-efficacy (Bandura, 1977, 1997):

1. *Experience of mastery*, or what Bandura refers to as "enactive attainment," is the most important factors. Experience of success will raise self-efficacy, whereas experience of failure will lower it.

2. *Modeling*, or what Bandura refers to as "vicarious experience," is effective when we see ourselves as similar to the model. We feel that if they can do it, so can we.

3. *Encouragement*, or what Bandura refers to as "social persuasion," is effective at increasing self-efficacy. *Discouragement*, however, is more effective at decreasing self-efficacy.

4. *Physiology*, especially signs of physical distress such as fatigue, fear, nausea, or getting "the sweats or the shakes" can markedly alter self-efficacy.

Perceived Self-Efficacy (PSE)

The client's level of perceived self-efficacy (PSE) is critical to the attainment of goals, expectations, and outcomes (Hoffman, 2013; Rogus-Pulia & Hind, 2015). Marks, Allegrante, and Lorig describe three components of PSE, all interrelated: knowledge and insight about one's condition, skills to complete a specific task, confidence, and the motivation to perform the tasks (2005).

The following are suggested strategies for enhancing client self-efficacy as part of your therapy program (DiMatteo, 2004; Hibbard & Mahoney, 2010; Rogus-Pulia & Hind, 2015):

1. Use a variety of learning modalities and strategies, such as demonstration and practice.
2. Facilitate self-monitoring/evaluation strategies in small steps.
3. Apply encouragement and support along with reinforcement.
4. Allow for self-pacing.
5. Encourage reflection about actions and feelings.
6. Involve family caregivers.

2. UNDERSTANDING CHANGE

Principles of Change

Information is there to be learned, and learning is reflected by a change in behavior due to our experience with information. The change can be internal or external, but must be observable in some fashion (Ormrod, 1999; Papir-Bernstein, 2012). In order for change to occur, clients need to commit to *three preconditions*: they must accept *responsibility* for current and future behaviors, they must be *motivated* to change something about their behavior, and they need to *know how* to facilitate the change process (Goldberg, 1997).

A.R.T.: Cute Speech

In my private practice, one young man of 12 years (we shall call him M.) exhibited very complex articulatory distortions, compounded by factors related to his oral myology. He seemed highly motivated, as he was very bright, socially adept, and enrolled in a prestigious private school. Both of his parents were high-powered attorneys, and anxious for me to help remediate M.'s infantilisms. We worked together for three months, twice a week. When I left him his exercises to practice and instructions for the weekend, on Mondays the story was always the same. His productions were back to what his family affectionately called "Bugs Bunny." On this particular day, his Mom, who was usually present, was not, and his dad was home. I decided to broach M.'s lack of carryover with dad. He listened to everything I had to say, and then responded with, "But don't you think M's speech is cute? Even at school they like the way he sounds."

Change is a process by which we move from one point to another. The definition is quite simple, however, the actual change event could not be more complex (Goldberg, 1997). Change is often assumed and not clearly understood. We usually either take it for granted, or believe that people never really change. Yet, we are all in the business of change. The belief in change is the foreground and background of our profession. Without it, nothing occurs.

Responsibility assumes conscious commitment, and may be impacted by the client's beliefs, upbringing, and cultural frames. We tend to isolate things that happen within our work setting from our personal lives, but it helps to remember that what we experience in our role of practitioner is sometimes not all that different from any of the other roles we assume during the rest of the day. As we talk about change, it is helpful to self-reflect about changes that took place in your own life and new learnings that came your way in the process.

Cycles of Change

The *cycle of change* model has been researched and is used to facilitate specific behavioral change. It evolved from the field of psychoanalysis and contains three stages (Prochaska & DiClemente, 2005). In the first stage, *precontemplation,* clients tend to resist change. They do not see themselves as having a problem. This might apply for clients referred to us for reasons of poor academic achievement or poor job performance, and do not think they need our help. They are simply being compliant by showing up. Our focus is to increase their awareness about the communication issue, as perceived by others (Finlay, 2015).

The second stage, or *contemplation,* is the beginning of acknowledging that change may be in the best interests of the client. However, the client may still be ambivalent. Once the client is in the *action* phase, they are committed to change and will be fully engaged in therapy. In the final stage, or *maintenance*, the practitioner steps back and enables the client to assume ownership (Finlay, 2015).

Joint Agreement

Clients do need a voice in determining the type of communication change they consider worthwhile. Before a therapeutic approach is decided upon, the clinician must know what is important to the client (Manning, 2010; Ylvisaker, 2006). Changes that are important to the clinician are not necessarily the changes that are meaningful to the client or parent.

> **A.R.T.: I Love You**
>
> One of the practitioners, (R.), under my supervision was a former pastry chef. In the years of our supervisory relationship, we talked about her former life, and she told me that she had loved her field and profession largely because she knew that she was providing a product that truly made people smile. She decided to change careers, but never forgot those early lessons about addressing what makes others happy.
>
> Shortly after a parent-teacher meeting, R. told me of an experience that changed her perspective about her work and reaffirmed the importance of teaming with parents and formulating joint agreements. At that meeting, R. asked the mother of one of her young students who uses AAC, "What would you like your daughter to be able to say to you?" The mother thought for a moment, and replied, "I just want to hear her tell me that she loves me." R. realized that with

> all of the category boards and curriculum related vocabulary displays, nowhere did she have that. During the same meeting with the parent, the decision was made to make up a "tickle" board as motivation and reinforcement, because the student loved to be tickled.

Normalization Process Theory (NPT)

Practice takes place in the interaction between a client and a practitioner. Normalization Process Theory (NPT) offers one structure for understanding the processes underpinning client care and the behavioral changes that occur. These processes can enable or undermine the integration of our practices into routine everyday care for our client, through the significant efforts and continuous investment by all parties involved (May & Finch, 2009).

The integration of intervention into everyday practice depends on collaborative action within each of four domains (Reeve et al., 2013):

1. *Sense-making:* how people make sense of the intervention, including a shared understanding of objectives and benefits. People need a sense of why it matters.
2. *Engagement and Participation:* the relationship work that helps sustain engagement through collectively defining necessary actions.
3. *Collective Action:* the operational work people do to make practices happen, including management, accountability, and trust.
4. *Reflexive Monitoring:* understanding and assessing the intervention, including collecting data on effectiveness and modifying the intervention in light of reflections.

Facilitating Client Agency

Client agency refers to clients actively making and enacting choices regarding their therapy. It may include motivation, understanding the goals, the value of accomplishment, and the experience of progress in therapy (Hoener et al., 2012). Client agency is sometimes promoted by *encouraging clients to self-reflect*. Questions such as, "What do you want to do today?" or "What would be of value to you?" can assist their introspective process (Frank, 1968; Levitt, 2011). A second way of promoting client agency is to help them decide *what is in their power to change*, and what is not (Gergen, 1994).

A third suggestion is to increase the client's awareness of how and why they are inhibiting change (Clairborn & Strong, 1982; Levitt, 2011). It has been suggested by Fourie that practitioners sometimes have "progress anxiety," because they think that progress will be made all the time, and if they don't see it, something is wrong. Fourie talks about "inexperience anxiety," which gives rise to client anxiety (2011).

One effective strategy when a client is not making progress is to assume responsibility for the lack of success. Remember to hand over the reins to the client once again, by agreeing to make it better together (Manning, 2010). What about *team power?* We do want the client to be the driver, but at the same time, we need not imply that the client is navigating alone. Rather, the process of change is a partnership. We are the coach and guide, there to help connect the pieces and motivate. This approach has been called by some *"client-centered therapy"* (2011).

Clinical Wisdom Related to the Change Process

In Tibetan Buddhism the word "bardo" refers to a transition or gap between the completion of one situation and the beginning of another, between who we once were and what we are becoming (Goldberg, 2012; Rinpoche, 1993).

In a 2011 presentation to speech-language pathologists at the ASHA convention, Levitt talked about psychotherapy research that gathered information, from interviewing psychotherapists who were nominated to the "wise therapist" category of practitioners from leadership organizations, doctoral programs, psychotherapy groups, and research affiliations. Practitioners were asked to explain their understanding of the workings of *clinical wisdom within their practice* and how it impacted client agency and change. Their comments included the following:

- Relinquish your power to facilitate client empowerment.
- Create agency by advocating with, not for, your clients (Plexico, Manning, & DiLollo, 2010).
- Utilize agency in therapy and respect the values, preferences, and experiences of your clients.
- Rather than viewing your role within a deficit model (supply to the client what he or she is missing), see it within a *facilitative model* (calling forth from the client's vast well of knowledge and experience) (LeBon, 2007).
- Whenever possible, co-construct (Greenberg, 1986).

It is helpful to view approaches to human nature, change, and clinical interventions through the lens of diverse orientations, such as humanist, relational, cognitive-behavioral, and constructivist. Never turn down an opportunity, either on line or in person, to attend a training session about the relationship of psychotherapeutic approaches to our work with clients (Levitt, 2011). These approaches reinforce for us the following essential points that have already been touched upon in earlier chapters and will be continued in Chapter 16, when we discuss working with others (Levitt, 2011; Plexico et al., 2010): First, the *empathic connection* is essential to our work, but we also must learn about the dangers of caring too much. Second, although a caring relationship is essential, it becomes a slippery slope when it facilitates client dependence, oversteps the clients' "agency," or allows clients to manipulate the practitioner. Finally, we must acknowledge the parts of therapy that are our responsibility, and the parts that are the responsibility of the client.

3. CRITICAL THINKING AND CLINICAL REASONING

What Is Critical Thinking?

The ability to think critically is one of many goals of higher education, yet progress has been slow in improving overall higher-order intellectual skills for students in undergraduate and graduate educational programs (Borja, 2006; Groopman, 2007; Willingham, 2007). It has been proposed that critical thinking, rather than being an isolated set of skills, is a type of thought process that is dependent on content domain knowledge, repetitive practice, and employing the right type of thinking at the right time (Koslowski, 1996; Willingham, 2007). The learning of metacognitive strategies facilitates the likelihood that critical thinking will be used.

As we discussed in the previous chapter, perspectives and frames of references have limitations, based upon gaps in perception, experience, and knowledge. The same is certainly the case for our process of reasoning and rational or critical thinking (Finn, 2011; Halpern, 1998; Kamhi, 2011). Personal beliefs and style of thinking will undoubtedly influence our

decision-making process, however our greatest safeguard against potentially unbalanced decisions will be our ability to think rationally and critically (Finn, 2011).

Critical thinking, or applied rationality, involves a set of skills that are learned and implemented within the context of our everyday personal and professional lives (Finn, 2011; Stanovich, 1999). It's conceptual roots evolved across the fields of education, psychology, and philosophy, and similarity of definitions vary primarily based upon disciplinary perspective (Jenicek & Hitchcock, 2005). A working definition of critical thinking often contains the following features and involves (Finn, 2011; Jenicek & Hitchcock, 2005; Wade & Tavris, 2008):

- *Motivation* as well as ability
- *Assessing claims* and making objective judgments
- *Distinguishing* between well-supported evidence and emotional claims with no scientific support
- *Understanding* that criticizing an argument is different than criticizing the person
- *Engaging* in debate
- Coming up with creative, constructive, and *alternative explanations*
- *Applying new knowledge* to both global community–based and individual client-based problems

A Process of Continuous Improvement

Critical thinking has been defined as the process of *continuous improvement* in our ability to think about problems and solutions (Paul & Elder, 2001). Grillo, Koenig, Gunter, and Kim (2014) identified critical thinking as having five parameters: knowledge, creativity, analysis, integration, and systematicity (Crist, 2001; Gunter & LeJeune, 2003). *Knowledge* is familiarity with practice standards, literature and laws as they relate to the presenting problem. *Creativity* is the ability to create alternative and less obvious solutions to problems. *Analysis* is the ability to identify an issue (including implications), and to evaluate pros and cons of potential solutions. *Integration* is the ability to relate elements of the problem and potential solutions from multiple sources. *Systematicity* is the ability to describe a critical thinking task in an organized, structured and systematic fashion.

A Set of Mental Activities

From the perspective of cognitive scientists, critical thinking is a subset of mental activities composed of reasoning, making judgments and decisions, and problem solving. There are three key features: effectiveness, novelty, and self-direction (Willingham, 2007). Critical thinking is *effective* because you need to avoid pitfalls such as only seeing one side of an issue, or discounting evidence because it conflicts with your ideas. Critical thinking is *novel* because you just cannot simply remember solutions to other similar solutions without evaluating effectiveness. Critical thinking is *self-directed* because the thinker is calling the shots.

Most frameworks that describe critical thinking include three sets of skills: *interpretative, evaluative, and metacognitive* (Finn, 2011; Fischer & Spiker, 2000).

1. *Interpretative:* The goal of interpretation is to determine your understanding of the argument that is being presented. In a critical thinking context, the argument consists of the proposed question, the conclusions, and the reasons that support the conclusions (Browne & Keeley, 2010). The interpretation of an argument includes examining the value of the claim, identifying available reasons for supporting the claim, and assessing clarity of the available information.

2. *Evaluative:* The goals of evaluation are to determine how acceptable you believe the argument is relative to the quality of the evidence, and the possibility of alternative recommendations (Finn, 2011).

3. *Metacognitive:* The goals of metacognition are to monitor and evaluate your own thinking as you interpret and evaluate the argument (Nickerson, Perkins, & Smith, 1985). This includes checking your assumptions, perspectives, and biases.

Thinking Dispositions

Critical thinking consists of more than a set of skills. Cognitive styles, or thinking dispositions, will also influence the direction and strength of your thinking, and are therefore considered *moderators* of critical thinking (Finn, 2011; Stanovich, 2009). Our style of thinking will not necessarily deter us from thinking critically, but may lead us to maintain our current beliefs and status quo as we remain fixed on our preferred and comfortable practice patterns (Finn, 2011). Open-mindedness, fair-mindedness, and reflectiveness are examples of thinking dispositions that facilitate our ability to consider alternative conditions and diverse perspectives necessary for improved client outcomes (Nickerson, 2008).

We are all subject to errors in our thinking that may ultimately influence our professional beliefs, clinical philosophies, or decision-making process (Finn, 2011). They happen for a variety of reasons: we prefer the comfort of status quo, we favor claims that support rather than question our beliefs, we underplay the influence of our personal frames of reference, perspectives and expectations, and we want to believe the accuracy of our senses in perceiving the world as it is (Kida, 2006).

Errors in our thinking often happen automatically and without our explicit awareness, and are therefore difficult to avoid (Pohl, 2004). What we can hope to accomplish is increase our self-awareness about the role that expectations and bias play in our thinking dispositions. Learning how to think critically is a core skill of education, and should be considered a required goal of our professional training programs (Finn, 2011; Moore & Montgomery, 2008).

Cognitive Skepticism

It is only human to think that we act objectively and rationally, but in truth, we work hard to validate our prior knowledge, prove right our past decisions, and sustain our prior beliefs. It is in our nature to work to satisfy our egos, but in the process, we may deny ourselves intellectual opportunity and growth. Critical thinking may not come naturally to us, but it is an essential skill to learn. It infers a type of *cognitive skepticism* and employs (Kurkland, 1994):

- Rationality, and relies on reason rather than emotion
- Self-awareness, and considers the influences of biases, assumptions, and points of view
- Honesty, and recognizes selfish motives
- Open-mindedness, and evaluates all inferences and alternative perspectives
- Discipline, and avoids snap judgments
- Judgment, and recognizes the extent and weight of evidence
- Inclusion, and appreciates the stories, beliefs, perspectives, and goals of others

Kamhi discusses the certainty and uncertainty behind our clinical practices and decisions as related to our encouragement of and skepticism for new ideas (Kamhi, 2011). Traditional ways of thinking and confident mindsets drive our *certainties*, and our belief in the need for change is what drives our *uncertainties*. Ultimately, our clinical decisions are influenced and driven by our belief systems and clinical philosophy (epistemology). However, the balance between skepticism and openness is a slippery slope, and will bring us to the edge of the mountain where we must examine and question our beliefs and assumptions.

Education builds confidence. It is the nature of professional training programs to educate students to believe that they are being taught the best courses of action in the field of speech-language pathology. Confidence is a powerful elixir, and the effect of clinician factors can sometimes be equal to or greater on clinical outcomes than the effect of the actual therapy approach (Kamhi, 2011; Wampold, Lichtenberg, & Waehler, 2005). Whereas certainty may give us a false sense of security, uncertainly can paralyze action. Admitting uncertainty, however, may enhance treatment effectiveness because it models honesty and commitment and keeps the door open to alternative treatments (Kamhi, 2011).

Rational Thought

Intelligence and *rational thinking* have been demonstrated to involve two distinct cognitive processes, and are not necessarily related to each other as one might naturally think. This research began in the early 1980s by psychologists Kahneman and Tversky (1982), and continues through the present (Hambrick et al., 2014; Hambrick, Macnamara, Campitelli, Ullen, & Mosing, 2016). Some highly intelligent people are prone to bouts of irrationality when making decisions. This has been coined as *dysrationalia,* and measured with a proposed rationality quotient or R. Q. (Stanovich, 2010). A test of R.Q. would measure the ability to step back from your own way of thinking to correct its biases and faulty tendencies—better known as the propensity for reflective thought (Hambrick et al., 2016).

While clinical expertise is difficult to explain, no model or clinical approach will ensure that practitioners are able to use all of the evidence and research to arrive at the best decisions. In an article from the Canadian Medical Association, Horton talks about the skill that physicians often lack: their ability to successfully reason (1995). He describes reasoning as the ability to interrogate a clinical argument to discover weaknesses or the basis for its validity.

Without reasoning and the ability to think critically and logically about a particular proposition, we render the evidence powerless (Horton, 1998). The process of questioning our claims and assumptions in clinical decision-making has become embedded in the interpretive turn in medicine, one that stands as complementary to evidence-based practical (Horton, 1995; Sackett, 1997). In fact, a reliance on evidence alone forces us to stop too soon in our clinical reasoning.

Whereas models do provide a framework to assist with the decision-making process, clinical decisions are influenced most by the practitioner's clinical philosophy and critical thinking ability (Kamhi, 2011). Kamhi refers to the practitioner's propensity for critical or rational thinking, and supports his viewpoint with the research of Stanovich (2009). Stanovich discusses the following tendencies that have been associated with *rational thought*:

1. Gathering information before making up one's mind
2. Seeking a variety of perspectives before reaching a conclusion
3. Reflecting extensively about a problem before responding
4. Balancing the strength of one's opinion with the degree of evidence present
5. Thinking about consequences before acting

Clinical Reasoning

Clinical reasoning has been described as an intangible and rarely explicit thought process, and thus is not often studied in our field (Ginsberg et al., 2016). It has been reported that there are fewer than 12 studies in the last 15 years that have examined the clinical reasoning skills used by SLPs as part of their decision-making processes (Ginsberg et al., 2016). The value of understanding how practitioners make decisions is important for both client care and client outcomes (Wainwright & McGinnis, 2009).

What we do know is that clinical reasoning seems to be based upon a series of interactions between domain-specific knowledge, contextual experience, and intuition (Forsberg et al., 2014; Ginsberg et al., 2016). It is through these interactions that a *cognitive prototype* is developed, an abstract mental model for a concept that includes characteristics associated with that specific concept (Harjai & Tiwari, 2009). Experienced practitioners rely on their professional memory to connect new clients with past prototypes (Forsberg et al., 2014; Ginsberg, Friberg, & Visconti, 2016). Less experienced clinicians have prototypes and schemas limited in depth and applicability due to more limited contextual and intuitive experiences. Strong prototypes can lead to the development of flexible schemas, which assists us in our evaluations and diagnostic capacities.

Ginsberg and colleagues, in their study about diagnostic reasoning used by practitioners and students, used a qualitative method of data collection called "think-aloud" (TA) (2016). The TA is a method of learning about cognitive processes that has participants verbalize their thinking as it is happening. The TA studies have been used in a variety of disciplines, including health and political sciences, and help us understand how we process information (Forsberg et al., 2014).

In a qualitative study such as this one, data must be coded and analyzed for descriptive patterns or themes. A total of eight themes were developed that reflected cognitive patterns of thinking and orientation: hypothesizing, summarizing, rationalizing, seeking outside input, differentiating among possible interpretations, deferring based upon lack of knowledge or experience, comparing, and planning. This was the case for both novice and experienced practitioners, and suggestions were made for increased use of cognitive hierarchies, authentic activities that focus on collaborative learning, and reflective practices (Ginsberg et al., 2016).

The Science of Practice

Clinical reasoning has been referred to as *the science of practice*. The focus on the science behind evidence and evaluation is not intended to rule out other crucial aspects of our practice: the art, the creativity, the values and the philosophy. Fischer and O'Donohue describe the *scientific practitioner* as having four critical components in his or her practice (2006):

1. *Using research* to select interventions that have evidence of effectiveness, which is the heart of evidence-based practice
2. *Using systemic monitoring and evaluation* of every case, which is the heart of evaluation-informed practice
3. Having the *skills, attitudes, and commitment* to keep learning, searching and growing
4. *Sustaining the ethics and values* supporting the helping professions, including sensitivity about the well-being, rights, and dignity of clients

Each component encompasses the scientific, the ethical, and the practice elements and reinforces each other. None can be minimized in favor of the other without detriment to the whole. However, even the selection of the best available evidence may not lead to effective outcomes with each and every client. Research shows that characteristics of both clients and practitioners can have profound effects on outcomes (Clarkin & Levy, 2004). A host of demographic and interpersonal variables —such as culture, socioeconomics and ethnicity—may keep what seems in the research to be "the perfect intervention" from doing its job (Fischer, 2009).

The field of psychology refers to an evaluation-informed practice approach complementing an evidence-based practice approach. The evaluation-informed approach uses ongoing monitoring, guiding, and evaluating client progress. The *science of practice* can be best described as professional action that is informed by the best available information, guided by techniques of demonstrated effectiveness, combined with objective evaluation components, and all provided within the context of sound professional values.

Reflection, Framing, and Problem Setting

Reflection-in-action is a major component in the process of critical thinking. What is the central role of reflection-in-action from a workplace-oriented perspective? Reflective conversations allow us to *frame and re-frame* situations through new discoveries, on-the-spot hypothesizing and experimentation, and changes in our perceptions based upon new situational meaning. In a sense the situation talks to us, we listen and appreciate what we hear, reframe the situation and make the necessary changes (Schön, 1983; Schön & Wiggins, 1992). It is like problem solving, except that problem solving is generally considered to be the handling of *problems as givens*. When we do that, we ignore the important process that Schön calls "problem setting" (1983, 1987).

When we start with problems as givens, decisions are made from available choices best suited to already-established solutions. However, in real world settings problems do not simply present themselves as "givens." *Problem setting* is a preliminary practice during which we actively define the decisions to be made, the ends or solutions to be achieved, and the means with which to accomplish then (Visser, 2010). The problems we set, the strategies we employ, the facts we treat as relevant, and our actions are all bound up with our way of framing our role. We can choose to evolve a theory of action suited to the role and problems we have framed, rather than setting up the easier, more common and self-reinforcing system of framing our role and problems to suit our theory (Schön, 1987).

In Schön's words, "we *name* the things to which we will attend and *frame* the context in which we will attend to them" (1983, p. 40). Naming and framing are both central to reflection-in-action, which facilitates a type of *transformation of perspective* and opens the doorway to *unintended consequences.* As a result, we are reducing the limitations that "givens" impose and eliminating the belief that it is always possible to consider all components and consequences of our actions in advance of making a particular move (Schön & Wiggins, 1992).

Storytelling can substitute for firsthand experience in the process of reflection-on-action, and becomes a powerful tool for establishing vignettes of practice and opportunities for learning within the process of thinking critically and rationally (Schön, 1987; Visser, 2010).

Metacognitive and Self-Reflective Models

Reflective practices were discussed in detail in Chapter 4, and we will continue the dialogue here as they relate to critical thinking. Self-reflective practice involves active noticing of what one is doing as one is doing it, and improves both independence and overall competency (Hill, Davidson, & Theodoros, 2012). It may be predicated on a well-developed metacognitive system of knowledge, which Flavell describes as the ability to possess knowledge about one's own capabilities by tapping into higher level cognitive processes in order to critically appraise the self (1979; Procaccini, Carlino, & Joseph, 2016).

Metacognitive teaching methods may play a role in developing self-reflective practices. Journaling, blogging, self-directing learning, and self-evaluating audio or video performance are all suggested metacognitive means of promoting self-reflection. These methods stimulate critical thinking in students, practitioners and the clients they serve (Chabon & Lee-Wilkerson, 2006; Hill et al., 2012; Procaccini et al., 2016).

Grillo and colleagues suggest the following growth strategies for each of the five parameters of critical thinking (2014).

1. *Enhance knowledge* by accessing and utilizing information provided from ASHA knowledge and skills documents, preferred practice standards documents, State and Federal laws, and rules and protocols from your local educational agency (LEA). Use this information to reframe your principles of practice and approach to meeting standards.
2. *Enhance creativity* by brainstorming treatment options with peers and supervisors, focusing on treatment efficacy.
3. *Enhance analysis* by being able to defend treatment choices using principles from evidence-based practice (EBP) and practice-based evidence (PBE).
4. *Enhance integration* by incorporating comprehensive research from translational and interdisciplinary fields of practice. Identify common themes, and the reasons those themes apply to our field.

5. *Enhance systematicity* by practicing presentations and use of visual learning materials to explain your critical thinking process for approaching this clinical problem.

Inquiry-Based Instruction (IBI)

Although critical thinking is a well-acknowledged prerequisite to sound decision making, the teaching of it within a clinical context is no simple task (Procaccini et al., 2016). One of the proposed reasons for this challenge relates its definition and implicit relationship to metacognitive processes, conscious exertion of mental effort, an attitude to recognize when it is needed, and a motivation to apply it (Halpern, 1998; Procaccini et al., 2016).

In an article written by Procaccini and colleagues, several teaching methods, termed *inquiry-based instruction* or IBI, were proposed to stimulate and foster the development of critical thinking and metacognitive abilities (2016). These methods are adaptable for professors and their students, as well as for practitioners who are trying to foster its development with their clients.

An IBI is a method that views the learner as active and central to the learning process, while the teacher is viewed in the role of facilitator (Mehahem & Paget, 1990). Inquiry-based strategies, which target applying concepts rather than memorizing facts, are sometimes used to stimulate and facilitate critical thinking skills (O'Donoghue, McMahon, Doody, Smith, & Cusack, 2011). This type of instruction discourages the *research and practice divide* that sometimes exists in the minds of students and practitioners (McCabe, Purcell, Baker, Madill, & Trembath, 2009).

Inquiry-based instruction includes *four types of learning environments* that exist on a continuum of learner support, from least to most: problem-based learning (PBL), case-based learning (CBL), concept mapping, and guided discovery (Procaccini et al., 2016).

- *PBL* originated from the field of medicine, and requires the use of functional problem-solving abilities for issues that mimic the clinical setting demands (Jin & Bridges, 2014; Procaccini et al., 2016).
- *CBL* includes the use of independent learning in a collaborative format, as learners gather information and find evidence relevant to a proposed problem (McCabe et al., 2009).
- *Concept maps* are visual representations that facilitate one's ability to organize and represent knowledge (Mok, Whitehill, & Dodd, 2014). They are sometimes referred to as cognitive maps, mind maps, graphic organizers or visual organizers.
- *Guided discovery* evolved from the constructivist philosophy of teaching, and students learn by doing by progressing through a sequenced series of steps, moving from simpler to more difficult (Spencer & Jordan, 1999). After receiving introductory information, students are presented with a general learning frame and series of more self-directed tasks (Procaccini et al., 2016).

4. DEVELOPING A CLINICAL PHILOSOPHY

Understanding Your Worldview and Lifeworld

What is our framework or paradigm for viewing the events that take place in our world? The *worldview* of every person is composed of many dimensions of knowledge and experience, including dimensions that are tacit and unacknowledged, as well as those dimensions that are consciously affirmed (Sellon, 1983). People of different cultures share worldviews, as do people of different ages in history. Our views about the world drive our perspectives about all that is important to us, and that, of course, includes our work.

Our worldview provides for us a context, a scientific orientation, a philosophical position, a prescription for individual and social action, and a motivation for personal growth and transformation. Metaphors provide the language of interpretation, and are useful for extracting personal meaning from ancient truths (Lakoff & Johnson, 1980). In order to integrate professional principles into our contemporary worldview, we need to have knowledge and experience of both.

Lifeworld is the ground and horizon for all shared human experiences in the sense that it is on that background of earth and sky that our experiences all appear as meaningful and significant for each of us (Husseri, 1970). Nothing can appear in our lifeworld, except as it is perceived to be lived. It is a dynamic horizon that both lives within us and within which we live. According to Kraus, life conditions describe the person's actual circumstances in life, however lifeworld describes a person's subjectively experienced construction of reality, formed under the conditions of his life's circumstances (2015).

Our Philosophies, Beliefs, and Attitudes

Philosophy, beliefs, and attitudes are the underpinnings of our practice, and it is important that we be aware of them. When we bring our practice philosophy to a conscious level, we reinforce and strengthen our decisions and collaborations. This is the beginning of the self-reflective process, and helps us identify a framework of the most important factors directing our role in the therapeutic process. Our philosophies, beliefs, and attitudes will impact our clinical practices—even if they

take place below our levels of awareness. They are integral components of our path-building process, and especially important for the development of clinical wisdom (Grundman, 2006).

Developing a philosophical statement or *practice philosophy* can serve a variety of functions (Muma, 2008). It can provide a mechanism for reflecting on your practice, serve as a framework for guiding clinical decisions, act as a vehicle of expression about your work that can be communicated to others, and help synthesize your professional vision and mission statement

According to Ormrod, we store knowledge in many different ways, and some of the main storage systems have been called concepts, prototypes, schemas, and personal theories (2010). A *concept* is a system of grouping and categorizing information for the purpose of sorting and storing it. A *prototype* is a mental example of a concept, which expands as we compare new objects and experiences with that original prototype. An organized set of knowledge becomes a mental model and is called a *schema,* which influences our perception and interpretation of new experiences. A schema is like a script, and has an implicit order and sequence. Ultimately, we form *personal theories* to explain how everything makes sense to us in our world. Our theories are based on observation and fact, but they grow and change as we do as individuals.

A Clinical Philosophy

A philosophy allows us to reflect on roles, synthesize personal beliefs, provide a framework for justifying and supporting clinical decisions, and in general, helps illuminate our professional path (Mitchell & Audet, 2005). All clinicians, students as well as seasoned practitioners, may benefit from the development process that goes into formulating a clinical philosophy statement. The *following guiding question themes* were used in the study by Mitchell & Audet to help graduate students assess the importance of crafting such a statement (2005): the purpose of therapy; motivation for selecting the profession; variables influencing client progress; best practice skills; and professional development needs.

Research cites numerous reasons that practitioners in the field of speech-language pathology would benefit from constructing a clinical philosophy (Mitchell & Audet, 2005; Muma, 2008):

- It provides a mechanism for ongoing reflection about current and future roles in clinical practice.
- It helps synthesize an individual perspective regarding key professional beliefs.
- It serves as a framework to guide and justify clinical decisions.
- It provides a vehicle of expression regarding the nature of clinical work, which can be communicated with clients, families, co-workers, administrators, and other professionals.
- It serves as a guidepost for continued professional development.

A Historical Way of Thinking

In 1947, Kenneth Scott Wood wrote an article entitled, "A Philosophy of Speech Correction" for ASHA's then *Journal of Speech Disorders.* He makes a case for balancing research with practice, philosophy with evidence, and having "even the public school correctionist" compile data about outcomes, and let other professionals know about their research through publications (p. 260).

He talks about the need to have a *working philosophy* of justification, a professional *raison d'etre,* that helps give us "an over-all sense of direction, relationship, and purpose" (p. 257). A philosophy must include knowledge about

the fields of biology, psychology, physiology, medicine, sociology, and draw together elements from many fields that apply to our own. We must be ready "to benefit from all the thinking and findings" of other workers in other fields (p. 261). Was this article the precursor to what we know call translational research and inter-professional education? The article ends with the following mantra:

> The important thing is that the speech correctionist must have a rationally sustained belief in his work. He should not become professional by accident. He must have well-conceived purposes, a direction of movement, and awareness of relationship to other professions, and a determination to get results. (p. 261)

Evidence-Based Practice and Clinical Philosophies

Evidence-based practice drives our clinical decisions, and the decision making process demands that we actively integrate three factors: external *scientific evidence*, client-caregiver *values and preferences*, and *clinical expertise* (ASHA, 2005). As students, we are *groomed to look outside* of ourselves for the answers. We look at the research, listen to the presentations, and rely upon online tools, evidence maps, and practice portals to support our clinical decisions (Hoffman, 2014).

It is, however, the clinical choices and decisions made on an ongoing moment to moment basis that truly drive the success of our therapy programs. Each choice is influenced by the philosophy, orientation, attitudes, and experience of the practitioner. Each choice requires that we reflect open our potential biases and implicit beliefs, and that we examine our own preferences, values, and practice tendencies. Although it is true that the potential of an intervention approach can be supported by external scientific evidence, the quality of intervention is determined by the delivering practitioner (Hoffman, 2014). Clinician expertise, that often ignored third leg of the EPB triangle, is an internal affair.

REFLECTIVE SUMMATIVE QUESTIONS

1. As you begin to think about your clinical philosophy and the stories that shaped your choices, construct a narrative to answer the following question: Why did you choose speech-language pathology as your field of interest?

2. How do you understand the process of change within your own coursework or practice? How do you experience and overcome fear of mistakes and self-criticism as a developing or practicing professional?

3. As a student or practitioner, how do you facilitate client agency?

4. Think of a situation where you were learning a new skill, and try to remember your feelings of self-efficacy. What strategies were used to increase your motivation and confidence?

5. How would you describe your cognitive style or thinking disposition as it relates to your ability to think critically?

REFERENCES

American Speech-Language-Hearing Association (ASHA). (2005). *Evidence-based practice in communication disorders* [Position statement]. Retrieved from http://www.asha.org/policy

Bandura, A. (1977). Self-efficacy: Toward a unifying theory of behavioral change. *Psychological Review, 84*, 191-215.

Bandura, A. (1997). *Self-efficacy: The exercise of control*. New York, NY: Freeman.

Berry, J. M. (1987, September). *A self-efficacy model of memory performance*. Paper presented at the meeting of the American Psychological Association, New York, NY.

Borja, R. R. (2006). Work skills of graduates seen lacking. *Education Week, 26*, 9–10.

Browne, M. N., & Keeley, S. M. (2010). *Asking the right questions: A guide to critical thinking.* (9th ed.). Upper Saddle River, NJ: Prentice Hall.

Chabon, S., & Lee-Wilkerson, D. (2006). Use of journal writing in the assessment of CSD students' learning about diversity: A method worthy of reflection. *Communication Disorders Quarterly, 27* (3), 146–158.

Clairborn, C. D., & Strong, S. R. (1982). *Change through interaction*. New York, NY: Wiley.

Clarkin, J. F., & Levy, K. N. (2004). The influence of client variables in psycho-therapy. In M. L. Lambert (Ed.), *Handbook of psychotherapy and behavior change*. New York, NY: Wiley.

Crist, O. (2001, March). Issues in fieldwork: Promoting critical thinking in students. *Advance for Occupational Therapists*, p. 4.

Csikszentmihalyi, M. (1990). *Flow: The psychology of optimal experience*. New York, NY: Harper and Row.

Csikszentmihalyi, M. (2014). *Applications of flow in human development and education: The collected works of Mihaly Csikszentmihalyi*. Dordrecht, Holland, Netherlands: Springer.

DiMatteo, M. R. (2004). Evidence-based strategies to foster adherence and improve patient outcomes. *JAAPA: Official Journal of the American Academy of Physician Assistants, 17*(11), 18–21.

Finlay, L. (2015). *Relational integrative psychotherapy: Engaging process and theory in practice*. E. Sussex, UK: Wiley.

Finn, P. (2011). Critical thinking: Knowledge and skills for evidence-based practice, *Language, Speech, and Hearing Services in Schools, 42*, 69–72.

Fischer, J. (2009). *Toward evidence-based practice: Variations on a theme*. Chicago, IL: Lyceum.

Fischer, J. E., & O'Donohue, W. T. (Eds.). (2006). *Practitioner's guide to evidence-based psychotherapy*. New York, NY: Springer.

Fischer, S., & Spiker, A. (2000). *Application of a theory of critical thinking to Army command and control*. Alexandria, VA: U.S. Army Research Institute for the Behavioral and Social Sciences.

Flavell, J. H. (1979). Metacognition and cognitive monitoring. A new area of cognitive-development inquiry. *American Psychologist, 34*(10), 906–911.

Forsberg, E., Ziegert, K., Hult, H., & Fors, U. (2014). Clinical reasoning in nursing, a think-aloud study using virtual patients. *Nurse Education Today, 34*(4), 538–542.

Fourie, R. J. (Ed). (2011). *Therapeutic processes for communication disorders: A guide for clinicians and students.* New York, NY: Psychology Press.

Frank, J. D. (1968). The influence of patient and therapist on the outcome of psychotherapy. *British Journal of Medical Psychology, 41,* 349–356.

Gergen, K. (1994). *Realities and relationships.* Cambridge, MA: Harvard University Press.

Ginsberg, S., Friberg, J., & Visconti, C. (2016). Diagnostic reasoning by experienced speech-language pathologists and student clinicians. *Contemporary Issues in Communication Science and Disorders, 43,* 87–97.

Goldberg, S. (1997). *Clinical skills for speech-language pathologists.* San Diego, CA: Singular.

Goldberg, S. (2012). *Leaning into sharp points: Practical guidance and nurturing support for caregivers.* Novato, CA: New World Library.

Greenberg, L. S. (1986). Change process research. *Journal of Consulting and Clinical Psychology, 54,* 4–9.

Grillo, E., Koenig, M., Gunter, C., & Kim, S. (2014, November). *Teaching students to think critically, apply evidence and write professionally.* Presented at the Annual Convention of the American Speech-Language-Hearing Association, Orlando, FL.

Groopman, J. (2007). *How doctors think.* New York, NY: Houghton Mifflin.

Grundman, H. G. (2006). Writing a teaching philosophy statement. *Notices of the AMS, 53*(11), 1329–1333

Gunter, C. D., & LeJeune, J. B. (2003, November). *Assessment of critical thinking skills in clinical practitioners.* Presented at ASHA Convention, Chicago, IL.

Halpern, D. F. (1998). Teaching critical thinking for transfer across domains: Dispositions, skills, structure, and metacognitive monitoring. *American Psychologist, 53,* 449–455.

Hambrick, D. Z., Macnamara, B. N., Campitelli, G., Ullen, F., & Mosing, M. A. (2016). Beyond born versus made: A new look at expertise. *Psychology of Learning and Motivation, 64,* 1–55.

Hambrick, D. Z., Oswald, F. L., Altmann, E. M., Meinz, E. J., Gobet, F., & Campitelli, G. (2014). Deliberate practice: Is that all it takes to become an expert? *Intelligence, 45,* 34–45. http://dx.doi.org/10.1016/j.intell.2013.04.001

Hanks, J., & Headley, D. (2015, April). *Infusing EBP with self-efficacy principles to prepare SLP clinicians.* Council of Academic Programs in Communication Sciences and Disorders 2015 Annual Conference. Retrieved June 12, 2016, from https://2015capcsd.sched.org/event/2niI/infusing-ebp-with-self-efficacy-principles-to-prepare-slp-clinicians

Harjai, P. K., & Tiwari, R. (2009). Model of critical diagnostic reasoning: Achieving expert clinician performance. *Nursing Education Perspectives, 30*(5), 306–311.

Hibbard, J. H., & Mahoney, E. (2010). Toward a theory of patient and consumer activation. *Patient Education and Counseling, 78*(3), 377–381.

Hill, A. E., Davidson, B. J., & Theodoros, D. G. (2012). Reflections on clinical learning in novice speech-language therapy students. *International Journal of Language and Communication Disorders, 47*(4), 413–426.

Hoener, C., Stiles, W., Luka, B., & Gordon, R. (2012). Client experiences of agency in therapy. *Person-Centered and Experiential Psychotherapies, 11*(1), 64–82.

Hoffman, A. J. (2013). Enhancing self-efficacy for optimized patient outcomes through the theory of symptom self-management. *Cancer Nursing, 36*(1), E16–26.

Hoffman, L. (2014). Prologue: Improving clinical practice from the inside out. *Language, Speech, and Hearing Services in Schools, 45,* 89–91

Horton, R. (1995). The rhetoric of research. *British Medical Journal, 31,* 985–988.

Horton, R. (1998). The grammar of interpretive medicine. *Canadian Medical Association Journal (JAMC), 159*(3), 245–249.

Husseri, E. (1970). *The crisis of European sciences and transcendental philosophy.* Evanston, IL: Northwestern University Press.

Jenicek, M., & Hitchcock, D. L. (2005). *Evidence based practice: Logic and critical thinking in medicine.* Chicago, IL: AMA Press.

Jin, J., & Bridges, S. (2014). Educational technologies in problem-based learning in health education: A systematic review. *Journal of Medical Internet Research, 16*(12), e251.

Kahneman, D., & Tversky, A. (1982). Variants of uncertainty. *Cognition, 11*, 143–157.

Kamhi, A. G. (2011). Balancing certainty and uncertainty in clinical practice. *Language, Speech, and Hearing Services in Schools, 42*, 59–64.

Kida, T. (2006). *Don't believe everything you think: The 6 basic mistakes we make in thinking.* Amherst, NY: Prometheus.

Koslowski, B. (1996). *Theory and evidence: The development of scientific reasoning.* Cambridge, MA: MIT Press.

Kraus, B. (2015). The life we live and the life we experience. *Social Work Society, 13*(2), 2–4.

Lakoff, G., & Johnson, M. (1980). *Metaphors we live by.* Chicago, IL: University of Chicago Press.

LeBon, T. (2007). *Wise therapy: Philosophy for counselors.* Los Angeles, CA: Sage.

Levitt, H. (2011, November). *Principles of change used by expert therapists.* Presented at ASHA Convention, San Diego, CA.

Manning, W. (2010). Evidence of clinically significant change: The therapeutic alliance and the outcomes-informed care. *Seminars in Speech and Language, 31*(4), 207–216.

Marks, R., Allegrante, J. P., & Lorig, K. (2005). A synthesis of research evidence for self-efficacy-enhancing interventions. *Health Promotion Practice, 6*(1), 37–43.

Marsh, H. W., Walker, & Debus, R. (1991). Subject-specific components of academic self-concept and self-efficacy. *Contemporary Educational Psychology, 16*, 331–345.

May, C., & Finch, T. (2009). Implementation, embedding and integration: An outline of normalization process theory. *Sociology, 43*(3), 535–554.

McCabe, P., Purcell, A., Baker, E., Madill, C., & Trembath, D. (2009). Case-based learning: One route to evidence-based practice. *Evidence-based Communication Assessment and Intervention, 3*(4), 208–219.

Menahem, S., & Paget, N. (1990). Role-play for the clinical tutor: Towards problem-based learning. *Medical Teacher, 12*(1), 57–61.

Mitchell, P., & Audet, L. (Fall, 2005). Development of a clinical philosophy by graduate students in speech-language pathology. Council of Academic Programs in *Communication Sciences and Disorders, 32*, 134–141.

Mok, C. K. F., Whitehill, T. L., & Dodd, B. J. (2014). Concept map analysis in the assessment of speech-language pathology students' learning in a problem-based learning curriculum. *Clinical Linguistics and Phonetics, 28*(1–2), 64–82.

Moore, B. J., & Montgomery, J. K. (2008). *Making a difference for America's children: Speech-language pathologists in public schools.* Austin, TX: Pro-Ed.

Muma, J. (2008). *Scholarship in communication disorders.* Hattiesburg, MS: Natural Child.

Nickerson, R. S. (2008). *Aspects of rationality: Reflections on what it means to be rational and whether we are.* New York, NY: Psychology Press.

Nickerson, R. S., Perkins, D., & Smith, E. E. (1985). *The teaching of thinking.* Mahwah, NJ: Erlbaum.

O'Donoghue, G., McMahon, S., Doody, C., Smith, K., & Cusack, T. (2011). Problem-based learning in professional entry-level therapy education: A review of controlled evaluation studies. *Interdisciplinary Journal of Problem-Based Learning, 5*(1), 54–73.

Ormrod, J.E. (2010). *Educational psychology: Developing learners.* New York, NY: Pearson.

Pajares, F. (1992). Teachers' beliefs and educational research: Cleaning up a messy construct. *Review of Educational Research, 62*, 307–332.

Pajares, F. (1996). Self-efficacy beliefs in academic settings. *Review of Educational Research, 66*, 543–578.

Papir-Bernstein, W. (2012). The artistry of practice-based evidence (PBE): One practitioner's path —Part I. In R. Goldfarb (Ed.), *Translational speech-language pathology and audiology.* San Diego, CA: Plural.

Paul, R., & Elder, L. (2001). *Critical thinking: Tools for taking charge of your learning and your life.* Upper Saddle River, NJ: Prentice Hall.

Plexico, L., Manning, W., & DiLollo, A. (2010). Client perceptions of effective therapeutic alliances during treatment. *Journal of Fluency Disorders, 35*(4), 333–354.

Pohl, R. F. (Ed.). (2004). *Cognitive illusions: A handbook on fallacies and biases in thinking, judgment and memory.* New York, NY: Psychology Press.

Procaccini, S., Carlino, N., & Joseph, D. (2016, April). Clinical teaching methods for stimulating students' critical thinking. *ASHA Perspectives SIG 11*(1), 3–17.

Prochaska, J. O., & DiClemente, C. C. (2005). The transtheoretical approach. In J. C. Norcross & M. R. Goldfried (Eds.), *Handbook of psychotherapy integration* (2nd ed., pp.147–171). New York, NY: Oxford.

Reeve, J., Blakeman, T., Freeman, G. K., Green, L. A., James, P. A. Lucassen, P., . . . Martin, C. M. (2013). Generalist solutions to complex problems: Generating practice-based evidence—the example of managing multi-morbidity. *BMC Family Practice, 14*, 110–114.

Rinpoche, S. (1993). *The Tibetan book of living and dying.* New York, NY: HarperCollins.

Rogus-Pulia, N., & Hind, J. (2015). Patient-centered dysphagia therapy-the critical impact of self-efficacy. *SIG 13 Perspectives on Swallowing and Swallowing Disorders (Dysphagia), 24*, 146–154.

Runne, C. (2012). *Self-efficacy in people with speech or language disorders: A qualitative study* (Unpublished master's thesis). University of Washington, Seattle.

Sackett, D. (1997). *Evidence-based medicine.* New York, NY: Churchill Livingstone.

Schön, D. A. (1983). *The reflective practitioner: How professionals think in action.* New York, NY: Basic Books.

Schön, D. A. (1987). *Educating the reflective practitioner.* San Francisco, CA: Jossey-Bass.

Schön, D. A., & Wiggins, G. (1992). Kinds of seeing and their functions in designing. *Design Studies, 13*(2), 135–156.

Schunk, D. H. (1983). Developing children's self-efficacy and skills: The roles of social information and goal setting. *Contemporary Educational Psychology, 8*, 76–86.

Sellon, E. (1983, July). Some reflections on a theosophical world-view. *American Theosophist.* The Theosophical Society of America.

Spencer, J., & Jordan, R. (1999). Learner centered approaches in medical education. *British Medical Journal, 318*, 1280–1283.

Stanovich, K. E. (1999). *Who is rational? Studies of individual differences in reasoning.* Mahwah, NJ: Erlbaum.

Stanovich, K. E. (2009). *What intelligence tests miss: The psychology of rational thought.* New Haven, CT: Yale University Press.

Stanovich, K. E. (2010). *Rationality and the reflective mind.* Oxford, UK: Oxford University Press.

Visser, W. (2010). *Schön: Design as a reflective practice* (pp. 21–25). Collection, Parsons Paris School of Art and Design, 2010, Art + Design & Psychology.

Wade, C., & Tavris, C. (2008). *Psychology* (9th ed.). Upper Saddle River, NJ: Prentice-Hall.

Wainwright, S. F., & McGinnis, P. Q. (2009). Factors that influence the clinical decision-making of rehabilitation professionals. *Journal of Allied Health, 38*(3), 143–151.

Wampold, B., Lichtenberg, J., & Waehler, C. (2005). A broader perspective: Counseling psychology's emphasis on evidence. *Journal of Contemporary Psychotherapy, 35*, 208–220.

Willingham, D. T. (2007, Summer). Critical thinking: Why is it so hard to teach? *American Educator*, 8–19.

Wood, K. S. (1947). A philosophy of speech correction. *Journal of Speech Disorders, 12*, 257–262.

Ylvisaker, M. (2006). Self-coaching: A context-sensitive, person-centered approach to social communication after traumatic brain injury. *Brain Impairment, 7*(3), 246–258.

CHAPTER 8

Detachment

1. WHAT DO WE MEAN BY DETACHMENT?

Why Is It Important?

Sages have talked throughout the ages about the *law of detachment* and the spiritual quality of nonattachment. Nonattachment or detachment often gets confused with a smug aloofness or cold indifference to the welfare of others. Detachment involves letting go of attitudes as well as the enormous amount of "stuff" we cart around (Hawley, 1993). As we unload stuff, we feel emancipated. We know the feeling of freedom and space we get when we empty out our closets. In this chapter, we will see how this philosophical pillar specifically applies to our work with regard to our beliefs about service longevity, facilitation of independent functioning, and appropriate use of clinical methodologies.

The Wisdom of Uncertainty

With detachment comes a sense of freedom, of space, of creativity, of belief that anything is possible. To be grounded in detachment is to be grounded in the wisdom of uncertainty. In Chapter 6, we talked about the balance of certainly with uncertainly as a vital component of science and clinical practice. Detachment creates opportunity for uncertainty, which in turn creates opportunity for change and, ultimately, growth through new learning.

When we are attached to a specific mind-set, we lose fluidity, creativity, and spontaneity. With an attitude of detachment, you don't need to have an exact idea of what to do or where to go next, because you are open to so many possibilities. You still have a goal, but know there are an infinite number of ways of getting there. Detachment within the field of uncertainty creates an internal state of alertness and focus on the present (Chopra, 1994).

Practicing Detachment in Our Work

Professionally, we develop patterns of dependence on too many things. It's an addiction in our society as well as most fields. Detachment facilitates a type of freedom, and makes space for a new energy, a different spirit. It allows us to accomplish more with less, and opens up the space for more instantaneous change. Our work involves risk. We need to take chances, to try new approaches and new ways of thinking. The very nature of hypothesizing is risky, because you don't know if something is going to work. We stop believing in trial and error, so we hold back. Detachment involves trust in the art and spirit of our field as well as the science. Do our clients learn to trust us because we have open hearts or good scientific minds?

Here are some simple exercises you can implement during your work day that drive home this particular philosophical pillar:

- *You don't have to fill empty space with the sound of your voice.* Increase your comfort level with *silence*. Allow more time for initiation of student responses. In sales and education, we are renowned overtalkers. Increase student talk time by decreasing our own talk time. Say less, and you will provide greater opportunity for response. Who knows, you may even give your students opportunity to initiate rather than to simply respond.
- *Simplify your materials.* Choose simple and less. Materials are sometimes distracters and may control the session or even overwhelm the student. Practice developing activities with fewer materials, and use materials creatively to accomplish numerous activities. We talk more about materials and activities in Chapter 11.
- *Be spontaneous.* Learn to balance planning with flexibility. Detach from your need to always be in control of what is happening during the therapy period. Listen to your students—they sometimes tell us all we need to know.
- *Acknowledge that "change and letting go" is the one constant in your therapy program.*

2. THE ULTIMATE PURPOSE OF OUR WORK

The Purpose of Education

A.R.T.: Related Service

In one of my undergraduate classes, an early discussion point concerns the purpose of education. I assume the students get some of this information from their education courses (as they are planning on working in the school setting), but they rarely get opportunity to reflect on the definition through the lens of speech-language pathologist. As practitioners, how can we, and how do we prepare our clients and students for independent functioning? We discuss this more fully later in this chapter, but our first task is to understand the concept of "related service," which defines most of the service that we provide to students in the educational setting.

The debate about the purposes of education never seems to end. Do we prepare our students to enter the workforce, or should education be focused more on social and cultural development so that students can become engaged citizens? The answer is both: education prepares people for both productive work and engaged citizenship. The ability to think critically and creatively, develop interpersonal and emotional competence, function independently, and assume a sense of social responsibility all influence success in life, work, and citizenship (Sayres, McKay, & Camins, 2015).

Early philosophers such as Aristotle, Plato, Locke, and Confucius shared common ideas and unique perspectives about what schools are supposed to accomplish in society. In modern times, John Dewey, George Counts, and Mortimer Adler stated that the primary purpose of education is to prepare students to live a useful and pragmatic life, both independently and as productive members of society (Noddings, 1995). Any education is an outgrowth of the needs of the society in which it exists (Dewey, 1934). Education should equip individuals with skills necessary to participate in the social life of their community, and to give back by contributing philosophies, viewpoints, skills, and services to the betterment of society (Adler, 1982; Reed & Johnson, 1996).

Our Beliefs About Our Service Longevity

A.R.T.: Our Purpose

As a staff developer and supervisor, I worked in a New York City Department of Education school district that served the speech therapy needs of students in programs with severe to profound disabilities, called District 75. At a principal's meeting, the superintendent was discussing the vision and mission statement of the district. She talked about the fact that if we all did our jobs really well, we would, in fact, not have jobs because the students would all be in the mainstreamed districts with regularly educated students. Of course, we knew that would never happen, not because we were not doing our jobs well, but rather because more and more of these students were appearing on our rosters.

The discussion did get me thinking about the overall purpose of education, and of speech therapy. We provide a service so that ultimately, our students can succeed without it.

We must continue to reflect on ways to insure that, we are building in and fading out prompts and supports to increase opportunities for independent functioning. One year, we decided to collect data from our more than 500 practitioners regarding terminations that occurred during that school year. The data reflected terminations—but only when students left the system or turned 21 and graduated from their high school program. The speech supervisors knew we had our jobs cut out for us, and data in future years included many more genuine terminations and other types of service delivery changes that reflected we were making strides in student gains in independence.

According to the U.S. Department of Education and the Individuals with Disabilities Education Act of 2004 (IDEA, 2004), speech-language pathology service in the special educational setting is a *related service.* Related services assist a child with a disability to benefit within their primary special educational placement (which is usually considered to be their instructional classroom). However, in fact, speech and language services are unique from the viewpoint of IDEA, because our services can be viewed as both special education and as related services (Power-de Fur, 2011). In order for disorders to be considered a disability, they must have an adverse effect on the child's educational performance (USDOE, 2004).

A.R.T.: The Definition of Speech Therapy

When I think about the practitioner's *beliefs and practices* as they relate to the purpose of our work, one story comes to mind. Leslie Faye Davis, neurodevelopment treatment (NDT) specialist, was hired to do training for those practitioners in my school district working with students with severe-to-profound motor disabilities (1987). During the training session, she conveyed to us the best definition of speech therapy I had ever heard: *you get in there as early as you can, do as little as you have to, and get out as quickly as possible.* If only we would remember those wise words, we would probably fade prompts more often than we do and actually terminate students from our service before they graduate.

Years ago, someone referred to speech therapy in the educational setting as "the Roach Motel: you check in and never check out" (Black Flag, 1972). Our services were never intended to be forever.

3. PROMPTS, CUES, AND CHAINS

What Is a Prompt?

A prompt is a stimulus that facilitates a particular response, and increases the chances that it will occur. It is a type of assist, hint, or help (Alberto & Troutman, 2003). It makes the response easier, and after all, that is why our clients need our services. Prompts are often defined as *auxiliary or extra* stimuli that are presented by the practitioner because our client needs them (Foxx, 1982; MacDuff, Krantz, & McClanahan, 2001; McClannahan & Krantz, 1999). They can be gestures, verbal directions, demonstrations, or other techniques we use to increase the likelihood that clients will respond correctly and thus *allow us to move on* (McClannaham & Krantz, 1999).

A *stimulus prompt* includes any way we change materials to help give the student a better opportunity to give the correct response (Reeve & Kabot, 2012). When we change the way *materials look* (size, color, continuity of lines, type of picture, type of font) or are *displayed* on a surface we are using a stimulus prompt. Positional prompts can include order of materials or even distance from the student.

Response prompting procedures are systematic strategies we use to increase the probability of correct response through positive reinforcement and prompt fading. Response prompting is sometimes called *errorless learning*, because when we use these techniques, it results in few errors by the student (Kabot & Reeve, 2010).

A.R.T.: Our Responsibility

As I write about the behaviorist aspect of our work, I think about a dialogue I have with students at the beginning of the semester in one of my classes. It is about the context of "responsibility," as it pertains to *stimulus* and *response*. It is our role to figure out the complex configuration of stimuli, or what is needed by our clients in order for them to produce the targeted response. We cannot assign external blame if no progress is made. I use the expression, "when you point one finger out there you are pointing three at yourself." It is not the fault of the parents (no carryover) or the client (no motivation). We have a huge responsibility, and we must keep analyzing clinical variables to figure out why outcomes have not been achieved.

Cues and prompts follow a general hierarchy of support from low level or least intrusive to high level or most intrusive. For the purpose of this chapter, we are not differentiating between the term *cue* and *prompt,* but there is sometimes a difference in how cues and prompts are understood and implemented. A *cue* refers to an action that encourages a student to initiate or continue a task previously performed (McIntosh, Vaughn, & Zaragoza, 1991). A cue is generally less intrusive than a prompt, and is more prevalent when we are giving less support to facilitate outcomes. It is like a hint or a nudge in the right direction. A *prompt* is an action taken when we are assisting the student with completion of a task (Zaragoza, Vaughn, & McIntosh, 1991). We use prompts more when introducing new skills. A prompt takes the student through each step of the task to its final completion, and, therefore, a breakdown or task-analysis is extremely helpful for its execution.

Prompts Increase Students' Ability to Self-Regulate

McCloskey and colleagues suggest that prompts cue students to self-regulate as they perceive, feel, think, and act in relationship to things happening in their environment (2014).

- Prompts incorporate instructions, such as "look," "listen," "feel," and cue the use of *sensory and perceptual* processes to input information from the external environment.
- Prompts incorporate reminders to "start describing" or "tell me now" and cue *initial engagement.*
- Prompts such as "if you listen to" or "think carefully about" cue *modulation and regulation of intensity* of mental energy.
- Prompts, such as "consider what you have to do," cue *identification of the task demands.*
- Similar phrases can be constructed to sustain engagement, inhibit impulses, shift or alter attention, anticipate conditions, organize information, and store and retrieve information from memory.

Prompt Classification

Prompts can be classified in a number of ways, and prompting procedures are often organized by *modality,* such as verbal prompts, gestural prompts, picture prompts, physical or manual prompts, textual prompts, and models (Luyben, Funk, Morgan, Clark, & Delulio, 1986; MacDuff et al., 2001). *Verbal prompts* are the most commonly reported type, and include words, instructions, step-by step directives, or questions that direct a client to engage in a targeted response. A verbal prompt is different from an initial instruction. An *initial instruction* is first offered to let the student know what is required or expected. All additional added instructions, offered as help or guidance, are considered verbal prompts (Alberto & Troutman, 2003). Verbal prompts are more difficult to fade, and should be replaced as quickly as possible with a different type of prompt. such as visual, gestural. or positional (Grandin, 2006).

Gestural prompts include pointing, motioning or nodding to indicate an action is to be performed. *Visual or picture prompts* include photographs, line drawings, or other graphics that are often combined with other types of prompts. *Physical or manual prompts* involve physical contact or guidance that is designed to facilitate the behavior of interest. *Textual prompts* include written or digital cues such as checklists, scripts, and written instructions. *Demonstrative prompts or models* are the second most common type of prompt procedure and require an imitative response. Modeling by another student is often more effective than adult modeling due to identification factors. *Other types of prompts* include tactile variables, light, sound, and colors.

General Prompt Guidelines

Instructional effectiveness and efficiency may be affected by prompt characteristics, and preferred sensory modalities (MacDuff et al., 2001). Another factor that may impact effectiveness is ease or difficulty of prompt implementation (Billingsley & Romer, 1983). One of the most critical, yet often ignored, elements in the therapeutic process is the fading of prompts, which if not implemented, might lead to learned helplessness and prompt dependence (Jahr, 1997). MacDuff and colleagues summarize some practical guidelines for integrating prompts and prompt-fading procedures as part of your therapeutic approach:

- Prompts should be used to provide opportunities to reinforce correct responses, but should be faded systematically and as quickly as possible.
- Increasing assistance procedures (least-to-most) are best used for assessment purposes, because you will see what students can do independently and with minimal assistance.

- Decreasing assistance procedures (most-to-least) are best used for teaching new skills with few errors and little prompt dependence.
- When errors occur, it is advisable to return to the previous level of prompting.
- Ultimately, prompting and prompt-fading techniques should be selected as a result of direct observation and assessment of responses.

Effective Use (and Fading) of Prompts

The effective use (and fading) of prompts will help the client initiate behaviors, maintain them, and eventually generalize them to functional and naturalistic settings. Prompting, fading, and data collection all impact student growth and independence. Any resource from *Applied Behavioral Analysis (ABA)* will provide more extensive explanations of the following six techniques that are used for applying and fading prompts (MacDuff et al., 2001; Miltenberger, 2008).

1. *Increasing assistance* by incorporating *least to most* prompts: If we provide minimal assistance, more help is needed if the client does not respond correctly within a specified period of time (usually 5 seconds or less). We generally increase assistance until the correct response is obtained.
2. *Decreasing assistance* by incorporating *most-to-least* (MTL) prompts: The amount of assistance is gradually reduced until no prompts are provided. This MTL procedure removes prompts by moving through a hierarchy, from most restrictive to least restrictive.
3. *Time delay:* A brief additional period of time (one or two seconds) is imposed between presentation of stimulus and delivery of a prompt (a second stimulus).

4. *Graduated assistance:* This is accomplished with manual or physical prompts when they are faded by changing intensity or location of the prompt.
5. *Fading of the physical stimulus:* A physical dimension of the stimulus is faded, such as color, size, or intensity. This technique works best when target behaviors are discrete responses, such as pointing or naming, rather than lengthy and more complex responses. Another way to accomplish this is with vocal volume.
6. *Stimulus shaping:* The physical characteristics of the prompt stimuli are gradually altered, which also facilitates generalization and carryover. This technique is especially useful when working on any type of discrimination.

Prompt Hierarchies

Prompt levels move from least assistive or intrusive, to most assistive or intrusive, as they move along the *social prompt* hierarchy, from verbal or gestural model, to partial physical, to full physical (White, 2016). Prompts can also be *environmental,* such as visual stimuli or auditory cues, which direct the student to the correct response.

Verbal prompts explicitly state the behavior that needs to occur. A *gesture prompt* includes pointing, looking at, moving toward, or touching to facilitate a correct response. *Modeling* is acting out the desired behavior to encourage initiation of that behavior by the student. You are saying or doing exactly what you expect the child to say or do. A *physical prompt* is manually guiding the student to make the correct response (McIntosh et al., 1991; Zarogoza et al., 1991). In summary, *levels of support* can progress in the following way: I do and you watch; I do and you can help; you do and I can help; you do and I watch (White, 2016).

Prompt Dependence and Learned Helplessness

Most of us who work with people with special needs are familiar with the term "learned helplessness." *Learned helplessness* is sometimes associated with *prompt dependence*. What we may not know is that the concept of learned helplessness evolved when Martin Seligman and his colleagues were doing research on classical conditioning, or the process by which one thing becomes associated with another (1974). The condition of *learned helplessness* is described as *not* attempting to get out of a negative situation because the past has taught you that you are helpless with regard to changing your circumstances.

The way in which we view events will have an impact on whether or not we feel helpless (Peterson, Maier, & Seligman, 1993; Seligman, 1974). As we view events, we attribute different reasons that the event occurred. Each attribution becomes a *blame factor*, and attributions can be both negative and positive. The *attributions* most likely to facilitate learned helplessness are internal, stable, and global.

An *internal attribution* relates the causal factor to the person, as opposed to something outside of the person's control. A *stable attribution* is one that never seems to change over time or across situations, as opposed to one that depends on a variety of explanatory factors. A *global attribution* is one that generalizes to other situations (Peterson et al., 1993). *Self-efficacy increases* when you are able to see the cause as external rather than internal (it's not my fault), believe the situation is unstable rather than stable (time will change things for the better), and believe that the situation is specific rather than global (it is just a very difficult time) (Branden, 1994).

How do we get past learned helplessness, especially with children? The *power of choice* is the key because we all have the inborn drive to be independent with a strong sense of self (Buckhart, 1993). When we provide choices, we enable the client to feel in control. When a client makes choices, it facilitates *cognitive engagement* and reduces passivity. More on this is discussed in Chapter 14, "Best Practices." One of the most important things to remember about *prompting* is that when we help a student by providing prompts and assists when they can do the action without the prompt, we are creating learned helplessness and overly dependent behavior (White, 2016).

Fading Prompts

Fading is defined as the gradual reduction of cues and prompts as the student demonstrates the desired behavior (White, 2016; Zaragoza et al., 1991). Our efforts to fade prompts must be intentionally and systematically planned by varying the amount of support and collecting data. Ultimately, we try to replace our more intrusive prompts with visuals and natural environmental supports. Data drives student learning and helps us monitor progress. Independence and self-sufficiency are promoted as we resist the urge to step in and overhelp.

Research and experience have taught us that all learners of new behaviors need the same things: frequent practice, feedback, and opportunities for functional implementation (Cooper, 1987; MacDuff et al., 2001). Ultimately, there must be demonstration that the new behaviors can be performed independently, and without cues or prompts (Berkowitz, 1990; Demchak, 1990). Research in areas related to children with autism and developmental disabilities has paved the way for us to understand the importance of using and fading prompts.

Prompts are like training wheels, because they provide extra support but must be faded out (Kabot & Reeve, 2010). As important as it is to understand the types and use of prompts, it is equally as important to understand the necessity of *prompt fading.* We can consider fading prompts to be aligned along the following three dimensions (Earles, Carlson, & Block, 1998):

1. *Force or degree of help:* This goes, for example, from full touch to partial touch, and eventually to a pointing gesture or eye gaze in the direction.
2. *Timing:* This is related to the amount of time between the instruction and the prompt, moving to longer periods of time between prompts.
3. *Spatial distance:* This is moving from very close to the student and increasing distance over time.

Chaining

Chaining is an approach that breaks down targets, such as words or sentences, into small parts, and teaches the beginning (or end) of the part first. Thus, chaining is a methodology for learning anything that involves sequence, such as syllables, words, sentences, or activities. The chain is broken down into steps, or links, using a task analysis. It begins with part of a desired response, then keeps that response while adding another part, then keeps those two parts of the response, while adding another part, and so on, continuing until the larger target is learned (Johnson & Hood, 1988). There are two main types of chaining used: forward chaining and backward, or reverse, chaining.

Chaining is sometimes used as a phonological or articulatory tool, as we teach one phoneme or syllable of a word at a time and then pull them together in sequence (Marshalla, 2011). An example of forward chaining of the word "telephone" would be: "say /te/ . . . Say /te le/ . . . say /te le fon/." An example of backward chaining would be: "say /fon/ . . . say /le fon/ . . . say /te le fon/" (Edwards & Schriberg, 1983). Chaining as a language therapy tool has been demonstrated to be effective, and it seems to carry a large untapped potential. With chaining, you're basically using successive approximation, or gradually increasing the length and complexity of an utterance (Hodson & Paden, 1983).

The chaining approach has been found to improve both unintelligible speech and delayed language skills, and capitalizes on the presence of coarticulation of speech first noted by Eugene McDonald. Forward chaining is sometimes used in teaching speech articulation, such as with multisyllabic words, and backward chaining is often used in teaching naturalistic language as part of self-help skills, such as brushing teeth or making a bed (McDonald, 1964).

When conducting backward chaining, you are reinforcing links in the chain beginning at the back end of the chain and working toward the front. In essence, you are teaching the last part of the progression first. You provide as much prompting as is necessary, then fade the prompts and move to the previous step (Brandon, 2003). The expectation is that you will need to offer fewer and less intensive prompts at earlier steps of the task analysis.

---

4. CARRYOVER AND GENERALIZATION

A.R.T.: How to Generalize

My philosophy about carryover and generalization goes something like this: just remember the basic definition of *a noun* that you learned about in elementary school. A noun is defined as a word used to identify *a person, place, or thing.* Just keep changing around and adding people, places and things (materials and activities), and you will be working on carryover.

> One of the practitioners under my supervision put together an approach called "hallway communication." There are so many things to communicate about and people to communicate with as you walk with the students through the hallways. Bulletin boards provide lots of language content, as do decorations on doorways. Walking and talking always seems to stress our systems more than simply sitting and talking, so it provides perfect carryover opportunity. Students are not accustomed to using their best communication strategies when walking in the hallway, so that technique challenges, and ultimately stretches, their comfort zone.

From Initial Learning to Carryover

There is a world of difference between learning something new, using it in a controlled and limited context, and integrating it in a more natural and functional environment. Moving past initial learning to integration of the new behaviors into *the stories of our life* presents many challenges for us as practitioners, and for our clients (Gagné & Jennings, 2000). It is helpful for our clients to construct narratives about how the new behaviors make them feel, share their stories, and listen as we retell them back (DiLollo, DiLollo, Mendel, English, & McCarthy, 2006). Any carryover or generalization documents that are given out should be cocreated by both practitioner and client, or entirely created by the client (Payne, 2000).

Breaking Out of Your Comfort Zone

Most of us prefer to operate within our *comfort zones* where stress and risk are minimized and emotional security keeps us feeling safe. However, in truth, growth occurs outside the comfort zone, and only when we are being challenged to take a risk or feel as though we are being asked to push our boundaries and do something new. It doesn't feel comfortable because it's new and different for us (Henry, 2013). There is an uncertainty about being outside of your comfort zone—maybe we will succeed and maybe we will not.

Comfort zone is defined as a behavioral space where your activities and behaviors fit a routine (Henry, 2013). Over a century ago, the relationship between levels of comfort and performance was explored in a study by two Harvard psychologists, Yerkes and Dodson (1908) (Henry, 2013). Their research indicated that a moderate amount of discomfort, called *optimal anxiety*, is where the magic of learning occurs.

The brain learns best when stress hormones are mildly elevated to a state of *productive discomfort*. Arousal enhances learning, but only to a point. When anxiety gets too high, performance suffers (Beck, 2012). How do we encourage our students to stretch their boundaries, fight auto-drive, and expand their comfort zones by taking controlled risks? That is most often how learning new behaviors will occur.

> **A.R.T.: Reinforcement of a Lisp**
>
> One of my most challenging cases regarding *environmental reinforcers* pertained to a student with a severe lateral emission lisp. Together, we successfully worked on redirection of airflow and adjusting lingual positions. Although this was in the days before we differentiated articulatory from phonologically based disorders, looking back, I know this was a pure motor speech disorder, and was not part of a larger speech or language issue. The student, N., was extremely

> motivated and so we worked, made progress, felt successful, always up, until a point of long weekend or holiday period. Whenever N. returned to school, his speech sounded as if we had never worked together.
>
> We discussed his home carryover routines, and they always included lots of practice time with his Mom. One evening during parent-teacher conference, I discovered the problem—N.'s Mom had the identical LE lisp.

Attitudes and Motivation

Principles of carryover evolve from learning theory, and one of the key principles pertain to reinforcement (Engel et al., 1966). As my earlier example illustrates, a boy is unlikely to be motivated to change his speaking patterns if he gets attention because people in his environment think his way of speaking is "cute" (Van Riper & Irwin, 1958). Whatever environmental factors maintain the old patterns, they need to be identified, controlled, and eliminated if possible.

The student's desire to improve his communication abilities is a powerful force in obtaining carryover, and should be encouraged and developed as soon as therapy begins (Engel et al., 1966). Young children sometimes are able to adapt their behavior simply to gain approval, and the approval of the practitioner provides easy motivation. Most often, motivation is not so clear-cut.

Many students approach therapy passively, and wait for the practitioner to do something *to* them to make their communication better. All they think they need to do is "make an appearance" and sit in the chair (Engel, Brandriet, Erickson, Gronhoud, & Gunderson, 1966). They are accustomed to their parents telling them what to do, and

their teachers issuing them instructions to complete their school activities. Even with children, we need to explain the active responsibility they have in the change process, and that change will occur because of their efforts and our guidance.

New responses must be stable enough to occur in *emotional situations* (Van Riper & Irwin, 1958). Emotion is introduced only after the student can handle the new behavior under ideal conditions. This is true for other variables as well—introduce something new to challenge routines and create a state of "optimal anxiety."

5. INCREASING INDEPENDENCE

We Are Overhelpers

We are overtalkers, and overhelpers. We are most comfortable giving advice, and telling our clients what to do—this, we think, is our job. We talked earlier in the chapter about "learned helplessness," and too much helping does just that. It is easy for us to try to "rescue" our client from feelings of defeat, failure, or sense of inadequacy. This creates a dependent client who then accepts a more passive role, and expects us to "fix" the communication issue. We are *responsible to* rather than *responsible for* our clients (Luterman, 2010). One of our most important roles is to enhance the client's self-esteem, thus *creating an independent client* who no longer needs us (Luterman, 2010).

Facilitating the Client As Change Agent

It is not unusual to begin treatment with clients expecting to be *passive recipients* rather than *active change agents*. Therefore, from the very first clinical session, the practitioner needs to explain to the client that they are the ultimate decision-makers, the navigators on their road, the drivers of their treatment program (Preston, 2015). Van Riper was one of the early pioneers who valued the role of clinician as a guide and coach, showing the client how best to assume responsibility for their outcomes through our establishment of a positive bond and working alliance (Blood, Blood, McCarthy, Tellis, & Gabel, 2001; Erickson & Van Riper, 1996; Preston, 2015). As we actively listen, our clients will reveal all we need to know.

Much has been written in our field about *client-centered therapy*, especially when viewing the intersection of counseling and principles of practice. We have touched on this in Chapters 5 and 6, and will revisit again in Chapter 14. Luterman reminds us that even when we remain client-centered, and balance against the *therapeutic equator* of support versus independence, there is a tendency to overhelp (Preston, 2015). It is important to remain devoted to maintaining a *sense of responsibility to the client*, not *for* the client (Luterman & Kurtzer-White, 1999; Ylvisaker & Feeney, 2000). When we overhelp, we create opportunities for client dependence and facilitate learned helplessness (Ciccia, 2015; Luterman, 2010).

The WHO ICF

The World Health Organization's (WHO) International Classification of Functioning, Disability and Health (ICF) promotes and supports the importance of our work related to clients' independent functioning (2001, 2006). The International Classification of Functioning, Disability and Health (ICF) is a conceptual framework that captures the multidimensionality of human functioning, from the biological through the social. Ability and disability are viewed on a continuum of

human functioning, and, therefore, disability is an intrinsic feature of the universal human condition (Campbell & Skarakis-Doyle, 2007).

Our profession of speech-language pathology was one of the earliest to adopt the ICF framework in their policy documents. The ASHA did this in 2001, the same year that the ICF was published (Threats, 2012). When WHO defined "health" in its original 1948 "constitution," their use of the term *well-being* indicated that health has a subjective and functional component as well (Brown & Hasselkus, 2008). We will see how this very document encourages the phasing-out of supportive services.

It is interesting to note one particular component of this latest 2006 philosophical ICF framework that focuses largely on the functional aspects of communication disorders: activity/participation (Threats, 2012; WHO, 2006). The *activity/participation* component related to communication disorders deals with conversations, narratives, using nonverbal communication, reading and writing for information and pleasure, involvement with educational and community activities, interpersonal relationships, and learning. Most of these can be best accomplished in a group setting. There is also a distinction made between the capacity to perform a given behavior in a structured setting, such as a therapy session, and the performance of such behaviors outside of the therapy setting, such as in the client's actual life when the therapist is not present (McLeod & Threats, 2008; Threats, 2012).

Group Therapy

Santo Pietro and Goldfarb suggest that specific techniques used to increase self-efficacy will also serve to decrease *learned helplessness* (1985). These techniques are more easily incorporated when working with groups, and include codeveloping home practice schedules, functional activities, such as ordering in a restaurant, craft activities such as making picture frames for a holiday gift, and role-playing activities, such as describing a problem with the student.

Yalom (1995) defined *therapeutic factors* as those mechanisms effecting change in the client. He identified numerous factors that influence the process of change among clients receiving group therapy. They can be summarized as:

1. *Universality and cohesion*, or feeling that you are not alone because someone else has a similar problem and valuing the group experience.
2. *Altruism*, or being able to help and support others, and feel hopeful about change
3. *Developing interpersonal social skills*, by learning new ways to talk about feelings and find out about others
4. *Imitative behaviors*, by modeling and imitating change strategies for others

Peer Cooperative Learning and Social Groups

When children work in small groups, we have a natural advantage that is sometimes called a buddy system, communication partners, or speech and language pals (Marquardt, 1959). Group work is founded on the premise that children learn more rapidly when behaviors are modeled by their peers rather than the adults (Engel et al., 1966). This type of *cooperative learning* is an alternative way to facilitate carryover (Dell Hazel, 1990).

Cooperative learning is a type of positive interdependence, and is characterized by individual accountability and face-to-face interactions among students (Johnson, Johnson, Roy, & Holubec, 1984). The students' efforts

will support each other's academic achievements, which lead to increased individual effort (Marquardt, 1959; Wang, Cui, & Parrila, 2011). We will talk more about the importance of group interaction in the section that follows.

Much of the research on *social groups* has taken place in areas related to adult clients with aphasia and children with autism spectrum disorders. However, social skill programs have similar objectives relating to play, conversation, joint engagement, executive function skills, role-playing, and peer modeling (Vickers, 2004; Williams, 2015). The following are some examples of social and pragmatic targets that can more easily be facilitated through group work (Koning, Magill-Evans, Volden, & Dick, 2013; Williams, 2015):

- Peer turn-taking, including turn initiation, turn-release, and turn-exchange
- Eye contact, including initiation, release and mutual regard
- Adopting the listener's perspective and expressing emotions
- Initiating and maintaining conversation
- Using appropriate body language and facial expressions
- Appropriate use of humor in conversations

6. THERAPEUTIC CHANGE

A.R.T.: Adult Change

In my university classes, when I talk about "change," I usually begin asking the students to recount a recent experience they had learning a new activity. As stories begin to unfold, we talk about the difficulties, the strategies that finally worked, and their attempts to integrate and carry over the new learnings into their mainstream lives. For example, learning to serve a tennis ball is thought of not only as an isolated movement for that sport, but as an awareness of coordination and timing that can be used during other activities as well. The students reflect on their own experiences, which gives them a greater understanding of how much we take for granted about our abilities to communicate at will, and how challenging it is for us to not only learn something new but to use it effectively.

Ownership and Locus of Control

Ownership and its relationship to therapeutic change has been studied as it relates to our work in the fields of speech and language pathology, audiology, and psychology (DiLollo et al., 2006; Kricos, 2000; Yalom, 2002). One aspect of our counseling approach that needs to be considered is *client ownership*. Our counseling skills are considered a *work in progress* that requires ongoing attention, adjustment, monitoring and reflection (DiLollo et al, 2006). *Client ownership* relates to both the problem and the solution, and either one—if missing—can impact therapeutic change. Another factor that must be considered, independent but related to ownership, is called *locus of control*. Locus of control refers to whether clients believe their behavior is actually under their own control (American Heritage, 1995; DiLollo et al., 2006; Yalom, 2002).

Whereas locus of control is based upon beliefs and expectations, ownership implies the motivation and ability to assume responsibility for the problem and solution. The first step in the therapeutic process is assumption of responsibility on the part of the client (Yalom, 2002). Acknowledgment of the problem must occur as the first part of the ownership journey. Ownership of the solution, however, is an equally important factor when dealing with communication disorders (DiLollo et al., 2006).

The assumption of responsibility for change in communication abilities and change in outcomes is part of the *empowerment process* we help to facilitate (Luterman, 2008). Luterman states that clients must realize that *they are responsible* for accomplishing clinical change and outcome transformation within their communicative abilities, and that the practitioner assists them with that process (2008). One of the reasons that change, in any context, is so difficult relates to our fears about *letting go* of who we are or the way we were in preparation for the way we will be (Shames, 2006). For some clients, therapeutic change occurs less consciously, more automatically, and is thus an easier process due to combinations of familial, environmental, and personality variables (DiLollo et al., 2006).

As we discussed in Chapter 7, at some point there must be a conscious decision to change, because without that commitment change is unlikely to occur. Some clients, both children and adults, feel *victimized*, and may shift responsibility for their behavior onto other people or events. Victimization will interfere with assumption of responsibility (Goldberg, 1997; Klein & Moses, 1994). For example, a student who failed to execute the carryover exercises at home may try to blame it on parents or too much other homework.

The Technology of Change

Every specialist that deals with human behavior has the opportunity to work on behavioral change. What is the *technology of change* that unites us all? It is the process of change, how change occurs, and the means used to affect it (Goldberg, 1997). We help our clients become their own *change agent*. We work with them so that they will no longer need our services. We facilitate their growth as they transition for needing environmental supports to being self-supportive. We provide as much environmental support, assistance, and guidance they need in order to progress. We then fade and ultimately withdraw support so that they can exert more internal control and self-support for continuing the behaviors. We do this by minimizing their effort and "pain" and by helping them gradually change behaviors (Goldberg, 1997).

A.R.T.: The Best Exercise

Our bodies are smarter than we are sometimes—they always choose the easiest route with the least effort. I tell my students that we are naturally lazy in that regard, and use the principle of coarticulation to illustrate the point. If allowed to, we will always shortcut. It is a factor of human energy—we conserve it when we can. In other words, don't expect your clients to work harder than they have to. The easier and more natural it feels, the more likely it will be used. The *best exercise* is the one that gets done.

Minimize Effort and Pain

Most human beings will not engage in activities that are too painful or difficult to implement unless the potential rewards far outweigh the efforts. That is true for us, and for our clients. Although motivation may be present, and the knowledge about and benefits of using the new behavior understood, "a method that is too effortful may be disregarded before it becomes effective" (Goldberg, 1997, p. 46).

It is usually easier to maintain status quo than to change something about us. There is a natural resistance to change that must be reduced, and we do this by gradually increasing the difficulty and reinforcing each step as it gets closer to the desired response. *Shaping* is the process of ongoing reinforcement of a series of *successive approximations* to an ultimate *target behavior* (Miller, 2006; Skinner, 1953). In other words, behaviors are gradually shaped through successive approximations to a specified target behavior. Shaping is a behavioral term that refers to gradually molding a specific response by reinforcing any responses that come close to the desired response. Each behavior that comes closer is called a successive approximation (Miltenberger, 2012).

Resistance to Change

New communicative behaviors constitute an unknown, even though they may be highly desirable. The greater the uncertainty, the greater will be the resistance to implementation (Gagné, 1970). Goldberg summarizes four aspects of this phenomenon that are observable in most of the human behavioral sciences (1997):

1. The greater the change, the more the resistance
2. The less the change, the less the resistance
3. The greater the resistance, the more likely failure will result
4. The less the resistance, the more likely success will result

Functional Outcomes

Traditionally, one of the drivers for determining curriculum was the belief that learning outcomes for young children should be based on mastery of skills that follow a developmental sequence. A modification of this perspective is based on functionality, whereby skills are chosen based upon their function in allowing the student to participate more fully in a variety of activities and settings. Skills would be targeted that are immediately useful across settings, people, materials, and environments (Horn & Banerjee, 2009).

Ylvisaker and Feeney present strategies for increasing likelihood of successful functional outcomes, with the hope that eventually the strategic behaviors would become routinized and finally internalized (1994, 2000). The following strategies are viewed as supports and other modifications of everyday routines that will facilitate opportunities for meaningful participation in valued and chosen activities. They all begin through observation and identification of the following (Ylvisaker & Feeney, 1998, 2000):

1. What is working and not working for the client in everyday routines?
2. What environmental and behavior changes hold potential for transforming unsuccessful effort into successful effort?
3. How can those changes become motivating for the client and critical for other people in the client's environment?
4. Build in necessary supports for practice.
5. Systematically withdraw supports.
6. Expand contexts.
7. Build in supports in new contexts as necessary
8. Systematically withdraw supports as soon as possible.

Motivational Factors

Myth and metaphor provide motivation, and the incorporation of role models and power heroes is a familiar theme when working with identity and motivational issues in children and adolescents with communication disorders (Czikszentmilhalyi & Larson, 1984). In the introduction to this book, I talked a bit about the importance of our stories, and how myth is still a very active part of our culture and what historically has lived and thrived throughout the ages. We all need to get back to our stories, to our mythologies (Campbell, 1988). Mythology is the expression of profound tendencies in the nature of man, and are expressed in stories about the wisdom of life.

The main themes of myths have always been the same, and they are historical as well as psychological. In comparative mythology, the hero's journey, or the monomyth, is the template of stories that involve a hero who goes on an adventure, goes through crisis, initiation and ultimately comes out victorious, and than comes home transformed (Campbell, 1949; Orias, 2016). This concept was introduced in 1949 in *The Hero with a Thousand Faces* (Campbell).

A mythology derives its life from the vitality of its metaphoric symbols delivering the narrative, which supply both the idea and sense of actual participation in a universe much larger than the individual (Campbell, 1986). Whether in the discovery or creation state, mythology serves to open the mind to commonalities, to shared experiences, to social supports (Campbell, 1988).

A metaphor is simply one thing representing something else, and which brings to light that other image. It can communicate something nonsensical, or even impossible. It is the stuff of our imagination, our art, our poetry and our dreams. The perspective that views metaphors, both explicit and implicit, as controlling much human thinking, emotions, and behavior has a long tradition in philosophy and linguistics (Lakoff & Johnson, 1980; Ylvisaker & Feeney, 2000). In fact, the ancients believed that truth lives in metaphor (Campbell, 1988). Metaphors, as symbols of meaning and the building blocks of mythology, are pervasive in thoughts and actions about everyday life (Lakoff & Johnson, 1980). It has been suggested that our entire conceptual system—including the way we think, what we perceive, how we get around in the world, and how we relate to others—is largely metaphorical (Campbell, 1986; Lakoff & Johnson, 1980; Waggoner, Messe, & Palermo, 1985). Tacit metaphors operate below our level of conscious awareness.

Ylvisaker and Feeney talk about the use of a popularized cartoon about a despondent Doberman pinscher (and a socially appropriate poodle) in the social rehabilitative process of adolescents with brain injury to illustrate the importance of metaphor in our work (2000). Metaphoric characters and stories can serve as compelling images that facilitate motivation and beacons of incentive for clients who are guiding themselves through potentially complex remediation territory. For example, personal heroes provide inspirational visions of success and self-direction while modeling the strength and courage that supports and motivates the client's progress. Individualized motivational metaphors can include personal heroes or simply role-plays. They might include, for example, basketball talk for social exchanges and journalism lingo for pragmatic functions (Ylvisaker & Feeney, 2000).

From External to Internal Transitions

Transitions are times for self-renewal, but often involve a disorientation and reorientation that mark key points in the growth process (Bridges, 2009). Bridges differentiates between *external change* from *internal transition*, a reaction to the change that involves a restructuring and eventual ownership of our new identity (Deutsch, 2015). He presents a three stage model for internal transition which is very similar to *the hero's journey* described by mythology scholar Joseph Campbell (Bridges, 2009; Campbell, 1986; Deutsch, 2015):

1. *Ending and letting go* of the old way and old identity (the hero's *departure*)
2. A neutral zone of *uncharted territory*, at which time we begin to cultivate our new identity (the hero's *initiation*), and
3. The *new beginning*, infused with optimism and confidence (the hero's *return*).

7. TERMINATION FROM SERVICE

Beginning at the End

Finishing well at the end of therapy is dependent on the quality of the relationships developed at the start of and throughout the process. Discharge from therapy is not a concept to be discussed for the first time at closure, and may be perceived as a type of negotiation. The process needs to promote client responsibility, shared decision-making, and ongoing self-management strategies (Hersh, 2010; Roulstone & Enderby, 2010).

Most endings require delicate timing and careful negotiation. Endings can be mutual, forced, or unilateral (Finlay, 2015). *Mutual endings* may be built into the therapy contract, or emerge over long-term therapy. *Forced endings* may occur when the decision is out of the control of both practitioner and client due to health issues, financial issues, moves, organizational changes, or loss of funding. *Unilateral endings* happen sometimes because clients stop coming. Maybe they weren't finding therapy helpful, or no longer felt the need. Abrupt endings may leave both the client and practitioner handling residual feelings of disappointment or rejection (Finlay, 2015).

Factors to Consider

There are many factors that influence the decision to dismiss, discharge, or terminate a client from therapy. Primary of course are the needs and desires of the client and/or caregiver, but this must be balanced with other considerations: practices of the work setting, available resources such as reimbursement, communication status and functional outcome data, and the beliefs and practices on the part of the practitioner (McNamara, Hindenlang, & Cascella, 2004). Discharge decisions require that the practitioner, in conjunction with parents and administrators, balance and triangulate client needs with the service delivery system and functional outcome data (ASHA, 2004a, 2004b; McNamara et al., 2004).

One of the most complete sources of information about discharge decision issues and guidelines is the American Speech-Language-Hearing Association (ASHA) document relating to admission and discharge criteria (2004a). The ASHA criteria are consistent with other reports in the professional literature, and discuss three areas for consideration: the client's behavioral status, the client's goals and choices, and the likelihood of treatment benefit. In a 2004 study, these and additional criteria were further divided into five subgroups based upon how discharge might be decided (McNamara et al., 2004):

1. *Deficit remediation factors:* whether the communication issue was remediated including, prognosis for continued improvement, the degree that objectives had been met, and the extent to which communication abilities are commensurate with developmental abilities.
2. *Client behavior factors:* behavior characteristics that influenced discharged including the degree to which treatment is tolerated, the level of motivation, consistency of attendance, and the ability to overcome interfering behaviors that negatively impact treatment outcomes.
3. *Client and context-centered factors:* client's opinions and circumstances including, the effect of communication issues on academic, social, emotional, and vocational performance or health status, functional skill actualization within the context of daily routines, and the degree of available family support.
4. *Client transfer:* availability of services if client left one setting for another setting.
5. *Organizational factors:* service delivery parameters that exist such as reimbursement, case management issues, and limitations in service provision.

A.R.T.: Pick and Choose

In ASHA's Admission and Discharge Guidelines (2004a), the following statement merits a tale: "In some situations, the individual, family or designated guardian may choose not to participate in treatment, may relocate, or may seek another provider if the therapeutic relationship is not satisfactory" (p. 5). In one of my high school programs, there were seven speech practitioners, all highly trained but with diverse cultural backgrounds and areas of expertise. Most of the parents had wonderful relationships with the practitioners however, in one instance a parent went to the principal and requested a change. Fortunately, the principal called me to consult (as the speech supervisor) before granting it. When I spoke with the practitioner, she was quite upset because the parent had somehow found out that this particular person did not have the level of certification that some of the others had obtained (simply because it was not required when this professional began her work some 20 plus years prior). We decided not to grant the parent her request, as it would start an inappropriate precedent of "picking and choosing." We did, however, use this as an opportunity to pull the speech team together, and do a "morale boost" session by reflecting on everyone's individual expertise, strengths, and tacit experiential knowledge base.

Thinking About Ending Therapy

The process of ending treatment is rarely explored in professional literature from our field, and that has implications for training programs as well as professional staff development activities (Hersh & Cruice, 2010). One of the first steps to making a change is to raise awareness and thus *make the implicit explicit* about how intervention ends by talking about it and sharing experiences (Baker, 2010; Hersh, 2010). We have learned from psychiatric and psychoanalytic fields that practitioners experience rewards and losses in therapeutic relationships, and they all become part of the complex process of endings (Baker, 2010).

Quattlebaum and Steppling (2010) suggest that discussions about dismissal become easier when therapy approaches include certain ongoing components:

- Collaborative goal-setting
- Transparency of assessment results
- Ongoing discussions about progress
- Mechanisms for monitoring change (Kambanaros, 2010)
- Planning for carryover and the end of therapy

A.R.T.: Private Endings

As I think about *endings*, I remember an experience with my private practice involving a family with three children who needed intervention. I was working through private insurance, and the parents preferred for most of the sessions to be provided individually. I abided by their wishes, except in cases where I felt the "group" interaction was essential. Needless to say, I was working with this family for several years. As I was nearing the end of the last session with the third of the children, the first one I worked with, now 7 years old, came into the room and said, "We no longer need you—this house is clean." This was mimicking the voice of the psychic from the then famous movie *The Poltergeist* as she cleared out the last of the evil spirits. I must say, I was close to tears.

Another memorable ending came also after years of working privately with a young man, moving along with him from an unintelligible 3-year-old to a 7-year-old with no discernable speech or language issues. The parents adored me, and asked me to continue and assist him with his homework. I explained to them that I could no longer justify the services, even though they were paying me privately. As I was leaving, the father said, "Well wait a minute—what else can you do? Didn't you say you like to decorate?" I smiled, left, and stayed in touch with them for years to come. My former client recently graduated from Harvard Law School.

After All Is Said and Done

With all this being said, it is still a difficult task for the practitioner and educational team to dismiss students from speech and language therapy. Opinions and agendas are often conflicted. Parents sometimes feel their children should be eligible for our services throughout their educational career simply because they have a disability. Administrators sometimes choose to back the wishes of their parents.

We must remember that eligibility of our service is based upon a student having a communication disorder that interferes with and/or adversely affects educational performance (ASHA, 2011). Education performance relates to functional performance in areas of academic impact, social impact, emotional impact, and vocational impact (Moore & Montgomery, 2008). The goal of speech and language therapy is to improve the student's communication so that the student is able to benefit from his educational placement and the disorder no longer deters educational achievement. Many states have adopted the Common Core State Standards in language arts and mathematics (CCSS, 2010). The ability of students to master academic content information requires high levels of academic vocabulary, syntactic and morphological proficiency, and the metalinguistic competence to use language to think about language (Marzano, 2004; Power-de Fur, 2010).

A student may be considered for *release, termination, exit or dismissal* from speech and language therapy for one of the following reasons (ASHA, 2004a, 2004b, 2011). Please note that even after exit, some students may continue to have communication goals that can be addressed within the context of their classroom instruction or another type of service.

- The student has met all speech and language objectives on the IEP with no additionally noted areas of concern in communication.
- The parent requests release from services.
- The student has developed compensatory or functional skills that allow access to the curriculum and participation within the educational program.
- The student's communication deficit areas can now be managed through classroom accommodations or modifications.
- The student's communication deficit areas can now be better managed through a difference type of service.
- The student has received treatment for a certain number of years, and treatment is no longer resulting in any measurable benefits.
- The student is unwilling or unable to tolerate treatment because of a medical, emotional, behavioral. or psychological condition.

As we think about ending therapy with a particular client, we juggle with the tensions brought on by real versus ideal endings and with the difficulties of breaking a close therapeutic relationship after months and perhaps years of building it. In addition, we may have to balance bureaucratic demands with our beliefs and client autonomy (Hersh, 2010). Endings are important, and with a bit of reflection we can raise awareness and develop strategies for successful discharge experiences for ourselves, as well as for our clients (Ahmad, 2010).

REFLECTIVE SUMMATIVE QUESTIONS

1. How have you practiced *detachment* in your personal life, and how might you integrate the same philosophy with your work?
2. How do you facilitate independent functioning using prompts?
3. What are the most challenging factors to consider when thinking about dismissal?
4. How would you deal with a parent who insists that her child still needs your services?

REFERENCES

Adler, M. J. (1982). *The Paideia proposal: An educational manifesto.* New York, NY: Collier Macmillan.

Ahmad, K. (2010). Discharging patients from speech-language pathology: A perspective from speech-language pathologists working in public hospitals in Malaysia. *International Journal of Speech-Language Pathology, 12,* 317–319.

Alberto, A. A., & Troutman, A. C. (2003). *Applied behavior analysis for teacher* (6th ed.). Upper Saddle River, NJ: Merrill Prentice Hall.

American Heritage Stedman's medical dictionary. (1995). Boston, MA: Houghton Mifflin.

American Speech-Language-Hearing Association (ASHA). (2004a). *Admission/discharge criteria in speech-language pathology* [Guidelines]. Retrieved from http://www.asha.org/policy

American Speech-Language-Hearing Association (ASHA). (2004b). *Decision making in termination of services.* Retrieved from http://www.asha.org/NJC/Decision-Making-in-Termination-of-Services/

American Speech-Language-Hearing Association (ASHA). (2011). *Eligibility and dismissal in schools.* Retrieved from http://www.asha.org/SLP/schools/prof-consult/eligibility/

Baker, E. (2010). The experience of discharging children from phonological intervention. *International Journal of Speech-Language Pathology, 12,* 325–328.

Beck, M. (2012, June). Anxiety can bring out the best. *Wall Street Journal.* Retrieved January 1, 2016, from http://www.wsj.com/articles/SB10001424052702303836404577474451463041994

Berkowitz, S. (1990). A comparison of two methods of prompting in training discrimination of communication book pictures by autistic students. *Journal of Autism and Developmental Disorders, 20,* 255–262.

Billingsley, R., & Romer, L. T. (1983). Response prompting and the transfer of stimulus control: Methods, research and a conceptual framework. *Journal of the Association for the Severely Handicapped, 8,* 3–12. Retrieved from http://journals.sagepub.com/doi/abs/10.1177/154079698300800201

Black Flag "Roach Motel" Commercial. (1978). Retrieved from https://www.youtube.com

Blood, G. W., Blood, I. M., McCarthy, J., Tellis, G., & Gabel, R. (2001). An analysis of verbal response patterns of Charles Van Riper during stuttering modification therapy. *Journal of Fluency Disorders, 26*(2), 129–147.

Branden, N. (1994). *The six pillars of self-esteem.* New York, NY: Bantam Books.

Brandon, B. (2003, October). Last things first: The power of backward chaining. *Learning Solutions Magazine.* Focuszone Media. Retrieved from http://www.focuszone.com

Bridges, W. (2009). *Managing transitions: Making the most of change.* Philadelphia, PA: Da Capo Press.

Brown, J., & Hasselkus, A. (2008). Professional associations' role in advancing the ICF in speech-language pathology. *International Journal of Speech-Language Pathology, 10,* 78–82.

Buckhart, L. (1993). *Total augmentative communication in the early childhood classroom.* Volo, IL: Don Johnston.

Campbell, J. (1949). *The hero with a thousand faces.* Princeton, NJ: Princeton University Press.

Campbell, J. (1986). *The inner reaches of outer space: Metaphor as myth and as religion.* New York, NY: Alfred van der Marck Editions.

Campbell, J. with Moyer, B. (1988). *The power of myth.* New York, NY: Doubleday.

Campbell, W., & Skarakis-Doyle, E. (2007, November). *Innovations in collaborative service delivery for school-age children with SLI.* Presented at ASHA Convention, Boston, MA.

Chopra, D. (1994). *The seven spiritual laws of success.* San Rafael, CA: New World Library.

Ciccia, A. (2015). TBI: The stealthy school stressor. *The ASHA Leader, 20,* 36–37.

Common Core State Standards Initiative (CCSS). (2012). *About the standards.* Retrieved August 5, 2014, from http://www.corestandards.org/

Cooper, J. O. (1987). Stimulus control. In J. O. Cooper, T. E. Heron, & W. L. Heward (Eds.), *Applied behavior analysis.* Columbus, OH: Merrill.

Czikszentmilhalyi, M., & Larson, R. (1984). *Being adolescent.* New York, NY: Basic Books.

Davis, L. F. (1987). Respiration and phonation in cerebral palsy: A developmental model. *Seminars in Speech and Language, 8*(1), 101–106.

Dell Hazel, E., L. (1990). Peer-assisted carryover alternatives. *Language, Speech, and Hearing Services in Schools, 21,* 185–187.

Demchak, M. A. (1990). Response prompting and fading methods: A review. *American Journal on Mental Retardation, 96,* 603–615.

Deutsch, M.P. (November, 2015). The dragon slayer in you. *The ASHA Leader, 20,* 38–44.

Dewey, J. (1934). Individual psychology and education. *The Philosopher, 12,* 8–9.

DiLollo, L. D., DiLollo, A., Mendel, L. L., English, K., & McCarthy, P. (2006). Facilitating ownership of acquired hearing loss: A narrative therapy approach. *Journal of the Academy of Rehabilitative Audiology, XXXIX,* 49–67.

Earles, T., Carlson, J., & Bock, S. J. (1998). Instructional strategies to facilitate successful learning outcomes for students with autism. In R. L. Simpson & B. S. Myles (Eds.), *Educating children and youth with autism: Strategies for effective practices* (pp. 55–111). Austin, TX: Pro-Ed.

Edwards, M. L. & Shriberg, L. D. (1983). *Phonology: Applications in communicative disorders.* San Diego, CA: College-Hill Press.

Engel, D., Brandriet, S., Erickson, K., Gronhoud, K., & Gunderson, G. (1966). Carryover. *Journal of Speech and Hearing Disorders, 31*(3), 227–233.

Erickson, R. L., & Van Riper, C. (1996). *Speech correction: Principles and methods.* Englewood Cliffs, NJ: Prentice Hall.

Finlay, L. (2015). *Relational integrative psychotherapy: Engaging process and theory in practice.* E. Sussex, UK: Wiley.

Foxx, R. M. (1982). *Increasing behaviors of severely retarded and autistic individuals.* Champaign, IL: Research Press

Gagné, J., & Jennings, M. B. (2000). Audiological rehabilitation intervention services for adults with acquired hearing impairment. In M. Valente, H. Hosford-Dunn, & R. J. Roeser (Eds.), *Audiology treatment.* New York, NY: Thieme Medical.

Gagné, R. M. (1970). *The conditions of learning.* New York, NY: Holt, Rinehart & Winston.

Goldberg, S. (1997). *Clinical skills for speech-language pathologists.* San Diego, CA: Singular.

Grandin, T. (2006). *Thinking in pictures: My life with autism.* New York, NY: Knopf.

Hawley, J. (1993). *Reawakening the spirit in work.* New York, NY: Simon & Shuster.

Henry, A. (2013). *The science behind breaking out of your comfort zone (and why you should).* Retrieved February 14, 2016, from: http://www.lifehacker.com/the-science-of-breaking-out-of-your-comfort-zone-and-w-656426705

Hersh, D. (2010). Finishing well: The personal impact of ending therapy on speech-language pathologists. *International Journal of Speech-Language Pathology, 12*(4), 329–332.

Hersh, D. & Cruice, M. (2010). Beginning to teach the end: The importance of including discharge from aphasia therapy in the curriculum. *International Journal of Language and Communication Disorders, 45*, 263–274.

Hodson, D., & Paden, E. (1983). *Targeting intelligible speech.* San Diego, CA: College-Hill Press.

Horn, E., & Banerjee, R. (2009). Understanding curriculum modifications and embedded learning opportunities in the context of supporting all children's success. *Language, Speech, and Hearing Services in Schools, 40*, 406–415.

Jahr, E. (1997). Current staff training. *Research in Developmental Disabilities, 19*, 73–87.

Johnson, D., Johnson, R., Roy, P., & Holubec, E. (1984). *Circles of learning: Cooperation in the classroom.* Alexandria, VA: Association for Supervision and Curriculum Development.

Johnson, H., & Hood, S. (1988). Teaching chaining to unintelligible children: How to deal with open syllables. *Language, Speech, and Hearing Services in Schools, 19*, 211–220

Kabot, S., & Reeve, C. (2010). *Setting up classroom spaces that support students with autism spectrum disorders.* Shawnee Mission, KS: AAPC.

Kambanaros, M. (2010). Discharge of speech-language pathologists working in Cyprus and Greece. *International Journal of Speech-Language Pathology, 12*, 296–300.

Klein, H., & Moses, N. (1994). *Intervention planning for children with communication disorders.* Englewood Cliffs, NJ: Prentice-Hall.

Koning, C., Magill-Evans, J., Volden, J., & Dick, B. (2013). Efficacy of cognitive behavior therapy-based social skills intervention for school-aged boys with autism spectrum disorders. *Research in Autism Spectrum Disorders, 7*(10), 1282–1290.

Kricos, P. (2000). The influence of nonaudiological variables on audiological rehabilitation outcomes. *Ear and Hearing, 21*(4), 9S–14S.

Lakoff, G., & Johnson, M. (1980). *Metaphors we live by.* Chicago, IL: University of Chicago Press.

Luterman, D. M. (2008). *Counseling persons with communication disorders and their families.* Austin, TX: Pro-Ed.

Luterman D. (2010). Ruminations of an old man—A 50-year perspective on clinical practice. *Audiology Today, 22*(2), 32–37.

Luterman, D., & Kurtzer-White, E. (1999). Identify hearing loss: Parents' needs. *American Journal of Audiology, 8,* 13–18.

Luyben, P., Funk, D., Morgan, Clark, K., & Delulio, D. (1986). Team sports for the severely retarded. *Journal of Applied Behavior Analysis, 19,* 431–436.

MacDuff, G. S., Krantz, P. J., & McClanahan, L. E.. (2001). Prompts and prompt-fading strategies for people with autism. In C. Maurice & G. Green (Eds.), *Making a difference: Behavioral intervention for autism* (pp. 37–50). Austin, TX: Pro-Ed.

Marquardt, E. (1959). Carryover with "speech pals." *Journal of Speech and Hearing Disorders, 24,* 154–157.

Marshalla, P. (2011). *Making speech targets salient: Tools for amplifying speech.* Retrieved from http://pammarshalla.com/docs/aud_salient_marshalla.pdf

Marzano, R. J. (2004). *Building background knowledge for academic achievement: Research on what works in schools.* Alexandria, VA: Association for Supervision and Curriculum Development.

McClannahan, L. E., & Krantz, P. J. (1999). *Activity schedules for children with autism: Teaching independent behavior.* Bethesda, MD: Woodbine.

McCloskey, G., Van Divner, B., & Perkins, L. (2014). *Self-regulation executive function definitions with examples of teacher prompts.* North Carolina Association for Middle Level Education. Retrieved from http://www.upsidedownorganization.org

McDonald, E. T. (1964). *Articulation testing and treatment: A sensory-motor approach.* Pittsburgh, PA: Stanwix House.

McIntosh, S., Vaughn, S., & Zaragoza, N. (1991). A review of social interventions for students with learning disabilities. *Journal of Learning Disabilities, 24,* 451–458.

McLeod, S., & Threats, T. T. (2008). Application of the ICF-CY to children with communication disabilities. *International Journal of Speech-Language Pathology, 10,* 92–109.

McNamara, K. M., Hindenlang, J., & Cascella, P. (Fall, 2004). Discharge practices in the university clinical setting. *Contemporary Issues in Communication Sciences & Disorders, 31,* 182–190.

Miller, L. K. (2005). *Principles of everyday behavior analysis.* San Francisco, CA: Cengage Learning.

Miltenberger, R. G. (2008). *Behavioral modification: Principles and procedures.* New York, NY: Thomson/Wadsworth.

Miltenberger, R. (2012). *Behavior modification, principles and procedures* (5th ed.). New York, NY: Wadsworth.

Moore, B. J., & Montgomery, J. K. (2008). *Making a difference for America's children: Speech-language pathologists in public schools.* Austin, TX: Pro-Ed.

Noddings, N. (1995). *Philosophy of education.* Boulder, CO: Westview Press.

Orias. (2016). *Monomyth: The hero's journey project.* Retrieved May 24, 2016, from http://orias.berkeley.edu/resources-teachers/monomth-heros-journey-project

Payne, M. (2000). *Narrative therapy: An introduction for counselors.* Thousand Oaks, CA: Sage.

Peterson, C., Maier, S., & Seligman, M. (1993). *Learned helplessness: A theory for the age of personal control.* New York, NY: Oxford University Press.

Power-deFur, L. (2010). The educational relevance of communication disorders. *The ASHA Leader, 15,* 20–21.

Power-de Fur, L. (2011). Special education eligibility: When is a speech-language impairment also a disability? *The ASHA Leader, 16,* 12–15.

Preston, K. (2015). Hands on the wheel. *The ASHA Leader, 20,* 38–43

Quattlebaum, P., & Steppling, M. (2010). Preparation for ending therapeutic relationships. *International Journal of Speech-Language Pathology, 12,* 313–316.

Reed, R. F., & Johnson, T. W. (Eds.). (1996). *Philosophical documents in education.* White Plains, NY: Longman.

Reeve, C., & Kabot, S. (2012). *Building independence: How to create and use structured work systems.* Shawnee Mission, KS: AAPC.

Roulstone, S., & Enderby, P. (2010). The end of an affair: Discharging clients from speech-language pathology. *International Journal of Speech-Language Pathology, 12,* 292–295.

Santo Pietro, M., & Goldfarb, R. (1985). *Target: Techniques for aphasia rehabilitation generating effective treatment.* Vero Beach, FL: The Speech Bin.

Sayres, J., McKay, M., & Camins, A. (2015). WaterBotics. In C. Sneider (Ed.), *The go-to guide for engineering curricula, grades 6–8*. Thousand Oaks, CA: Corwin Press.

Seligman, M. E. P. (1974). Depression and learned helplessness. In R. J. Friedman & M. M. Katz (Eds.), *The psychology of depression: Contemporary theory and research*. Washington DC: Winston-Wiley.

Shames, G. H. (2006). *Counseling the communicatively disabled and their families: A manual for clinicians*. Boston, MA: Allyn & Bacon.

Skinner, B. F. (1953). *Science and human behavior* (pp. 92–93). Oxford, UK: Macmillan.

Threats, T. (2012). Use of the ICF for guiding patient-reported outcome measures. *SIG 2 Perspectives on Neurophysiology and Neurogenic Speech and Language Disorders, 22*, 128–135.

U.S. Department of Education. (2004). *Building the legacy: IDEA 2004*. Retrieved June 6, 2016, from http://www.idea.ed.gov

Van Riper, C., & Irwin, J. W. (1958). *Voice and articulation*. Englewood Cliffs, NJ: Prentice Hall.

Vickers, C. (2004). Communicating in groups: One stop on the road to improved participation for persons with aphasia. *SIG 2 Perspectives on Neurophysiology and Neurogenic Speech and Language Disorders, 14*, 16–20.

Waggoner, J. E., Messe, M. J., & Palermo, D. S. (1985). Grasping the meaning of metaphor: Story recall and comprehension. *Child Development, 56*, 1156–1166.

Wang, S-Y., Cui, Y., & Parila, R. (2011). Examining the effectiveness of peer-mediated and video-modeling social skills interventions for children with autism spectrum disorders. *Research in Autism Spectrum Disorders, 5*(1), 562–569.

White, S. (2016). *System of least support: Prompting, fading and data collection*. Oak Brook, IL: Northwestern Illinois Association National Conference for Paraprofessionals.

Williams, B. (2015). Building a science of friendship. *The ASHA Leader, 20*, 50–54.

World Health Organization. (2001). *International Classification of Functioning, Disability, and Health*. Geneva, Switzerland: Author.

World Health Organization. (2006). *World Health Organization constitution*. Geneva, Switzerland: Author.

Yalom, I. D. (1995). *The theory and practice of group psychotherapy*. New York, NY: Basic Books.

Yalom, I. D. (2002). *The gift of therapy: An open letter to a new generation of therapists and their patients*. New York, NY: HarperCollins.

Yerkes, R., & Dodson, J. (1908). *The strength of stimulus to rapidity of habit-formation*. Retrieved March 3, 2016, from http://www.psychclassics.yorku.ca/Yerkes/Law/

Ylvisaker, M., & Feeney, T. (1994). Communication and behavior: Collaboration between speech-language pathologists and behavioral psychologist. *Topics in Language Disorders, 15*, 37–52.

Ylvisaker, M., & Feeney, T. (1998). *Collaborative brain injury intervention: Positive everyday routines*. San Diego, CA: Singular.

Ylvisaker, M., & Feeney, T. (2000). Reflections on Dobermanns, poodles, and social rehabilitation for difficult-to-serve individuals with traumatic brain injury. *Aphasiology, 14*(4), 407–431.

Zaragoza, N., Vaughn, S., & McIntosh, R. (1991). Social skills interventions and children with behavior problems: A review. *Behavioral Disorders, 16*, 260–275.

PART III

Following Our Path:
Guideposts and Stepping Stones

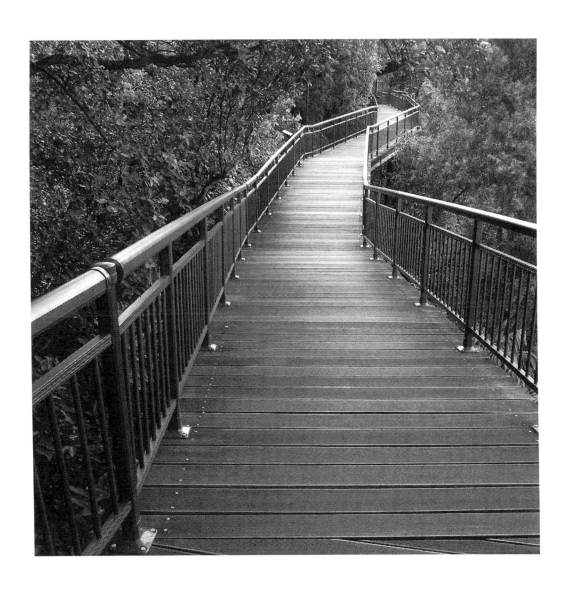

INTRODUCTION

What does it mean to be a *professional*, and how is a profession defined? Professions have become an essential component of our daily lives, and are held responsible and accountable for the workings of numerous systems within our society (DiLollo, 2010). Cruess, Johnston, and Cruess define a profession as having core elements based upon mastery of a complex body of knowledge and skills used in service to others (2004). All professionals must study, master, and integrate a complex set of principles and practices within the *daily workings* of their professional lives.

Part III begins our discussion about following the practitioner's path in speech-language pathology, with guideposts that direct and focus our thinking along our travels. It contains five chapters, with each chapter presented as a guidepost or stepping-stone on the path to clinical effectiveness and professional fulfillment. Principles from assessment and intervention practices that impact the therapeutic processes are highlighted throughout the chapters, and will serve as a field-guide to the *development of a professional attitude* (Cornett & Chabon, 1988). This will be communicated though narratives about my own work experiences, illuminating and assisting the reader with understanding the importance of that particular guidepost.

Travels along the practitioner's path are highlighted and strengthened by *professional pillars of practice* such as our ability to study different maps, implement materials and activities, measure progress, incorporate good and best practices, and work in community. Nothing that is done in therapy should be casual or haphazard. Goldberg states it well:

"Not only do clients and their families have the right to expect competent, efficient and caring interactions, but speech-language clinicians are ethically obligated to provide it" (Goldberg, 1997, p. 3). The quality of the intervention provided to students is only as good as the practitioner who is providing it. Each one of us can improve the quality of our services by attending to and reflecting about professional principles of practice, and variables related to performance and change. Our standards must be set high, and our actions as well as attitudes must be examined (Hoffman, 2014).

Guideposts and stepping stones help us navigate through an often perplexing field, filled with few absolute certainties and loads of exceptions. They provide us with rallying points for our travels as they mark *the differences that make a difference.*

REFERENCES

Cornett, B. S., & Chabon, S. (1988*). The clinical practice of speech-language pathology.* Columbus, OH: Merrill.

Cruess, S. R., Johnston, S., & Cruess, R. L. (2004). Profession: A working definition for medical educators. *Teaching and Learning in Medicine, 16*(1), 74–76.

DiLollo, A. (2010). Business: The crisis of confidence in professional knowledge: Implications for clinical education in speech-language pathology. *SIG 11-Perspectives on Administration and Supervision, 20,* 85–91.

Goldberg, S. (1997). *Clinical skills for speech-language pathologists.* San Diego, CA: Singular.

Hoffman, L. (2014). Prologue: Improving clinical practice from the inside out. *Language, Speech, and Hearing Services in Schools, 45,* 89–91.

CHAPTER 9

Studying Different Maps

1. PHILOSOPHICAL THEORIES AND FRAMEWORKS

A Knowledge and Skills Revolution

As students and learners, we are recipients of information and must transform ourselves to become generators of knowledge and implementers of wisdom. We all play an essential role, as we have been "cast" in the story about *behavioral change* related to speech, language, and communication. Some of us are professors, some learners, some students, some practitioners, and some—even clients. And although our roles shift around, overlap, and change, we are always part of the story.

All professional fields of knowledge are in a transformative phase resulting from a *skills revolution* in this *demanding cognitive age* (Brooks, 2008). We are faced with the challenge to not simply know *more*, but to *know differently*. The ability to know differently requires *experiencing learning* as contextual, reflective, translational, and integrative. Brooks reminds us that although information can travel thousands and thousands of miles in a second, the most important part of the journey is the last few inches—the space between the person's eyes or ears (2008).

What Do We Mean By a Philosophical Theory or Epistemology?

Philosophy is the study of the reality, values, and reason of any body of knowledge. The ancient Greek word was probably coined by Pythagoras and literally means "love or friend of wisdom" (Grayling, 1999; Teichmann & Evans, 1999). Ultimately, as discussed in Chapter 7, our clinical decisions are influenced and driven by our belief systems and clinical philosophy or epistemology. Epistemology actually means *knowledge and understanding*, and has come to represent a branch of philosophy concerned with the theory of knowledge as it relates to truth and belief (Bengson & Moffett, 2011).

A.R.T.: Lens and Frameworks

I have been interested in epistemologies and frameworks since I can remember. Early in my career, I became involved with research and development within my organization. In the mid- 1970s through the 1990s, I coordinated and conducted with extensive research and writing projects in the area of speech and language therapy for students with severe to profound disabilities, all published within the

New York City Department of Education. I worked within a huge bureaucracy, but usually had supportive and encouraging supervisors. They didn't always understand my drivers, but neither did I. I would get busy with enormous research undertakings, form a committee (that's another story), and proceed to develop an assessment or intervention packet. Each one presented a unique epistemological lens and organizational framework. We then constructed and presented training sessions for the speech practitioners throughout the organization, and anywhere from 300 to 500 practitioners received the information.

The Philosophy of Multiple Perspectives

In Chapter 7, we began a discussion about the development of clinical philosophies as they relate to professional growth. Why are philosophies and theories important for our work? We develop goals, objectives, and clinical targets from our understanding of the underlying philosophical and theoretical models of the disorder. However, our actual implementation is often rooted in much broader psychological and educational theories of development and principles of learning (Folkins, Brackenbury, Krause, & Haviland, 2016).

Many members of diverse and varied professions pride themselves in discussing, promoting, and facilitating "multiple perspectives." But we do have favorites, and each favorite perspective is driven by a particular philosophical model (Wankoff, 2005). How do we adapt a belief in a particular perspective or philosophy? What is the process that we go through that sells to us one over another? It is important that we look broadly and investigate many, because the philosophy drives the

theoretical model, which then drives the intervention tasks we use.

No single theory accounts for all aspects related to how children learn language and communication, so the understanding of different theories provide a more integrated view of different aspects of language learning (Kamhi, 1993; Klein & Moses, 1999). Multiple theoretical positions are useful for accounting for the acquisition, development and disorder of different facets of speech, language, and communication (Klein & Moses, 1999).

In Chapter 6, we talked about perspectives, frames, and lenses. Intervention planning assumes our ability to view communication events from a *multitude of theoretical perspectives* (Klein & Moses, 1999). According to Klein and Moses, three perspective variations that must influence our intervention choices are (1999, p. 275):

1. A child's *world view* is different from that of an adult.
2. *Different theories* of language, learning, phonology, for example, may all have merit.
3. The practitioner has a *personal and professional point of view* and clinical philosophy, which impact all choices that we make.

A.R.T.: Theories of the Day

Historically, the *theories of the day* will influence our beliefs, our perspectives, and the way we work. Hopefully, a *newly introduced theory* will *not* replace everything you once believed to be true about assessment and intervention practices for a particular communicative disorder. Such was the case with M., a very seasoned practitioner with whom I was working on an assessment project for children with language and learning issues. It was 1978, the year that Bloom and Lahey's red bible about language disorders was published. She wanted to discard every other resource, in favor of that one. I experienced with other professionals a similar "cognitive storm" two years later, when Lucas published her seminal text about semantic and pragmatic language disorders (1980). I came to call that process "the baby and the bathwater syndrome," when they both go down the drain as you eliminate the essential with the nonessential.

Philosophical Theories About Professional Content

As times change, attempts are made to categorize educational and clinical practices that sometimes call for new allegiance to a particular theory or paradigm (Kamhi, 1994). Those of us fortunate enough to be practicing in the 1980s and 1990s have experience this shift largely in the area of language and learning disorders. The term "paradigm" came into favor in the early 1970s with Kuhn's coin of the phrase "paradigm shift" and its use in popular culture (1970). Paradigms are much more encompassing than a single theory because they represent a way or seeing, or "worldview," which ultimately influences our thoughts and actions (Kamhi, 1994).

As an example of the role that philosophical viewpoints play in our understanding of professional content, Muma and Cloud review different *philosophies or paradigms about cognition and language* (2009; Searle, 1992). They include monism and dualism, materialism, behaviorism, functionalism, constructionism, reductionism, and quantification.

- *Monism and dualism* consider the mind-brain distinctions as they relate to cognition and language.

- *Materialism* focuses on neurochemistry and neuro-connections.
- *Behaviorism* relates cognition and language to stimulus and response relationships and positive and negative reinforcement.
- *Functionalism* considers the cognitive and communicative functions that language serve, including intent and content.
- *Constructionism* represents the view that we construct our knowledge of language, based upon our life experiences.
- *Reductionism* represents the perspective that all behavior should be reduced to elemental components, and we should begin our intervention with these components (similar to target behaviors within a task analysis).
- *Quantification* is the assignment of numbers to behavior, such as frequency counts or rating scales.

The Philosophy of Science: Rationalism Versus Empiricism

In a study about advanced training in our field, Muma and Cloud found there to be a paucity of academic readings related to the *philosophy of science* (2008). Both philosophy and theory should be essential components of our training. Philosophical perspectives establish our frameworks and points of view, whereas theoretical perspectives provide a more organized and disciplined understanding of professional arenas (Fodor, 1975; Muma & Cloud, 2009).

We are reminded that evidence-based practices should be grounded on rational evidence as an addendum to more commonly used empirical evidence (Muma & Cloud, 2008, 2009).

Rationalists claim that our concepts and knowledge are acquired independently of sensory experience (as in reasoning and intuition), whereas empiricists claim that sensory experience is the source of all knowledge (Carruthers, 1992; De Paul & Ramsey, 1998).

Often, research findings and evidence-based practices rely on empirical evidence to the virtual exclusion of rational evidence. Muma and Cloud state that rational evidence is comprised of philosophical views as well as theoretical perspectives, both of which support empirical evidence (2009).

A Philosophical Alternative to Technical Rationality

When Schön (1983) presented his idea of reflection-in-action, he was one of the pioneers in describing the "soft" knowledge of art and intuition that skilled practitioners bring to their practice in the form of problem setting, problem solving, and theory building. He did this through an examination of other professional fields, including architecture and engineering. Donald Schön (1983) started us thinking about the idea of *professional knowing* as unlike the kind of knowledge presented in *school knowledge*, academic books or scientific research papers, which he calls *technical rationality*. In fact, he advocated for the development of a formalized epistemology, validating the knowledge and scientific methodologies behind reflective practice (Vera-Barachowitz, 2003).

Following Schön's model, in reflection-in-action, *doing* and *thinking* are complementary. Reflection-in-action is the driver for the development of that essential tacit component of our knowledge base, *knowing-in-action* (Schön, 1990; Vera-Barachowitz, 2003). When we understand this idea, if helps provide an alternative way of viewing the developmental process for clinical knowledge, the integration of theory with practice, and the interaction of strategies, theories and frames within the process of critical thinking, problem setting (as distinguished from problem solving), and clinical reasoning (as discussed in earlier chapters).

Most of us educated in this country have been schooled in the positivist philosophy of science and education, emphasizing careful measurements and collections of quantitative data (DiLollo, 2010). As Schön has pointed out, the dominant driving *positivist philosophy* that has been adapted in many professions is one of "technical rationality," which places the practitioner in the role of *disorder-based and instrumental problem-solver*, and leaves little room for the emphasis on those softer skills that facilitate the *artistry of our practice* (Cruess et al., 2004; DiLollo, 2010; Schön, 1990). Goldberg uses an analogy to describe this difference (2012). He talks about the words "fix" and "serve." Fixing occurs when something is broken and needs to be mended, and in most cases, the person requiring the help is viewed as weak. Service, on the other hand, is a win-win, where both parties benefit.

2. THE PARADIGM DEBATE: MECHANISTIC VERSUS HOLISTIC

The Mechanistic Paradigm

This classic model for science (and speech therapy) was called forth from Descartes as a kind of separatism and disjunction between subject (practitioner) and object (client). It is rational, objective, analytical, logical, compartmentalized, reductionist, and ordered. All is dissected into as many parts as possible, closely examined and measured, and the whole is equal to the sum of the parts (Kahmi, 1994; Sampaio, 2014). This paradigm was termed *mechanistic* to honor the body as the ultimate machine.

The following principles from the mechanistic paradigm have been translated into implementation practices in the fields of education, special education, and speech-language pathology. At the same time, they are sometimes criticized (Kamhi, 1994; Poplin, 1988a):

- Knowledge is *quantifiable, measurable, and hierarchical.* However, earning chunks are sometimes isolated and segmented.
- Learning involves *sequences of behaviors* and mastery of *predetermined curriculum* outcomes. However when we sequence objectives we focus on the task rather than on the learner. In addition, by targeting curriculum you are targeting school goals rather than life goals.
- Behaviors are predictable through *stimulus control and reinforcement.* However, behaviors are not always predicable.
- Student *deficits* are the focus. However, intervention should be strength rather than deficit driven.
- Our intervention is directed by assessment and diagnosis. However, not everything is quantifiable.

The Holistic Paradigm

A more contemporary model evolved with the significant new age discoveries in quantum theory, when the concept of "absolute" just didn't seem to work anymore. As a result, new perspectives began to emerge that infiltrated all of the sciences and social sciences. Concepts were introduced focusing on uncertainty, complementary, integration, interrelationship, and holism. The nature of the whole is always different from the mere sum of its parts, and relationships are dynamic (Sampaio, 2014). Rather than looking at isolated elements, we look at patterns and principles. Holism focuses on the individual as a human organism rather than a machine-like mechanism (Kamhi, 1994).

The following principles from the holistic paradigm have been translated into implementation practices in the fields of education, special education, and speech-language pathology (Kamhi, 1994; Poplin, 1988b):

- Learning proceeds from *whole to part to whole.*

- We learn best from *interest, involvement, and experience.*
- Goals of instruction should be *life related, naturalistic, and functional.*
- *Reflection and interpretation* is more critical to learning than correct answers.
- *Life story narratives* indicating beliefs and values are drivers of treatment processes.

The Importance of Integration

Although there have been attempts to come up with one systemic perspective or paradigm for educational and clinical practices in our field, there are still largely two: the *mechanistic paradigm and the holistic paradigm* (Kahmi, 1994; Muma, 1998; Sampaio, 2014). We hope we can learn about each, and use the best elements of each one to serve the needs of our students. No one paradigm is better than the other; they are simply alternative lenses that highlight aspects of the learning process differently. Our job is to sort, cull, discard, and integrate.

Either paradigm becomes dangerous when viewed in isolation, because each is useful and necessary for understanding a broader and deeper viewpoint. The *integration* of the two highlights the *multidimensionality* of our profession, and that we are treating all aspects of a person when we treat communication disorders: the physical, social, cultural, emotional, psychological, and spiritual (Sampaio, 2014).

3. SYSTEMS THINKING

Systems Theory

Some of us learned about systems theory in our training programs. An understanding of system dynamics will allow us to differentiate the "component parts" from the "whole," and to examine the interrelationships between the two perspectives. Without an ability to think systematically, we will fall short professionally in our ability to break down clinical tasks into their component parts, or task analyze. Systems theory also helps us understand bureaucracies, within which many of us do or will work. In fact, practitioners working within the educational setting must place their decision making within a *systems theory framework* in order to meet policy driven requirements and help students meet statewide curriculum standards (Nelson, 2011).

In organizations, the *systems* consist of the people, the structure, and the processes that work together to make an organization healthy or unhealthy (Cabrera & Cabrera, 2015). The field of general systems theory began in the 1920s, and was further developed by members of Society for Organizational Learning at MIT. Peter Senge further defined systems thinking as the most important element in organizational development and learning, and the learning and development that individuals pursue within that system (1990). Systems thinking has been defined as one approach to problem solving that examines *each component part in relationship to the whole* (Ackoff, 2010).

Defining Characteristics of Systems

Systems have several defining characteristics, and our learning and "organization survival" will be smoother if we understand how systems operate (Ackoff, 2010; von Bertalanffy, 1968):

- Every system has a purpose that serves the larger system.
- All of a system's component parts must be present for the system to carry out its purpose.
- A system's parts must be arranged in a specific way for the system to function optimally.

- Systems change in response to feedback, and maintain their stability by making such adjustments. This is called homeostasis.

The Total Quality Management (TQM) Movement

An organizational learning movement of the early 1990s was TQM, pioneered by the early works of W. Edwards Deming (2000). Deming believed that *systemic transformations* were fueled by profound *knowledge about the system*, theories of knowledge and *mental models*, and what he referred to as psychology, or *knowledge of human nature*. This is discussed in more detail in Chapter 16 when we talk about *learning organizations*.

Deming described challenges embedded within bureaucratic structures that can lead to burnout. They are (Deming, 2000; Senge, 1990):

1. Management by *measurement:* The criterion can be short sighted, and often values the short term and devalues what cannot be measured.
2. *Compliance*-based cultures: The way to get ahead is to please the boss, and management is accomplished through intimidation.
3. *Right versus wrong:* There is little middle road, and technical, rather that process, problem solving is emphasized.
4. *Uniformity* is emphasized. Sameness rather than diversity of opinion is stressed, and conflict is suppressed as a type of control.
5. *Competition* and distrust are building blocks. Competition is created as a performance enhancer.

DSRP (Distinctions, Systems, Relationships, Perspectives)

The DSRP is a theoretical model that *blends cognitive science with systems thinking*, and was developed by two educational theorists and cognitive scientists (Cabrera, 2001; Cabrera & Cabrera, 2015). The DSRP model is helpful for building knowledge in any field, because knowledge and thinking are in a continuous feedback loop (Böttcher & Meisert , 2011).

According to this theory, there are *four patterns of cognitive behavior* that are universal to the process of structuring information: distinctions, systems, relationships, and perspectives.

- Making *distinctions*, which consist of *an identity and an other*. The guiding question would be, *What is _____ and what is it not?*
- Organizing *systems*, which consist of *part and whole*. The guiding question would be, *What is _____ a part of?*
- Recognizing *relationships*, which consist of something *in relationship to* something else, such as cause and effect. The guiding question would be, *What is _____ in relationship to?*
- Taking *perspectives*, which consist of *point and view*. The guiding question would be, *How would _____ appear from a different perspective?*

Graphic Organizers

The use of graphic organizers (sometimes called concept maps or relationship charts) are helpful in showing key elements of systems and how they connect (Senge, 1990). Graphic organizers are visual tools that enable learners to connect new information to existing information, and thus spot relationships more easily. Because they utilize grouping strategies, they also facilitate storage and retrieval. Graphic organizers depict information in a number of ways by using lines, boxes, circles, and other shapes to form images that are organized through linear sequences, hierarchies, or concepts such as cause and effect (Ellis & Howard, 2005).

Graphic organizers are also called visual road maps, mind maps, word webs, and semantic or conceptual charts. They provide a logical and sequenced visual aspect to information. The information generally contains a logically structured presentation, has a strong and appealing visual presence, and is sequentially related with respect to all parts and sub parts (Popp, 2006). Graphic organizers help structure projects, and assist with problem solving and decision-making (Anders & Beech, 1990). Any professional who is a fan of lists and outlines would find graphic organizers even more useful.

Children with language disorders and delays have difficulty processing material primarily presented in through auditory channels (Bloom & Lahey, 1978; Popp, 2006). However, we are all visual learners because when words and concepts are associated with images, we retain the information better. Visual learning helps us organize and analyze information, integrate new knowledge, examine relationships between concepts, and problem solve (Gardner, 1993; Inspiration, 2016).

Concept maps that illustrate relationships between concepts are linked together by words that are descriptive of their relationship to the concept. *Word webs* show how different categories of information relate to each other. *Mind maps* are represented with hierarchical information with a central idea surrounded by branches of associated ideas (Inspiration, 2016). If you have any doubt about the power of graphic organizers, keep reading.

Online resources and software applications provide some of the best resources for understanding the vast diversity and array of visual organizational strategies (Education Place, Inspiration, Enchanted Learning, CMap). There seem to be four general types of graphic organizers: those that show *relationships*, those that *categorize* information, those that show *order and sequence*, and those that *compare and contrast* words and concepts (Alshatti, Watters, & Kidman, 2011; DeWispalaere & Kossack, 1996; Ellis & Howard, 2005; Enchanted Learning, 2016; Inspiration, 2016).

1. *Relationship* graphic organizers include *cause and effect* and *fishbone*. *Cause and effect* is used to illustrate the problem solving process, and identifies a problem and a variety of solutions. *Fishbone* is used for details in complex ideas, such as main topics with subpoints.
2. *Categorization* graphic organizers include *concept maps* and *mind mapping*. *Concept maps* develop concepts by linking together information in shape-cells. *Mind mapping* is used to organize and classify information using a nonlinear format.
3. *Order and sequence* graphic organizers include *chains, cycles, flow charts*, and *story boards* or *ladders*. *Chains* are used for temporal sequences and cycles for continuity with no beginning or end. *Flow charts* are used to display sequences of events with directions and decision points. *Story boards and ladders* map out scenes in a story.
4. *Comparative* graphic organizers include *attribute charts, T-charts*, and *Venn diagrams*. *Attribute charts* compare attributes of at least two items, while *T-charts* specify two aspects of a topic, such as *pros and cons*. *Venn diagrams* specify similarities and differences between items, and is composed of overlapping shapes.

System theorists relate the use of graphic organizers to enhanced learning processes for a variety of reasons (Alshatti, Watters, & Kidman, 2011). First, learners are *involved actively* with constructing a visual representation of their comprehension of a concept. Visual thinking leads to a *deeper level of understanding*, and the use of visual strategies facilitates concept elaboration, *metacognitive skills*, self-regulation, *critical thinking*, and problem solving skills.

4. TYPES OF LEARNING

Trends in Human Learning

During the past decade, scholars have engaged in transdisciplinary and interdisciplinary research that relates the fields of cognitive psychology and neuroscience to all aspects of the educational process. Educational neuroscience integrates cognitive science, biology, and linguistics to inform and drive all aspects of teaching and learning (Swoboda, 2014).

As often happens with divergent lines of research and diverse philosophical perspectives, implications for practice are pattern driven, and the following consistencies have emerged: learners are in the center of the learning activity, learner outcomes are the most important, collaboration works better than competition or isolation, teacher reflection enhances learning processes, learning must be engaging and experiential and based on the most current research on human learning (Feden, 2012).

Double-Loop Learning

When data are transformed into information, patterns and relationships are formed. This transformation takes place through what cognitive scientists refers to as Single-Loop Learning. In essence, this type of learning involves action without reflection. At this stage, we focus on doing something in the most compliant and efficient way, but with no understanding or evaluation of the beliefs, assumptions or values that underlie the original intention for the action.

Through our experiences with the information, our self-reflection about the information enhances our knowledge, and *double-loop learning* takes place. We now are able to evaluate, choose between alternatives, and decide on the most effective action. The importance of adopting this expanded view of commitment and accountability is supported by cognitive science research in the areas of single-loop learning (SLL) and double-loop learning (DLL) (Argyris & Schon, 1974). Only with DLL is there potential for real change, because we evaluate assumptions through reflection, which better align ideas with actions and actions with outcomes (Kolb, 1984; Osterman & Kottkamp, 1993). In essence, we become more skilled at gathering information, and develop greater awareness of the impact of our actions.

One of the earlier distinctions between single-loop learning (SLL) and double-loop learning (DLL) was made by Argyris and Schon (1974). The first is a kind of quick fix, but does not address the underlying causes of the problem. DLL leads to greater alignment between ideas, actions and brings us closer to the four-stage experiential learning cycle at the heart of the reflective process: experience, observation and reflection, reconceptualization, and experimentation (Kolb, 1984; Osterman & Kottkamp, 1993).

Experiential Learning

Another type of learning is called *experiential*. Kolb's work in the area of experiential learning (1984) is grounded in the philosophical investigations of Dewey, and his belief that experience was essential for learning (1938). Experiential learning is a dialectical and cyclical process comprised of four interactive stages as part of a learning cycle: concrete experience, reflective observation, abstract conceptualization, and active experimentation (Hafler, 2011; Kolb, 1984). Learners need opportunities for engaging in concrete experiences, reflecting on these experiences from diverse perspectives, developing conceptual frameworks based on their reflections, and evaluat-

ing as they actively experiment and thus create new experiences.

In essence, experiential learning allows students to take greater responsibility for their own learning. Learning is most effective when the learner is actively involved in the learning process, when it takes place as a collaborative rather than an isolated activity, and when it takes place in a context relevant to the learner (Kolb, 1984). Although experience is the basis for learning, learning cannot take place without reflection. Conversely, although reflection is essential to the process, reflection must be integrally linked with action. Reflective practice, then, which integrates theory with practice and thought with action, creates a dialogue of thinking and doing through which we become more skillful (Schön, 1990).

Experiential learning is a concept closely related to reflective practices, both of which define conditions under which optimal learning takes place. There have been five actions identified in experiential learning operations (Jansen, 2015; Kolb, 1984):

1. The learner is motivated to partake in concrete, *novel experiences.*
2. Relationships are developed and nurtured: learner to self, learner to others, and learner to the world at large.
3. The learner engages with metacognitive and *reflective observation.*
4. New and *abstract ideas* are formulated as a result of the experience.
5. *Problem-solving strategies* are utilized through active experimentation.

When facilitating experiential learning approaches, practitioners need to recognize and encourage spontaneous and natural opportunities for learning; be aware of their own biases and how these influence the learner; and nurture opportunities for themselves and the students to explore and examine their own values (Jansen, 2015).

Meaningful Learning

According to the theories of cognitive learning and information processing, the acquisition and retention of knowledge is very much linked to the way new knowledge is related to what we already know (Ausubel, 1960, 2000). *Meaningful learning* refers to existence of a relationship that new knowledge has to previously stored knowledge. Meaningful learning is in contrast to rote learning, which happens when information is simply memorized and no effort is made to relate it to prior learning.

According to Ausubel, new material is only meaningful when it becomes attached to an internalized structure that already exists (1960). The most important principle in meaningful learning is that because knowledge has a tendency to be arranged hierarchically, concepts in the discipline need that same type of structure in order for efficient storage and linking to occur (Popp, 2006).

A.R.T.: Experiential and Meaningful

In my early years, I was working in a program called, School for Language and Hearing-Impaired Children (SLHIC). Many of the students were born of mothers who had contracted rubella in their first trimester of pregnancy, years before the rubella vaccine. They had very unique issues with all areas of language, some more severe than others. This population eventually evolved into a designation of Specific Language Impairment or SLI, but that designation did not yet exist. Specific language impairment is characterized by difficulty with language that is not caused by a known neurological, sensory, intellectual, or emotional deficit. Any aspect of receptive or expressive language may be affected, and sometimes very unevenly. Children with SLI may be intelligent and healthy in all other regards, and are often able to develop functional strategies for working around and compensating for their language dysfunctions.

I was meeting, for the first time, a bright and very language impaired 5-year-old. It was not unusual to include automatic or serial language as a component of our assessment. First, I asked for the alphabet—no problem. Then I asked for counting from 1 to 20—again, no problem. When I asked for the days of the week, she looked up at me with questioning eyes, so I said, "You know, Monday . . . " With that she responded, "Oh, I know, oneday twoday, theeday, fourday, fiday." She was very satisfied with herself, and wound up teaching me much about experiential compensatory strategies.

Effective and Enduring Learning

There are three types of learners: *surface learners, strategic learners, and deep learners.* Surface learners memorize the facts. Strategic learners analyze what the teacher wants, and do just that. Deep learners try to understand the meaning of the materials and assignments by reflecting on implications and applications (Bain, 2012; Folkins, 2013).

Schulman, past president of The Carnegie Foundation for the Advancement of Teaching, explains there are four principles for *effective and enduring learning* for us as well as our clients (2004):

1. *Meaningful activity:* Activities involve sharing information and challenging ideas. We know that active learning results in more authentic learning than passive learning.

2. *Metacognitive awareness:* For learning to occur, reflection must accompany activ-

ity. We learn by thinking about our activity, by engaging in *metacognition.*

3. *Passion and commitment:* Passion is the *emotional side of learning,* fueled by commitment and enthusiasm. It communicates the spirit and excitement that develops within individuals who are learning.

4. *Community:* We learn best when the processes of activity, reflection, emotion, and collaboration are legitimized and nurtured by members of a culture that values such experience. These are called *communities of practice,* and will be discussed more fully in Chapter 14.

Integrative Learning

A.R.T.: Integrative Learning

One of the biggest challenges we have as supervisors and professors is creating the environment so that our students and practitioners use the information they are exposed to. They attend continuing education seminars or staff development events at work, and few do more than simply "file" the information. One practitioner under my supervision came to my training sessions with Post-Its and a caseload list. As she listened, she would scan her caseload, making student specific notes on the Post-Its and stick them on the actual seminar materials. Now, of course, this can all be done digitally. What better way is there to practice integrative learning, immediately linking new knowledge from theory with students' needs in your actual practice.

Another example of integrative learning concerns content for evaluation/feedback protocols after attending a staff development event. As staff development coordinator for my organization, I had opportunity to make some changes in the information we collected from our practitioners. We asked them to include some ideas of how they would implement the information from the training session with specific students on their caseloads.

The most successful students and practitioners are those who are able to naturally integrate new knowledge from diverse sources into clinical contexts (Anema, 2014). This process-oriented approach to learning, integrative learning, although not new to pedagogy, is often poorly implemented by students and practitioners. Integrative learning is the ability to recognize and evaluate connects among diverse concepts and contexts, and stimulate individuals to relate to new information on three different levels: the abstract level, the disciplinary level, and the categorical level (Anema, 2014; Huber, Hutchings, Gale, Miller, & Breen, 2007; Ramsden, 2003). The *abstract level* stimulates students to improve general abilities to think critically and imaginatively. The *disciplinary level* stimulates students to consider information as it pertains to the specific profession. The *categorical level* stimulates acquisition of concepts and fundamental vocabulary related to a topic.

One of the most important goals of education is to foster student's abilities to integrate learning. First, we connect previous information to newly learned information. Individual disciplines serve as our foundation, but integrative learning extends beyond academic boundaries. Integrative learning experiences occur as students and practitioners solve real-practice problems with new information. Over time and with repeated opportunities, internal changes in the learner take place and enable us to adapt our intellectual skills to a diverse number of situations and clients (Greenwald, 2006; Seeley-Brown & Adler, 2008).

Palmer and colleagues describe education being truly integrative when it encourages and engages students to explore the relationship between their studies and the purpose, meaning, and aspirations of their lives (2010). It calls upon the following philosophical domains (McComas, Frank, Miller, & Wood 2012): *ontology* or ways of being (with ourselves and with the community); *epistemology* or ways of knowing (through engagement, imagination, and challenge); *pedagogy* or ways of learning (that are meaningful, experiential, emotional, metacognitive, social, and divergent); and *ethics* or ways of living (including choices, codes, and evidence-based practice). It requires us to integrate the worlds of inner experience with outer experience so that your way of knowing (epistemology) is implemented into your way of learning (pedagogy) and becomes your way of living (ethic) (Palmer, Zajonc, & Scribner, 2010). Integrative learning comes in many forms, and includes (Laird, Shoup, Kuh, & Schwarz, 2008; Palmer et al., 2010):

1. applying theory to practice
2. implementing diverse perspectives and philosophies
3. connecting information from a variety of fields, sources and experiences
4. understanding and explaining strengths and weaknesses of issues and positions
5. discussing ideas with others
6. learning something that changes how you understand an issue

5. LEARNING THEORIES

Behaviorism

Behaviorism is a theory about learning that focuses only on objectively observable behaviors, and discounts mental activities (Edelman, 1992). Behaviorists define learning as the acquisition of new, observable behavior. Behavioral theory is about observation, condi-

tioning, shaping behaviors, stimulus-response associations, motivation, reinforcement, and consequences of behavior (Glenn, Ellis, & Greenspoon, 1992; Klein & Moses, 1999). When it emerged as a dominant paradigm in the 1960s, practitioners began to re-examine the way they planned and implemented their therapy sessions. Behavioral and operant techniques have been found to be useful for strengthening or weakening observable behaviors.

According to behaviorists, learning is indicated by either a change in the form or frequency of observable performance, or a demonstrated appropriate response following a specific environmental stimulus (Schunk, 1991). The most critical factors for learning to occur are environmental, such as the arrangement of stimuli and consequences of the behavior. Behaviorism approaches are most useful for prescriptions of prompts, instructional design, practice schedules, and reinforcement, and least useful for development of problem solving and critical thinking (Ertmer & Newby, 1993; Winn, 1990). The *principles of behaviorism* that impact instructional design of therapy programs include (Ertmer & Newby, 1993):

- Producing observable and measure outcomes, including the use of behavioral objectives, task analysis and criterion-referenced assessment,
- Learner analysis through pre-assessment,
- Sequencing of instructional presentation and emphasis on mastery of earlier steps before progressing to more complex steps,
- Use of cues, prompts, and shaping techniques,
- Use of reinforcement and feedback to impact performance.

There is little doubt that intervention has been influenced by behaviorism. All one has to do is look at the way our IEP goals and objectives are being written, and how we are trained to write target behaviors for our intervention sessions. *Behavioral theory* has affected and shaped how Individualized Educational Plans (IEPs) and intervention plans are written for students with special education needs in the following ways (Klein & Moses, 1999):

1. *Annual goals and short-term objectives* refer to the performance of functional behaviors.
2. *Goals* should be analyzed and broken down into smaller and more *obtainable steps*.
3. *Objectives* should be task analyzed into a list of more *discrete target behaviors*, which provide the sequenced content for targeting intervention. More about this is discussed in Chapter 11.
4. Verbs used are *behavioral and measureable*.
5. *Consequences of behavior are engineered* so that practitioner's responses to the student's efforts are purposeful.
6. *Target behaviors are shaped* using principles of reinforcement.
7. Intervention *procedures are used across categories* of disorder and disability.

The following interrogatives need to be asked and answered during the IEP goal and objective-writing process to insure that this "legal document" has been operationalized to meet the accountability regulations of recent legislation (Moore & Montgomery, 2008). *Who* refers to the student. *Does what* refers to observable behavior. *When* refers to by what reporting date. *Given what* refers to the conditions. *How much* refers to mastery or criteria. And *how will it be measured* refers to performance data.

Developmental Psycholinguistics

The developmental psycholinguistic movement came along in the 1970s, and decades later morphed into a new discipline known as "cognitive science" (Klein & Moses, 1999). This movement focused on *developmental sequences of behavior* sometimes known as *schemas or taxonomies*. Each one used a predominant organizational construct, and one of the most famous was the *content-form-use paradigm* devised by Bloom and Lahey to describe child language (1978).

Developmental psycholinguistics also impacted the content of our intervention programs, and continues to do so. No graduate student has escaped coding content-form interactions that reflect a child's presumed language intent during the language sampling process. Every practitioner has written goals and objectives about the student "coding existence" or "eliminating the process of fronting," all emanating from developmental psycholinguistics.

Cognitivism

Cognitive science is the interdisciplinary scientific study of the mind as information processors and includes research on how learning takes place. Cognitive science consists of multiple research disciplines including, philosophy, psychology, neuroscience, linguistics, anthropology, sociology, and educations. Cognitive learning theories help us understand how one perceives, organizes, stores, and retrieves information (Bell-Gredler, 1986).

In the 1950s and 1960s, learning theory began its shift away from relying on observable behaviors to more complex cognitive processes such as concept formation and problem solving (Snelbecker, 1983). Learning is equated with changes in states of knowledge rather than observable responses, and address how information is received, organized, stored, and retrieved. Cognitivism is less concerned with what learners *do*, but with what they *know* and how they know it. The *principles of cognitivism* that impact instructional design include (Ertmer & Newby, 1993):

- Active involvement of the learner in the process of learning, including aspects of metacognition, such as self-planning and monitoring strategies,
- Cognitive task analyses that emphasis hierarchies to illustrate different types of relationships,
- Use of organizational strategies to facilitate optimal cognitive processing, such as outlines and cognitive organizers,
- Learning environments that encourage students to connect new information with previously learned material, such as examples, analogies, and tacit narratives.

Social Learning Theories

Social learning theories added components to our work and reminded us that our greatest therapeutic influence occurs when we work within a *zone of proximal development* (ZPD) (Wertsch, 1984). It was a concept introduced by Soviet psychologist Vygotsky as the difference between what a learner can do without guidance and what can be done with guidance (Crain, 2010). The ZPD is seen as a type of *scaffolding*, which is a *structure of support points* for facilitating performance of an action.

Social learning theory emphasizes the significance of peer interactions, adult modeling and verbal guidance and feedback in the language learning process. The following principles were formulated by van Kleeck and Richardson, and stress the importance of the role of children and adults (1986; Klein & Moses, 1999).

1. The relationship between child and adult must be perceived by the child as supportive and positive.

2. The adult must fill in help where needed, while giving the child as much control as can be comfortably handled.
3. Target behaviors should be modeled by adults, with scaffolds built in until the child has achieved some level of competence and confidence in task performance.
4. Children should be encouraged to interact with peers to facilitate goal achievement and generalize behaviors. The importance of classroom interactions and collaborative classroom-based therapy becomes apparent with social learning theory.

Constructivism

Constructivism is a theory about how people learn, and asserts that learning happens through observation and scientific study (Duffy & Jonassen, 1993). In essence, we construct our own understanding and knowledge about the world through experiencing things and reflecting on those experiences. Everything new has to be reconciled with our previous ideas and experiences through a process of including, adapting, and discarding.

In any type of learning environment (classroom or therapy room), the constructivist view of learning can facilitate different types of educational practices. They include active techniques such as real-world problem solving, reflection about changing comprehension, and teacher guidance to build on preexisting conceptions (von Glasersfeld, 1995). The student's role is transformed from a passive recipient of information to an active participant in the learning process. They learn to hypothesize, test their theories, and draw conclusions from their findings.

The teacher serves as a facilitator who coaches, mediates, prompts, and asks great questions. Both teacher and student think of knowledge as dynamic views of the world, as they learn to stretch and explore their viewpoints. The classroom is no longer a place where the expert teacher pours knowledge into the students' as if they were empty vessels waiting to be filled (Fosnot, 1989).

Like many other theories of learning, constructivism has its roots in philosophical and psychological constructs. It views learning and knowledge as a function of how the individual creates meaning from individual experiences (Jonassen, 1991). Constructivists believe that the mind filters input from the world to create a unique reality. What we know about the world stems from our own interpretation of our individual experiences and environmental interactions. Context becomes an essential component, just as learning new vocabulary is enhanced by relevance when embedded in a situation in which it is used.

The *principles of constructivism* that impact instructional design include (Ertmer & Newby, 1993):

- An emphasis on *meaningful contexts* in which the skills will be learned and implemented,
- The need for information to be presented from a *variety of perspectives* and for different purposes,
- A focus on *learner control* and active use of the information,
- Support of *problem solving skills* that facilitate going beyond the given information,
- Assessment of *transfer and carryover* of knowledge that differs from conditions of initial exposure.

Constructivist theories emphasize the *importance of intervention materials, contexts, and interactions* matching the developmental level, interests and experiences of the children. When that match occurs, children are more likely to attend to, remember, and reflect on the activities that take place during the intervention program (Bloom & Lahey, 1978; Klein & Moses, 1999).

A second constructivist principle relates to the *goals, strategies, and preferences children use* to accomplish their own goals—such as operating a toy car—and how those goals and strategies interact with the ones we set for them (i.e., coding action) (Klein & Moses, 1999). When we attend to their strategies and preferences, we are facilitating their active participation with the learning process. The third constructivist premise that impacts our work relates to how children's *problem solving activities* can advance their language learning, as they resolve challenges that interfere with the accomplishment of their own goals. As we design procedures that motivate children to notice new information and resolve problems, we are helping them advance their own communication development (Klein & Moses, 1999).

6. PRINCIPLES OF INSTRUCTIONAL DESIGN

Connecting Learning Theory With Intervention Practices

One of the common themes that spans across many professional fields is the need for a bridge between research and practice. Dewey called for the creation and development of a science linking the two (Reigeluth, 1983). The need for such a *middleman position* has been expressed in engineering terms as well (Ertmer & Newby, 1993; Lynch, 1945). How can we translate learning theories into optimal clinical and instructional actions? The answer lies with *instructional design.*

Instructional designers translate principles of learning into materials and activities (Smith & Ragan, 1993). The designer must understand the priorities and content of the practitioner's field, and the strategies, tactics, and techniques surrounding the process of learning. In essence, we must be instructional designers, and this part of the chapter is an attempt to fill in some of gaps in our knowledge base about learning theories.

As instructional designers, we need to be well versed in all theories and models of learning, because no design model works in all cases. The best approach for each client or student may not ever be the same as any previous approach, because there are so many personal and contextual variables to consider. *Theoretical eclecticism* becomes a strength, as no single theoretical premise could possibly provide complete prescriptive principles for each student with a speech, language or communication disorder (Smith & Ragan, 1993; Snelbecker, 1989).

Matching Learner With Content, Tasks, and Strategies

When considering learner knowledge and *type of content*, a behavioral approach often works best for facilitating the "know-what" or content mastery of the profession. Cognitive approaches are more useful for facilitating "know-how" or problem solving strategies (applying rules in unfamiliar situations). Constructivist strategies work best when reflecting-in-action because situations are unpredictable and task demands are in a state of flux. A second consideration will depend upon the *level of cognitive processing* that is required by the task.

Behavioral strategies work best with low level processing tasks, such as associations, discriminations, and memorization. As processing needs increase (as with classification of execution of procedures), cognitive strategies with strong schematic organizations work best. The highest level of processing, for problem solving, will call for constructivist approaches such as social interactions and situated learning (Ertmer & Newby, 1993).

Our exposure to these learning approaches helps us gain different competencies to use as part of our ongoing intervention programs. However, it is important to remember that learning is influenced by a multitude of factors from a variety of sources. The learning process is dynamic, changing as it progresses, so we will be using different approaches for different types of learning at different times (Shuell, 1990). We, too, will be learning new content as we progress from *knowing what* to *knowing how* and finally to *reflecting in action* (as discussed in Chapter 4) (Schön, 1987). We must consider the nature of the learning task and the proficiency level of the learner when formulating the *instructional design process*.

REFLECTIVE SUMMATIVE QUESTIONS

1. How does the process of studying various *epistemologies* help us with our professional content learning?
2. In which area of communication disorders for children and adults have you learned about *multiple perspectives*? Please describe your learning experience.
3. What is your familiarity with *systems thinking*, and how might it enrich your understanding of organizational dynamics?
4. Please describe your comfort with the diversity of *learning methodologies and theories* that impact our therapeutic approaches. How is this knowledge helpful?
5. What are your thoughts about your role with *instructional design*?

REFERENCES

Ackoff, R. (2010). *Systems thinking for curious managers*. Portland, OR: Triarchy Press.

Alshatti, S., Watters, J., & Kidman, G. (2011) Enhancing the teaching of family and consumer sciences: The role of graphic organizers. *Journal of Family and Consumer Sciences Education, 28*(2), 14–35.

Anders, G., & Beech, L. (1990). *Reading: Mapping for meaning: 70 graphic organizers for comprehension.* Kent, CT: Sniffen Court Books.

Anema, I. (Spring, 2014). Integrative learning and evidence-based practice: Mastering the process. *Contemporary Issues in Communicative Science and Disorders, 41,* 1–11.

Argyris, C., & Schön, D. (1974). *Theory in practice: Increasing professional effectiveness.* Oxford, UK: Jossey-Bass.

Ausubel, D. P., (1960). The use of advanced organizers in the learning and retention or meaningful verbal material. *Journal of Educational Psychology, 51,* 267–272.

Ausubel, D. P. (2000). *The acquisition and retention of knowledge: A cognitive view,* Boston, MA: Kluwer Academic.

Bain, K. (2012). *What the best college students do.* Cambridge, MA: Harvard Press.

Bel-Gredler, M. E. (1986). *Learning and instruction: Theory into practice.* New York, NY: Macmillan.

Bengson, J., & Moffett, M. (Eds.). (2011). *Essays on knowledge, mind and action.* New York, NY: Oxford University Press.

Bloom, L., & Lahey, M. (1978). *Language development and language disorders.* New York, NY: John Wiley & Sons.

Böttcher, F., & Meisert, A. (February 2011). Argumentation in science education: A model-based framework. *Science and Education, 20* (2), 103–140.

Brooks, D. (May 2, 2008). *The cognitive age.* Retrieved June 13, 2016 from, http://www.nytimes.com/2008/05/02/opinion/02brooks.html

Cabrera, D. (2001). *Remedial genius: think and learn like a genius with the five principles of knowledge.* Loveland, CO: Project N Press.

Cabrera, D., & Cabrera, L. (2015) *Systems thinking made simple: New hope for solving wicked problems.* Ithaca, NY: Odyssean.

Carruthers, P. (1992). *Human knowledge and human nature.* Oxford, UK: Oxford University Press.

CMap. (2016). *Graphic organizers.* Retrieved from http://www.cmap.ihmc.us/docs/learn/php

Crain, W. (2010). *Theories of development: Concepts and applications, (* 6th ed.). Upper Saddle River, NJ: Prentice Hall.

Cruess, S. R., Johnston, S., & Cruess, R. L. (2004). Profession: A working definition for medical educators. *Teaching and Learning in Medicine, 16*(1), 74–76

Deming, W. E. (2000). *Out of the crisis.* Cambridge, MA: MIT Press.

De Paul, M., & Ramsey, W. (Eds.). (1998). *Rethinking intuition: The psychology of intuition and its role in philosophical inquiry.* Lanham, MD: Rowman and Littlefield.

Dewey, J. (1938). *Experience and education.* New York, NY: Kappa Delta Phi. Touchstone.

DeWispelaere, C., & Kossack, J. (1996). *Improving student thinking skills through the use of graphic organizers* (Unpublished master's thesis). Saint Xavier University, Elk Grove Village, IL.

DiLollo, A. (2010, October). Business: The crisis of confidence in professional knowledge: Implications for clinical education in speech-language pathology. *SIG 11-Perspectives on Administration and Supervision, 20,* 85–91.

Duffy, T. M., & Jonassen, D. (1993). *Constructivism and the technology of instruction: A conversation.* Hillsdale, NJ: Lawrence Erlbaum.

Edelman, G. (1992). *Bright air, brilliant fire: On the matter of the mind.* New York, NY: Basic Books.

Education Place. (2016). *Graphic organizers.* Retrieved from http://www.eduplace.com/graphic organizer/

Ellis, E., & Howard, P. (2005). Graphic organizers: Power tools for teaching students with learning disabilities. *Graphic Organizers and Learning Disabilities, 1,* 1–5.

Enchanted Learning. (2016). *Graphic organizers.* Retrieved from http://www.enchantedlearning.com/graphicorganizers/

Ertmer, P. A., & Newby, T. J. (1993). Behaviorism, cognitivism, constructivism: Comparing critical features from an instructional design perspective. *Performance Improvement Quarterly, 6*(4), 50–72.

Feden, P. (2012). Teaching without telling: Contemporary pedagogical theory put into practice. *Journal on Excellence in College Teaching, 23*(2), 5–23.

Fodor, J. (1975). *The language of thought*. Cambridge, MA: Harvard University Press.

Folkins, J. (2013, November). *Student attitudes*. Paper presented at ASHA Convention, Chicago, IL.

Folkins, J. W., Brackenbury, T., Krause, M., & Haviland, A. (2016). Enhancing the therapy experience using principles of video game design. *American Journal of Speech-Language Pathology, 25*, 111–121.

Fosnot, C.T. (1989). *Constructivism: Theory, perspectives and practice*. New York, NY: Teachers College Press.

Gardner, H. (1993). *Multiple intelligences: The theory in practice*. New York, NY: Basic Books.

Glenn, S., Ellis., J., & Greenspoon, J. (1992). On the revolutionary nature of the operant as a unit of behavioral selection. *American Psychologist, 47*, 1329–1336.

Goldberg, S. (2012*). Leaning into sharp points: Practical guidance and nurturing support for caregivers*. San Rafael, CA: New World Library.

Grayling, A. C. (1999). *Philosophy 1: A guide through the subject*. New York, NY: Oxford University Press.

Greenwald, M. L. (2006). Teaching research methods in communication disorders: A problem-based approach. *Communication Disorders Quarterly, 27*(3), 173–179.

Hafler, J. P. (Ed.) (2011). *Extraordinary learning in the workplace*. New York, NY: Springer.

Huber, M. T., Hutchings, P., Gale, R., Miller, R., & Breen, M. (2007). Leading initiatives for integrative learning. *Liberal Education, 93*(2), 46–61.

Inspiration Software. (2016). Retrieved June 10, 2016, from http://www.inspiration.com/visual-learning

Jansen, L. J. (2015, June). The benefits of simulation-based education. *SIG 10 Perspectives on Issues in Higher Education, 18*, 32–42.

Jonassen, D. H. (1991). Evaluating constructivistic learning. *Educational Technology, 31*(9), 28–33.

Kamhi, A. G. (1993). Research into practice: Some problems with the marriage between theory and clinical practice. *Language, Speech, and Hearing Services in Schools, 24*, 57–60.

Kamhi, A. (1994). Research to practice: Paradigms of teaching and learning: Is one view the best? *Language, Speech, and Hearing Services in Schools, 25*, 194–198.

Klein, H. B., & Moses, N. (1999). *Intervention planning for children with communication disorders: A guide for clinical practicum and professional practice*. Boston, MA: Allyn & Bacon.

Kolb, D. A. (1984). *The experiential learning: Experience as the source of learning and development*. Upper Saddle River, NJ: Prentice-Hall.

Kuhn, T. (1970). *The structure of scientific revolutions*. Chicago, IL: University of Chicago Press.

Laird, T. N., Shoup, R., Kuh, G., & Schwarz, M. (2008). The effects of discipline on deep approaches to student learning. *Research in Higher Education, 49*(6), 469–494.

Lucas, E. V. (1980). *Semantic and pragmatic language disorders: Assessment and remediation*. Rockville, MD: Aspen.

Lynch, J. M. (1945). The applicability of psychological research to education. *Journal of Educational Psychology, 43*, 289–296.

McComas, K., Frank, S.T., Miller, B., & Wood, W. (2012, November). *Pedagogy of research in a community of practice*. Presented at ASHA Convention, Atlanta, GA.

Moore, B. J., & Montgomery, J. K. (2008). *Making a difference for America's children: Speech-language pathologists in public schools*. Austin, TX: Pro-Ed.

Muma, J. (1998). *Effective speech-language pathology: A cognitive socialization approach*. New York, NY: Psychology Press.

Muma, J., & Cloud, S. (2008). *Advancing communication disorders: 60 basic issues*. Hattiesburg, MS: Natural Child.

Muma, J., & Cloud, S. (2009). *Evidence-based practices: Rational evidence*. Presented at ASHA Convention, New Orleans, LA.

Nelson, N. W. (2011). Questions about certainty and uncertainty in clinical practice. *Language, Speech, and Hearing Services in Schools, 42*, 81–87.

Osterman, K.F., & Kottkamp, R. B. (1993). *Reflective practice for educators*. Thousand Oaks, CA: Corwin Press.

Palmer, P. J., Zajonc, A., & Scribner, M. (2010). *The heart of higher education: A call to renewal*. San Francisco, CA: Jossey-Bass.

Poplin, M. (1988a). The reductionist fallacy in learning disabilities: Replicating the past by reducing the present. *Journal of Learning Disabilities, 21,* 389–401.

Poplin, M. (1988b). Holistic/constructivist principles of the teaching/learning process: Implications for the field of learning disabilities. *Journal of Learning Disabilities, 21,* 401–417.

Popp, T. (2006, November). *Lovise: A visual, logically sequenced language program using graphic organizers.* Paper presented at ASHA Convention, Miami Beach, FL.

Ramsden, P. (2003). *Learning to teach in higher education* (2nd ed.). London, UK: Taylor & Francis.

Reigeluth, C. M. (1983). Instructional design: What is it and why is it? In C. M. Reigeluth (Ed.), *Instructional theories in action* (pp. 3–36). Hillsdale, NJ: Lawrence Erlbaum.

Sampaio, T. M. M. (2014). The afterthought of speech language and hearing science therapy in the contemporary scientific epistemology. *Revista CEFAC, 16*(6), 2029–2033. https://doi.org/10.1590/1982-0216201411513

Schön, D. A. (1983). *The reflective practitioner: How professionals think in action.* New York, NY: Basic Books.

Schön, D. A. (1987). *Educating the reflective practitioner.* San Francisco, CA: Jossey-Bass.

Schön, D. A. (1990). *Educating the reflective practitioner: Toward a new design for teaching and learning in the professions.* San Francisco, CA: Jossey-Bass.

Schunk, D.H. (1991). *Learning theories: An educational perspective.* New York, NY: Macmillan.

Searle, J. (1992). *The rediscovery of the mind.* Cambridge, MA: MIT Press.

Seeley-Brown, A., & Adler, R. (2008). Minds on fire: Open education, the long tail, and learning 2.0. *EDUCAUSE Review, 43*(1), 16–32.

Senge, P. (1990*) The fifth discipline: The art and practice of the learning organization.* New York, NY: Currency Doubleday.

Shuell, T.J. (1990). Phases of meaningful learning. *Educational Research, 60,* 531–547.

Shulman, L. S. (2004). *The wisdom of practice: Essays on teaching, learning, and learning to teach.* New York, NY Jossey-Bass.

Smith, P. L., & Ragan, T. J. (1993). *Instructional design.* New York, NY: Macmillan.

Snelbecker, G. E. (1983). *Learning theory, instructional theory, and psycho-educational design.* New York, NY: McGraw-Hill.

Snelbecker, G. E. (1989). Contrasting and complementary approaches to instructional design. In C. M. Reigeluth (Ed.), *Instructional theories in action* (pp. 321–337). Hillsdale, NJ: Lawrence Erlbaum.

Swoboda, D. (2014). Applying evidence-based principles of learning to teaching practice: The bridging of the gap seminar. In V. A. Benassi, C. E. Overson, & C. M. Hakala (Eds.), *Applying Science of learning in education: Infusing psychological science into the curriculum.* Washington, DC: American Psychological Association.

Teichmann, J., & Evans, K. (1999). *Philosophy: A beginner's guide.* Hoboken, NJ: Blackwell.

van Kleeck, A., & Richardson, A. (1986). What's in an error? Wrong responses as language teaching opportunities. *National Student Speech-Language Hearing Association, 14,* 25–50.

Vera-Barachowitz, C. (2003, June). Book nook: Review of the reflective practitioner. *ASHA SIG Administration and Supervision,* pp. 14–15.

von Bertalanffy, L. (1968). *General system theory: Foundations, development, applications.* New York, NY: George Braziller.

von Glasersfeld, E. (1995). A constructivist approach to teaching. In L. Steffe & J. Gale (Eds.), *Constructivism in education.* Hillsdale, NJ: Lawrence Erlbaum.

Wankoff, L. S. (Ed.). (2005). *Innovative methods in language intervention: Treatment outcome measures.* Austin, TX: Pro-Ed.

Wertsch, J. V. (1984). The zone of proximal development: Some conceptual issues. In B. Rogoff & J. V. Wertsch (Eds.), *Children's learning in the zone of proximal development: New directions for child development.* San Francisco, CA: Jossey-Bass.

Winn, W. (1990). Some implications of cognitive theory for instructional design. *Instructional Science, 19,* 53–69.

CHAPTER 10

Implementing Materials and Activities

1. MATERIALS VERSUS ACTIVITIES

What Is the Difference Between a Material and an Activity?

Many seasoned practitioners do not consider the difference between materials and activities. As a supervisor and professor, I explain it in a simple way: think of one material and 10 different activities to do with that same material. As long as you are including a verb, it is probably an activity. So if the material is a picture card, activities might include naming, placing in a sentence, pointing, describing, rhyming, and so forth. The more specific you are, the more activities you can come up with. Then, think of one activity and 10 different materials you might use. That type of reflection forces flexibility and creativity. If you go through it once, it will help you for years to come.

What are the overall differences between a material and an activity? A material can be thought of as a *noun*, and an activity as an *action verb*. Another way of thinking about it is that a material is *a thing*, and an activity is *what you can do* with that thing. An activity refers to any kind of *purposeful therapeutic procedure* that involves learners doing something that relates to the goals of the session. Companies generally *sell materials*, many of

which come with a set *activity*. For example, the game Monopoly is a material, and the "natural" activity that is described in the game directions would be the activity of *playing that game*.

Keep the Game, Change the Activity

Games are often used exactly the way they were designed. That is unfortunate because of the lost opportunities for new and exciting activities. Here are some guidelines for using games differently than the purpose for which they were designed:

- Children, if familiar with the game, will probably want to play it according to the rules. All you have to do is tell them you have a new way of playing, and most children will be open to that.
- Make up your own set of rules, and have the children contribute.
- Ask them what they like or didn't like about the original game.
- Nobody says that you must finish the game. Children do like to complete activities, however if you explain "the rules" before you get started, they will know when it is time to stop playing. Activities should have discrete end points, and timers help the process (Goldberg, 1987).

- Use parts of games that the children like from other activities.
- Always remind the children *why* you are playing that game/activity, and what you are practicing. That is important for obvious reasons, but it may also help "script" an alternative answer to that age-old question, "What did you do in speech today?"

A.R.T.: Spinners and Dice

As a young practitioner, I noticed that many of my students loved dice and spinners. I decided one day to rev up my activities by incorporation one of those in a variety of ways. My students loved the idea, and it didn't much matter what activities we were doing as long as they could throw the dice or spin that spinner. Those materials provided both motivation and reinforcement, so what could have been better?

Why Is That Difference Important?

It is important for many reasons. First, it is about *economics*. In 1952, an article was written describing the basic essentials of a "medicine bag" of materials and supplies for our work, which was then called "speech correction" (Bell & Pross). One of my early professors in undergraduate school used to say that the only materials we needed were a pencil and paper. That's a big responsibility, because it all rests with us. In those years, we didn't have all of the vendor companies that we now do so there was nobody to blame if the students were "bored."

When I began working, I had a few boxes of DLM cards (Developmental Learning Materials is a company long gone), a tape recorder, some "lick and stick" colored shapes of different sizes, index cards, and colored mark-

ers. I had this incredible sense of joy when I bought a new material, even if it was a new colored marker. I used everything I had, and got very creative thinking of new possibilities for my work with the students.

A second reason it is important is that it encourages us to be *practice-based, interdisciplinary and translational* with our approach. When we are less rigid about what we use and how we use it, we look for and find innovative materials and activities in highly unusual places.

A.R.T.: "This Is Not Speech Therapy"

In 1970, my first professional supervisor came back from a theatre arts staff development workshop, and her description of that workshop became my first memorable translational experience. It was at this training session that I learned theatre games such as *mirroring* and *vocal symphony*. My job was to figure out how to integrate these techniques with articulatory placements, repetitive production, and bombardment. No one talked about the research; we were imaginative, we were creative, and our enthusiasm sold success.

I continued to use these and other "unusual" activities in my speech therapy program. One day a student looked up at me with a brace-filled smile and in all of his lateral emission glory spurted out, "I don't know what this is, but it's *not* speech therapy." This student grew up to become a world-famous comedic film actor, lisp-less of course. And I was hooked on the glories of implementing research and discovering techniques with demonstrated success from other disciplines (Papir-Bernstein, 2012, pp. 51–52).

A third and probably most important reason that we need to think about the material-activity distinction pertains to our own *creativity and enthusiasm*. Nothing tests enthusiasm quite the same way as a child's response does when you pull out that same material again and again. Enthusiasm is that magic ingredient that can sell anything, especially to a child.

Creativity

In the introduction to Part II, we talked about *the therapeutic use of self as a tool of practice* (Kuhaneck, Spitzer, & Miller, 2010). As we become a *tool of practice*, every response and interaction can be potentially therapeutic in effect. Therapeutic use of self involves a high level of creative interaction. Creativity, as a tool, involves the intense integration of new knowledge and problem solving (Price, 2009).

Some of us are more naturally creative, and that certainly helps us with our work. However, everyone has the ability to become creative. Creativity is often viewed as an ongoing process of making intentional choices for materials and activities. To make those choices, we use deliberation, reflection, and mindfulness rather than opting for sameness and routine (Kuhaneck et al., 2010; Runco, 2007).

A.R.T.: Material Rotation

In our speech therapy programs many of the practitioners had storage closets for their therapeutic materials, as well as carts to move them from space to space during their classroom collaborations. Throughout my visits, it became commonplace to observe them using the same materials again and again. As a result, we began a new staff development initiative: each practitioner was asked to physically "rotate" their materials every two weeks and move them around in their storage closet. The ones in the front got used more often, so it

was important to go through this change of location. It worked.

A second part of this initiative involved setting up a "material exchange" at our meetings. Practitioners were asked to bring in materials they no longer used, with the hope that others would do the same and they would leave the meeting with new materials. This was especially effective when funding dried up, because they left my meetings with "new toys."

Ideas to Enhance Therapeutic Creativity (Kuhaneck et al., 2010)

- *Shake up your perspective* by changing your space or rearranging furniture and seating.
- *Apply an analogy* of how this situation is similar to something else, possible unrelated to the field.
- *Borrow* from a different aspect of the field, or from another field.
- Do something you have *never tried* before (an approach, a material, an interaction).
- *Question your assumptions* that seem to be holding you back by listing them.

---

2. PLAY

Play Is Not Simply Entertainment

Play can be defined as a voluntary activity that either takes us out of time or at least keeps us from tracking it (Brown & Vaughan, 2009). It also allows us a diminished capacity to sense self and therefore gives us reason and permission to be silly and goofy. Playfulness is not an escape from meaningful activity such as work, but rather gives us the pause that helps with innovation and creativity.

We know from neuroscientists, psychologists, and social scientists that play is a profound biological process that has evolved to promote survival by making us happier, smarter, and more social (Brown & Vaughan, 2009; Elkind, 2007). We get a great source of pleasure from watching our children and our pets play. Some of our happiest memories of our own childhoods come from remembering the joy we obtained from games and other types of play. As adults, we still need play, but the type and degree we need has changed.

Although we all play, some adults have never learned how to comfortably play with children. Some of us play as adult monitors rather than *play partners*. We have a great deal to learn about play and playfulness from our sister field, occupational therapy. Play is considered an "occupation" rather than a "means to an end" type of skill. Play is the work of childhood. The newest literature in that field suggests that play is an integral part of the human experience, rather than just a vehicle for enhancing other skills (Kuhaneck, 2010; Parham & Fazio, 2007). As such, it is important for enhancing the child's quality of life and state of health.

There are many definitions of play, and most of them contain the words "fun" or "enjoyment." In addition, play contains elements of flexibility, spontaneity, engagement, and motivation (Kuhaneck et al., 2010). Play can occur anytime, as long as the child feels relaxed and safe. Play and work are not mutually exclusive, but rather exist on a continuum (Bateson, 2005; Kuhaneck et al., 2010). One can play while working, and work when playing. Current theories of play report that play is preparation for adulthood, builds motor and social competence, and promotes creativity and flexibility (Burghardt, 2005).

Types of Play

Play theorists describe types of play by intertwining developmental patterns with categorization schemes. One of the most widely used categorization scheme is from the National Institute for Play, which lists seven patterns of play (Kuhaneck et al., 2010):

1. *Attunement play* is emotional and interactive play with caregivers.
2. *Body play* is movement-related play that helps a child learn about their body.
3. *Object play* is play with toys and other objects.
4. *Social play* is "rough and tumble" play or jump rope.
5. *Imaginative/pretend play* is symbolic play.
6. *Narrative play* is telling or acting out stories.
7. *Creative play* uses the imagination and emerging creativity.

Everyone Needs to Play

Play is something that we all do, whether child, adolescent, or adult. Although we use the term "play" more when talking about children, when talking about older children or adults, we often refer to leisure activities, recreation or hobbies (Sutton-Smith, 1997). It is through play that we adapt the world to ourselves and create new learning experiences (Csikszentmihalyi, 1996; Elkind, 2007). It has long been recognized that play is a vital human disposition and crucial to the human experience; however, it has often been discussed in isolation from work and rarely alongside of it.

For many adults, work is something they do to simply earn a living and affords them little creativity or emotional satisfaction. Philosopher-psychologist Csikszentmihalyi describes the special state experienced by adults when work and play unite into a state of *flow* (1990). He reports that regardless of profession, gender, age, or socio-economics, individuals described the *flow* experience in very similar ways and with many of these same features (Csikszentmihalyi, 1990, 1996; Elkind, 2007):

- Clear goals for every step
- Immediate flashbacks on actions
- A balancing between skills and challenges
- Awareness merged with action
- No distractions
- No concern about failure
- No self-consciousness
- Distorted sense of time
- The activity is the end to a means.

Playfulness has been defined as a style of approaching activities that transcends the actual activity (Kuhaneck, 2010). Skard and Bundy propose that in order for playfulness to exist, three elements must be present: intrinsic motivation, internal control, and freedom to suspend reality (2008). When there is *intrinsic motivation*, the focus of the activity is on the process. Choice is a vital component. The child wants to do the activity, and that activity has been chosen. *Internal control* allows the child to be in the driver's seat with regard to how to play. The play must be child directed. The final element, *freedom to suspend reality*, allows the child to pretend and take risks that would not be taken outside of the play activity.

Sending the Message of Play: This Is Fun

Play is not assumed by children to be a part of therapy, as the mere presence of adults can predispose children to view activities in school as more work than play (Howard, Jenvey, & Hill, 2006). Earlier in this chapter we talked about *the therapeutic use of self as a tool of practice* (Kuhaneck et al., 2010). *Playfulness* is communicated through *tools of self*, including engagement, physical orientation, vocal characteristics, and nonverbal communication style. Body orientation, head movements, eye movements, and facial expressions all impact the communication of playfulness (Taylor, 2008).

Our job is *not* to entertain our students through play; however, we can create a playful context for practice. Play and playfulness enhance our tools for motivation and reinforcement of activities. However, it is wise to remember that sometimes a "playful" atmosphere in the therapy room can signals a type of *false lightheartedness* as an avoidance of dealing with a serious matter that requires a more serious posture (Wilson, 2007).

The following strategies have been found to communicate playful attitudes (Kuhaneck,et al. 2010):

- *Eyes:* use reciprocal gaze, alternating between the child and the play object.
- *Face:* sustain positive emotional expressions, especially surprise and smiles.
- *Body:* turning toward the child, manipulating or pointing to objects.
- *Voice:* use a playful tone, varying pitch, loudness, and intonational contours.

There Is No Substitute For Play

In his 2007 book about play, Dr. Elkind tells us that children's play—or their inborn disposition for learning through curiosity and imagination—is being silenced in our high-tech, media driven, digital world. I wonder what he would say now, a decade later. Research has taught us of the consequences behind failing to engage in active, spontaneous, and self-initiated play. When children are in front of screens, they are not developing the mental tools required for success in higher level math and science—fantasy, curiosity, imagination, and creativity (Elkind, 2007). Our obsession with data and test-driven standards and curricula has put a strain on the importance of play integrated with educational practices. We know *how* to play; we simply have to remember to do it. Play is not a luxury, but rather a necessity.

The newest studies about "active learning" show that children act a lot like scientists doing experiments when they play with toys (Gopnik, 2002). They naturally chose to play with toys that teach them the most, and play with them in a way that gives them the most information about the world and how people act in the world (Gopnik, 2016). Although most children will gladly and effectively imitate what parents and teachers show them, their own manipulations are more conducive for creative innovation. In fact, imitation often runs counter to innovation. The most effective learning, especially for young children, happens when we engineer the environment and let them learn through their own manipulative play.

---

3. MATERIAL SELECTION

General Guidelines for Selection

Whenever possible, give *children* the opportunity to *choose* the materials and activities through which therapy will be provided. Responsibility and choice go hand in hand. By allowing them to make their own choices and then comply with circumstances, self-responsibility is nurtured (Goldberg, 1997).

Materials for young adolescents may involve similar games and activities used with children; however, they will be reluctant to engage if the similarities are too obvious. We tend to use more conversational discourse when working with older children and adults. The sources for content include music, TV shows, technology, sports, clubs, relationships with family, work, current events, politics, and leisure activities (Florsheim & Herr, 1990; Goldberg, 1997; Zarbatany, Ghesquiere, & Mohr, 1992). One source of information is

an "interest inventory," listing all types of possible activities and materials for consideration.

Most of the materials and activities you chose will hopefully meet the following suggested guidelines (Oregon Department of Education, 1995): contains activities that can be adapted to student-proficiency; appeals to a variety of learning styles; actively engages students in meaningful, interactive communication; allows for open-ended and creative use of language; requires higher order thinking skills; promotes a variety of language functions; and includes visuals of both genders, varied ages, and are representative of ethnic, racial, cultural, and ability diversities.

Interest Inventories

The purpose of an interest inventory is to identify the student's preferences, values, and interests and then match them with materials and activities during the therapy sessions. The information may be obtained in one of three different ways: have the student complete the inventory, interview the student directly, or obtain the information from parents, caregivers, or other staff members. In each case, the carrier phrase would be changed accordingly (do you/does your child/does the student). The following types of questions were used to gather interests for a speech therapy curriculum guide called *Activity-Based Language Experiences*, or ABLE (Papir-Bernstein, 1992):

● . . . watch a lot of TV? Which shows?
● . . . spend time on a digital device? Doing what?
● . . . have any hobbies? What are they?
● . . . play or watch sports? Which ones?
● . . . help with chores around the house? Which ones?
● . . . have a job? What kind?
● . . . like to read? What?
● . . . like to listen to or play music? What kinds?

- . . . like to work with hands? What activities?
- . . . enjoy going shopping? For what?
- . . . collection anything? What types of things?
- Is there anything your child would like to learn to do?
- Is there anything you would like your child to be able to do that she or he presently cannot?

Using Materials and Activities With Purpose

Everything we do with our clients is purposeful and should have a clear direction for us and for them. Our sessions usually need to begin by telling our client the purpose of the activity, how the activity is to be carried out, and why the activity is being done (Goldberg, 1997). These are called organizing statements. These very directed statements about *the what, the how, and the why* of our work will help our clients develop a sense of focus and purpose, both of which facilitate the learning and retention processes (Balluerka, 1995).

Research has shown that when we provide organizing statements before an activity, the *response time* between the presentation of the stimulus and the response diminishes (Goldberg, 1997). We also know that organizing statements increase the *success rate* for both easier and more difficult cognitive tasks (Snapp & Glover, 1990). In addition, direction and focus increases the *general retention* of information and the specific retention of items the client's attention is directed to (Goldberg, 1997).

Types of Materials

The choice of what to use in therapy is often dictated by what is available, what is easily accessible, what is motivating, and what is simple to set up. The following materials and activities are age appropriate, student directed,

functional, and naturalistic (all principles of best practices, which will be further discussed in a later chapter). Practitioners under my supervision working in elementary, middle, and high school programs commonly and often used them. Just recently, before writing this chapter, I found a blog listing many of these same materials (Eisenberg, 2014, 2015a, 2015b).

1. *Newspapers* target literacy, interrogatives, leisure and sport activities, and current events. They provide realistic content for most areas of communication remediation.
2. *Comic strips* receive special mention. They can be found in newspapers or comic books can be laminated, placed on index cards, and used over and over again. They can be used for expanding vocabulary, learning about semantic transformations and different types of humor, conversational turn-taking, literacy, and facial expressions and body language (Gray, 2015; Gray & Garand, 1993).
3. *Magazines* are always surprising for their articles and pictures.

A.R.T.: Collages

One activity done at the beginning of the school year was the *creation of collages*. Students would get to bring in *magazines* from home, and identify favorite pictures from specific vocabulary categories that helped define their preferences and personalities. Some of these vocabulary categories were foods, activities, places, clothing, and so forth. One young man grabbed magazines from a pile at home, and had probably not looked closely at what he had chosen until he was back for his next speech therapy session. Imagine the looks on the faces of the six 12- to 13-year-old young children, when he held up a copy of Good Housekeeping and *Playboy*!

4. *Grocery circulars* are wonderful for categorization, sequencing, and vocabulary. We also used them to make up shopping lists for community intervention, or speech therapy in the community.

5. *Store catalogs* serve the same purpose. Different students can bring in catalogs that cater to their individual interests: home décor, electronics, clothing, and so forth.

6. *Public transportation maps* are also free and functional for work on travel training, vocational training, problem solving, and literacy.

7. *Menus* are not only functional, but serve so many therapeutic purposes. You can work on vocabulary, categorization, problem solving (how do you even begin to find what you want?), sequencing, quantity concepts (math), attribution (adjectives and descriptive language), pragmatics, and literacy (just to name a few).

8. *Television show and cable guide listings* can be used for descriptions, interrogatives, and general literacy.

9. *Employment applications* provide excellent opportunity for building basic knowledge about personal information, memory work, and writing skills.

10. *Playing cards* can be used for matching, sentence building, turn-taking, memory work, making and following rules, and so forth.

Places to Find Materials

Listed below are categories of activities that can be used to generate ideas for *activity-based language experiences*, all linkable to curriculum standards: arts and crafts, shopping trips, hobbies, music and movement, sports, sports, play and leisure, work, grooming and personal hygiene, fashion, history, and current events. The specific activities within each category are in Appendix A. Most of the activities are motivating, fun to perform, and appeal to a wide variety of students with diverse interests, ages, developmental abilities, and cultural backgrounds. Each one of them has been field-tested by professionals working under my supervision (Papir-Bernstein, 1992).

Two of the most common ways to accumulate materials are to visit flea markets and ask for donations. The following is a partial list of the types of materials available, usually free, just for asking (Papir-Bernstein, 1987; Schwartz & Miller, 1996): *carpet stores*: carpet samples and scraps for floors, mobiles, and so forth; *fabric stores*: sewing notions, patches, remnants; *grocery stores*: boxes, cartons, displays, circulars; *garage sales*: toys, books, games, art supplies; *lumber yards*: wood scraps, building supplies; *paint stores*: paint color cards; *paper and greeting card companies*: damaged or outdated items; and *wallpaper stores*: outdated sample books, paper swatches.

A.R.T.: String Art

In my work supervising speech therapy programs for students with severe and profound disabilities, one very difficult setting was a high school program for students with severe emotional disabilities. Student motivation to attend school in general was at an all time low, and my team of practitioners was close to burned out. After attending a speech workshop on the use of *craft materials*, and a second one on *culturally diversifying* their therapy programs and their creative juices began to flow they came up with a fabulous project that became the model for many others like it. Using a world map and string art, students were able to track their countries of origin and construct national flags to attach to the string. Of course, it all connected with social studies and geography standards and later became one of the widely used multicultural themes in the entire district.

Art Experiences

Art experiences for children can focus on process, on product, or on both. When we focus on both, the benefits are overwhelming (Richards, 2015):

- There is no right or wrong way.
- The art is unique and original.
- The experience is relaxing and joyful.
- The art is in the child's individual voice
- The art is focused on exploration of tools and materials.
- There may be instructions and sequential steps to follow.
- There may be a visual sample to follow.
- There may be a product in mind.

Open ended, creative art experiences can be directed through the use of the following types of activities and materials (Bongiorno, 2004; Edwards, 2010): finger painting, use of a variety of discarded *household tools*, such as or potato mashers, exploring with clay and play dough, creating spin art with common objects, stringing beads or shells, making collages out of craft elements, such as pompoms, and creating string art.

> **A.R.T.: Pompoms**
>
> Pompoms hold a very special place in my heart, and I still wake me up giggling at 3:00 AM when I think of this story. Our staff development unit developed an interest in the use of craft materials, and so we ordered many different types for use in the field. We were an organization of over 500 speech practitioners, and our orders were quite large. An error had been made with the pompom order, and so instead of 500 bags we wound up with 500 dozen bags (with 150 pompoms in each bag). Because the product was on sale, no returns were accepted.

> We all became very creative with our use of pompoms, and to this day I shy away from that aisle in craft stores.

Critical Activity Features

What are critical features? For the student, they are the essential components that make the material worth paying attention to. For the practitioner, they help distinguish what is critical from what is unimportant or irrelevant. There are six critical features in materials and activities that children respond to (Goldberg, 1987). They are mobility, construction and destruction, material and activity movement, completion, flexibility, and surprise. Each material or activity you use should have at least one critical feature. The more of these features that an activity or material contain, the more likely will the child have a positive response to it (Goldberg, 1987; Kuhaneck et al., 2010).

1. *Mobility*, such as moving about the therapy space, reduces mental fatigue and improves engagement. Mobility also includes moving parts of the body. Children seem to stay on task longer when we alternate between cognitive and physical tasks, or combine them (Dunchan, Hewitt, & Sonnenmeier, 1994).

2. *Construction and destruction*, such as building or taking apart, adds a dimension of temporal progression and control. Construction is a natural activity for children, and putting things together to create something new is both exciting and intriguing. The opposite of construction is destruction, or taking apart, and affords children a sense of control (Piaget, 1972).

3. *Material and activity movement*, such as movable pieces in a game, engages the child and adds a dimension of forward

movement. Movement gives the activity a sense of dynamism that is not present when using static pictures in naming tasks. That is one of the reasons we love to use fishing games, which allow for integration of activity movement.

4. *Completion of activities* with discrete end points and minimal time requirements, provide a sense of fulfillment and achievement. Children like to complete activities, so guidelines should be clearly stated about when the activity will be considered complete for that session. That is one of the reasons that board games may not be the best choice, especially if the child is already familiar with the game. For them, the game is over when somebody wins. You are better off making your own board games that come with specific rules about "being finished."

5. *Flexibility,* such as materials that can be used for a variety of purposes, helps the child stay motivated by sustaining interest. Objects that are flexible hold the child's interest longer because they can become something new at the drop of a hat.

6. *Surprise,* such as guessing games, maintain attention. Most children like the unknown, whether it involves the outcome of a story or the next object that will be used in therapy. It is easy to incorporate the critical feature of surprise into a therapy session by hiding or covering objects and letting the child choose.

Interleaving

In Chapter 8 we discussed that generalization of learning is facilitated by using a variety of "people, places, and things." Current educational research continues to support the importance of varying learning conditions rather than keeping them constant and predictable. We do this by introducing a variety

of methods, materials, activities, contexts, and conditions of practice (Frazier & Hooper, 2012; Pan, 2015).

Traditionally, we thought the best way to learn a complex skill is to practice one skill at a time. Learning researchers call this "blocking," and it tends to dominate training programs and educational settings. *Interleaving* is an alternative, little known technique that is capturing the attention of cognitive psychologists and neuroscientists (Pan, 2015). If blocking is practicing one skill with one material before the next skill (AAABBBCCC), then interleaving practices several related skills together (ABCABCABC).

A growing body of research tells us that interleaving outperforms blocking in a variety of subjects, including learning foreign language, motor skills, math, and linguistic categories (Pan, 2015; Rohrer & Taylor, 2007). *Interleaving* seems to improve the brain's ability to discriminate between concepts and search for different solutions. It also strengthens memory associations because your brain is engaged at retrieving different types of responses and storing them into short-term memory. In short, integrate a variety of materials and activities within your therapy routines.

In summary, when looking for materials and activities, remember to look everywhere and implement everything that works. If you don't see it, create it. Find out what the student enjoys and include what you enjoy.

4. MATERIAL CAUTIONS

Preparation

Many materials are complex to use, and you must take the time to review the instructions, the components, and the set up. The first time you use a material may be a bit cumbersome and awkward, and you certainly do not want to do this in front of your student. You need to know how you are going to use the material before the session begins. Do not let the material "setup" take over the session.

Cleanliness

Therapy toys and materials must be cleaned and disinfected when appropriate (Drake, 2009; Grube & Nunley, 1995; Lubinski, 2007).

1. Use therapy materials that can easily be wiped clean.
2. Anything that has entered the client's mouth should be isolated and disinfected.
3. Avoid any toys or dolls with fur or fabric that cannot be easily washed or wiped clean.
4. For toys that can withstand heat, a dishwasher may be used.
5. A ratio of 96% bleach to 4% water may be used to disinfect therapy materials and furniture.

Age Appropriateness

Very few materials are so adaptable that they work comfortably for students of all ages. There is nothing more boring for a child and humiliating for an adult than age-inappropriateness when selecting materials (Goldberg, 1997).

A.R.T.: Material Choice

Not all of my stories reflect the use of best clinical judgment. There are two instances of material choice that best illustrate this principle *not* being used. The first was in a high school program for students with profound physical and cognitive disabilities. The speech practitioner was teaming with the occupational therapist, working on auditory aware-

ness through music. (One might question why *auditory awareness* was being targeted for high school-aged students, and the answer would include the fact that many of these students had come from the now closed Willowbrook State School. Their care had been more institutional than educational, and most students were neither toilet trained nor able to communicate.) Rather than musical instruments, infant rattles were used, to imitate maracas.

A second example took place in a middle school, and the practitioner was using books from the *Disney* collection, all of which had cartoon characters like Donald Duck and Mickey Mouse. Both of these practitioners had access to more appropriate materials, but both thought what they were using was fine because the students either didn't understand or would prefer cartoons because they had no literacy skills.

Safety

Be on the lookout for *sharp edges* and points. Stay away from toys and games with *small parts*, especially when working with young students. This applies to stuffed toy dolls or animals that have parts that can easily be pulled off. Toys that make *loud noises or have strong smells* (even pleasant) are undesirable for many reasons. We sometimes work with students who have diagnosed with sensory issues, but others may simply not respond well to that type of stimulation.

A.R.T.: Olfactory Play-Dough

Another disaster order involved what came to be known as "smell dough"—play dough that one could now order in various (some quite pleasant) fragrances:

> cookie dough, chocolate, cherry, vanilla, and so forth. Guess what the majority of our students did with it? That's right —into their mouths it went. Something similar happened when we order olfactory stickers, or what we called "stick and lick." We only made that mistake once, well—twice.

5. VISUAL LEARNING MATERIALS

Why We Use Them

Many of the students needing these types of visual displays are in regular education classrooms, or in classes with students needing some augmentative communication support. Communication displays make excellent teaching tools, and most materials used in therapy or in classroom teaching can be adapted to provide helpful visual cues for all students (Rouse & Murphy, 1999). The use of picture symbols will benefit the non-verbal child, as well as the verbal students, and the professionals who work with them. So remember, whatever adaptations you make can be used over and over again to benefit all of your students.

Visual displays and visual communication assists are effective for many reasons (Papir-Bernstein, 2002; Rouse & Murphy, 1999):

- The primary reason is that they provide different or additional cues so that learning weaknesses are minimized.
- At the same time, they support the learning strengths.
- Whereas speech is transient and therefore disappears quickly, visual symbols remain present for a long as needed to combat auditory processing issues.
- They also focus attention on highlighted details.

- They provide an additional cue for comprehending spoken information
- They provide an easy way to sequence information or activities.
- They show what we mean.
- They clarify information and expectations.
- They can tell us what to do and what to do next.

Visual Teaching Materials and Strategies

Three major resources for visual learning materials are the TEACCH program, Icon-Talk, and Mayer-Johnson Company. Icon-Talk is a company dedicated to visual learning strategies and supports for children with communication and learning challenges. Their resource guide is free and offers hundreds of helpful hints and websites for constructing visual learning materials. The TEACCH program was developed for children with autism, children with communication disorders, and children who need visual supports to enhance comprehension and predictability. Mayer-Johnson is a company that specializes in visual learning supports and materials.

There are many types of visual materials and teaching strategies that work well for students with special learning needs (Goossens', Crain, & Elder, 1992; Papir-Bernstein, 2002):

1. We use choice boards or various types of choice displays to *clarify and delineate* available *options* and facilitate *decision-making.* The also *encourage student-directed* materials and activities.
2. We buy or construct *Vocabulary Cue Books* for specific type of classroom activities. For example, a cue book for cooking might contain picture symbols for open, pour, cut, shake, and measure. Cue books help expand vocabulary and categorization skills.

3. We use *picture symbols* as communication response modes, as students are taught to indicate desires or needs by pointing or exchanging a picture for what they want, as in the PECS program (Frost & Bondy, 2002). Picture symbols, used in these ways, can provide both the content and form of communicating.

4. We use *picture prompt sequences* to help students learn social routines, such as when saying hello and goodbye, or exchanging turns. These displays usually contain photos of the people, in addition to the picture symbols and words.

5. We use large picture symbols to redirect behaviors. For example, Barbara Bloomfield's company IconTalk produces Super Symbols. They are simply large symbols bound together, tabbed, and easily accessed at times of need. (sit down, stay in line, hands down).

6. Another adaptation is the First—then strip of words, which also assists with sequencing, transitions and behavioral issues.

7. We use *picture sequences for task completion*. This is usually presented in a top down or left to right format. The TEACCH program popularized the "all done" board, which sequences the parts of an activity or various activities within a specific time frame (Mesibov, Rose, & Gordon, 2010).

8. We use *visual schedules*, to delineate daily activities and roles within each activity. This too was initiated by TEACCH, and like some of the others, adapted by other vendors.

Storing Visual Displays

When you construct and use pictures and visual displays, organization and storage becomes a major part of the process. Here are some tried and true strategies that have worked well. Use *slide sheet protectors* for storing 1-inch symbols, place in large loose-leaf, and separate with dividers by activity or curriculum area. This is especially useful if you want students to be involved with making up their own communication displays for particular activities. Store *commonly used* symbols as above, but organize alphabetically. Use *file folders*, Velcro symbols to the inside of the folder. Place the name of the activity or curriculum area on the folder tab. These folders can be easily stored in file drawers. Fasten symbols to foam board or to *laminated cardboard* (such as the once that comes with your laundered shirt), and store in your therapy room as a wall display or in the classroom. Put *fastener strips on existing backgrounds* so that individual symbols (or sentence strips containing several symbols) may be placed and displayed during lessons. Create *communication boxes* for symbol storage. Cigar boxes (when you can find them) or shoe boxes are often "donated" for this purpose.

A.R.T.: Communication Boxes

A practitioner under my supervision introduced the idea of communication boxes. She had a relative who smoked cigars, and while in the store noticed cigar boxes being disposed of. She asked if the shop would "donate" them to her school where many of the students were non-ambulatory and using picture symbols. She fastened a cigar box to the tray on each chair, which became an easy storage system.

From that idea, I began a staff development dialogue about developing a *Donation Resource Guide*. Each practitioner was to walk around his or her own neighborhood and discover a shop that had potential materials to donate for their students. I developed a format listing the type of shop, the materials donated, and the potential use of the materials. It was a big hit, and a win-win for all.

Symbols can be stored in *zip lock baggies*, with the baggies fastened to the back of closed doors. This is an effective storage system for literacy activities, with each baggie containing symbols for one book. Containers, boxes, trays, *cubbies, and bins* can be placed around the room for communication board storage.

Symbols can be *fastened to receptive surfaces* such as certain types of carpeting or felt. (Be sure to use the "correct" appropriate half of the hook-and-loop on the symbol by trying it out first.) Carpet samples are easy and inexpensive to come across, and plastic tablecloths from the dollar store often have a felt liner. This is an effective and creating way of maximizing room dividers and wall space. *Tempo loop aprons and gloves* provide wearable surfaces for symbol display during lessons or activities. Large, interactive *song and story displays* can be constructed from software obtained by Southeast Augmentative Communication Conference Publications. They can also be constructed free-hand, and this is a great subject for a staff development workshop. *Books are easily adaptable.* Symbols or modified word scripts can be taped to the pages. Books can also be scanned, rebound, and adapted that way. The can also be rewritten using *Picture This* software or *Writing With Symbols* software by Mayer-Johnson. Label things around the room, and use picture symbols to further *"communize"* the environment. Create bulletin boards and *adapt existing bulletin boards* (with permission, of course) with communication symbols. Create *communication bracelets*, belts, and necklaces. Adapt transitional items such as *lunch boxes* or backpacks (Papir-Bernstein, 2002; Rouse & Murphy, 1999).

A.R.T.: Bulletin Boards

Bulletin boards are commonly used in hallways and classroom, and teachers on a "rotational assignment" basis construct them the most. While visiting a practitioner working in an inclusionary program for her students with autism, we looked for opportunities to integrate her students with the regular education program. The hallway bulletin boards were quite extensive, and after discussing our idea with the building principal, we implemented a picture dictionary translation for several of the boards already posted. The students felt included, and shared their personalized way of communicating with the other students.

Laws of Organization

In 1910, psychologist Max Wertheimer had an insight about flashing lights at a railroad crossing that let him to develop a set of descriptive principles about how we visually perceive objects (Bradley, 2015; Wertheimer, 1959). These *principles of gestalt* and *laws of organizing visuals* provide the supportive structure for graphic designers, and can be considered by us, as well, when designing visual materials for our own use (Bradley, 2015; Popp, 2006):

1. *Law of Prägnanz or simplicity* states that we perceive and interpret complex images as the *simplest form possible.* We prefer to look at things that are simple and clearly ordered, because they seem predictable and thus feel safer.

2. *Law of Closure* states that we combine parts to form a simpler whole. It is the human tendency to *look for patterns.* The key to closure is to provide just enough information so that the eye fills in the rest.

3. *Law of Symmetry and order* states that we tend to perceive objects as symmetric shapes that *evolve around a center.* Symmetry offers a type of balance and solidity.

4. *Law of Figure/Ground* states that we perceive elements as either the figure in focus

or the background. They form the relationship between positive and negative space.

5. *Law of Uniform connectedness* states that elements that are *visually connected* are perceived to be more belated to each other than elements with no visual connection.

6. *Law of Common regions* states that elements are perceived to be members of a group if they are *located within some closed region.*

7. *Law of Proximity* states that elements that are *closer together* are perceived as more related than elements that are further apart.

8. *Law of Continuation* states that *elements on a curve or a line* are viewed as more related than elements not on that curve or line. Our eye tends to follow a river or a path, and we continue our perception beyond the ending point.

9. *Law of Synchrony or common fate* states that elements *moving in the same direction* are viewed as more related than elements that are stationary or moving in different directions. When we view things changing together, they become related.

10. *Law of Similarity* states that when elements *share similar features*, they are perceived as more related to each other than elements that do not.

11. *Law of Focal points* state that element that have a *point of emphasis or difference* will capture and hold the viewer's attention.

Universal Design for Learning (UDL)

Universal Design of learning employs a set of principles for developing methods and materials that give all individuals equal opportunities to learn (Meyer, Rose, & Gordon, 2014; National Center on UDL). Each of three principles is based on neuroscience research about how we learn. They focus our attention on the importance of presenting multiple means of *representation, actions and expression,* and *means of engagement.*

Representation relates to the way information is presented and displayed, and considers the learner's perception, use of abstraction (symbols), and comprehension. Multiple means of representation ensure that learning opportunities are provided at different complexity levels and within a variety of representational formats to match ability levels. *Action and expression* relates to the demonstration of knowledge and skills and includes the learner's physical actions, organization, and executive function. Multiple means of expression ensure that students have a variety of formats available for expressing their ideas and demonstrating what they know. *Engagement* relates to how learners stay engaged and includes, motivation, effort and persistence, and self-regulation. Multiple means of engagement ensure that various opportunities are presented for addressing a range of interests, preferences, and personal learning styles (Horn & Banerjee, 2009; Meyer et al., 2014; Rose & Meyer, 2006).

As we consider the *representation principle,* we can better match presentation features to learning. The perceptual features of display information can be varied in the following ways: by the size of text or graphics, the contrast between background and foreground, colors used for meaning and emphasis, the speed or timing of visual presentation, and the layout and organization of visual elements.

Create TLC Opportunities

Part of our creativity involves recognizing opportunities when they appear. Sometimes, though, we need to *engineer the environment* a bit and create opportunities for communication. The techniques we implement are sometimes called *communication enhancers, communication temptations, environment sabotage,* or *sabotage strategies* (Goossens', Crain, & Elder, 1992; Papir-Bernstein, 2002; Wetherby & Prisant, 1989).

- *Forgetfulness:* forget an item or action that is necessary for an activity or routine.
- *Choices:* offer two or three choices if the student is looking in the direction of something.
- *Novelty:* provide different or unexpected materials or actions.
- *Proximity:* purposely place items out of reach or in a container the student cannot open.
- *Pieces:* withhold necessary pieces of a multipart toy.
- *Expectations:* purposely make a mistake during an activity.
- *Insufficiency:* offer insufficient amounts of a material during an activity.
- *Silliness:* do something funny or silly when least expected.

Some practitioners (and parents) prefer not to use the word sabotage because it may lead one to focus on the potential "frustration" for the child. It is important to remember, when using these techniques, that they need to be child-friendly in a *fun and animated* way. The purpose is to engineer situations in such an obvious way so it is close to impossible for the student *not* to respond.

A.R.T.: TLC

When I use the phrase *TLC opportunities*, I do not mean tender loving care —although, relationship and social connections are implicit in all of these techniques. The TLC came to me one day when I was meeting with the practitioners under my supervision. We commonly used the phrase "speech, language, and communication" to describe our work,

and with a slip of my tongue we became "talking, language, and communication." Thus, TLC was born.

6. GAMIFICATION

What Is Gamification?

We are part *environmental engineer*, as we design interventions that encourage students to remain engaged in completing activities. We are part *behavioral scientist*, as we nudge interventions to transform themselves through the small contextual changes we make that hopefully result in improved outcomes. We look for approaches that catch our students' interest, and that result in longer-term adherence to a task at hand (Hsin-Yuan Huang & Soman, 2013). Gamification has become one such theoretical approach, and in this digital age its design principles have much to teach us about motivation and engagement.

Gamification has been defined as the implementation of game-based thinking and game design elements to facilitate motivation, learning, and problem solving in areas outside of gaming (Folkins, Brackenbury, Krause, & Haviland, 2016; Kapp, 2012). The concept is appealing to us in the field of communication disorders for several reasons (Brackenbury, Folkins, & Ginsberg, 2014; Kapp, 2012):

- Video game design principles enhance educational activities through *procedural learning.*
- Students are taught how to analyze different situations and act as *skilled participants.*
- Students react to games as if they were *truly meaningful experiences* (Knewton, 2016).
- It *emphasizes practice* instead of theory, a more appealing option to many adults and most children.

Principles of Contemporary Game Design

Six principles of contemporary video game design are proposed for consideration in "nongame contexts" such as clinical intervention (Folkins et al., 2016; Robb, 2012). These principles were selected by Folkins and colleagues as discussed in the gaming and educational literature for having positive impacts on learning outcomes. A more detailed discussion about some of these principles takes place in our next chapter about materials.

Thematic experiences evoke cognitive and emotional responses that immerse players in the game. *Discovery and experimentation* promotes focused attention and problem solving. *Risk-taking,* appropriate to skill level, seems to increase enjoyment. *Generalization* occurs naturally, as players advance to more challenging levels. *Reward systems* signals achievement, enhances skill development and provides entertainment. *Alternate identities* are assumed through presentation of diverse and complex characters, as players are encouraged to adapt their perspectives and points of view through changes of attitudes, behaviors, and actions.

Applying Gamification in Education

The gamification of a learning concept can be simplified by following a five-step process (Hsin-Yuan Huang & Soman, 2013). It is interesting to note that most of these steps are already familiar to us, so I will include only unfamiliar content:

1. Understand the *target audience and the context.* We do this automatically as we consider age, interests, group size, leaning abilities, and necessary skill sets. However, gaming theory adds an important component—we need to identify and work around the potential *"pain points"* in the learning program. We might call these pain points the *areas of challenge.* They might include focus, skill difficulty, physical and emotional factors, motivation, and something called "pride." *Pride* is considered a major potential pain point for adolescents and young adults in particular, and may manifest as thinking you already know what someone is trying to teach you.

2. Define the *learning objectives.*

3. *Structure* the experience by breaking down the objectives into small measureable steps or *milestones* and identify potential *pain points.*

4. *Identify gaming resources.* Resource terminology includes tracking mechanism, currency, level, rules, and feedback. The *tracking mechanism* is simply the tool used to measure progress. The *currency* is the unit of measure, which could be a point in time or a type of currency. The *level* is the amount of time or currency that is needed to complete the task on that level and move to the next one, and the *rules* are the boundaries for what a student can and cannot do in the program. *Feedback* is the mechanism for learning about progress and becomes an important ally. One of the reasons that games are so appealing is they give students immediate feedback if they do a task incorrectly, which allows them to try it again (Meister, 2013; Wang, 2011).

5. *Apply gamification mechanics.* Game mechanics are classified as either self-elements or social elements. *Self-elements* are points, badges, levels, or time changes that allow the players to compete with only themselves and recognize their own achievements. *Social-elements* are interactive and involve competition or cooperation. These elements place students in community

with others, and allow their achievements to become public.

Design Principles of Video Games Can Enhance Speech Therapy Experiences

Folkins and colleagues consider the benefits that *design principles of video games* have on enhancing speech therapy experiences as they relate to student motivation, engagement, and other learning variables (2016). Players of video games are engaged and motivated to continue playing because they find games personally meaningful and socially rewarding (Entertainment Software Association, 2014; Folkins et al., 2016; Kapp, 2012). Game players exhibit persistence, problem-solving, and attention to detail—all of which are behaviors strongly encouraged in educational settings (Knewton, 2016).

Gamification takes the essence of game attributes—fun, play, transparency, design, and competition—and applies them to real-world organizations and learning processes (Meister, 2013). In education, the gamification process comes down to the application of game mechanics in non-game settings (Hsin-Yuan Huang & Soman, 2013).

7. DIGITAL MEDIA

Reading From a Screen

As we look at the ratio of digital and traditional book sales, it looks as if digital book sales has started to taper off and will settle at about 15% of the total market (Milliot, 2014; Tanner, 2014). Advances in digital technologies will continue to enhance convenience and ease of accessibility; however, studies have begun to investigate how optical issues and comprehension (cognitive and metacognitive) might be impacted differently as we move from paper to screens.

Reading (on paper and computer screens) requires *visual focus*, which necessitates a reduction in the frequency of eye blinks. That in turn causes dry eye along with the possibility of fatigue, headache, and blurred vision. This type of ocular discomfort and perceptual difficulty can compromise one's ability to learn from information presented on a screen—more so than when presented on paper—due largely to angles and lighting (Barthakur, 2013; Benedetto, Drai-Zerbib, Pedrotti, Tissier, & Baccino, 2013; Conlon & Sanders, 2011; Tanner, 2014).

What about *cognition,* and the way texts are processed, stored, and retrieved? Tanner reminds us that the same cognitive structures that evolved for navigation in the physical world have been adapted to accomplish the learned behavior of "reading" (2014; Wolf, 2007). In other words, letters and words exist to the "reading brain" as physical objects. Text or context is a type of landscape. Preliminary experiments in academia show that methods of cognitive processing differ as we move from book to screen. The readers of printed text understood and remembered the material, whereas readers of digital text were not able to indicate comprehension. Without understanding, a newly learned concept resides in short term memory only and is unavailable for linkages with later learning (Jabr, 2013; Tanner, 2014).

In a reading comprehension test given to tenth-graders, students who read on paper scored higher than digital readers. It is easier to remember what you read on paper because paper gives spatiotemporal markers. Although touching paper and turning pages aids the memory, scrolling and tapping on a screen makes remembering more difficult (Mangen, Walgermo, & Brønnick., 2013; Myrbert & Wiberg, 2015).

The Physicality of Reading

There has also been investigation into subjective experiences of reading on paper versus screens. Gerlach and Boxmann coined the phrase "haptic dissonance" to describe a perception of an object that does not correspond to one's previous sense-experiences of that same object (2011). We have expectations of what an object should feel like, look like, and even smell like. When the expectations and current perception are at a mismatch, it creates a type of subjective distance. One of our initial paths to learning about the world is through manipulation of objects, and screen taping may not be a satisfactory substitution for page-turning (Margolin, Driscoll, Toland, & Kegler, 2013).

The physicality of reading has been shown to be important for comprehension and metacognitive skills. *Virtual reading* lacks the haptic qualities that readers enjoy about books. In terms of metacognition, digital reading provides limited opportunities for interaction. Print books remain the preferred medium for learning. Mueller and Oppenheimer have confirmed that note taking in cursive facilitates comprehension better than typing on a keyboard (Konnikova, 2014; Mueller & Oppenheimer, 2014). When we write, we tend to synthesize and restate in our own words, and when we type it is usually verbatim. Rephrasing leads to better comprehension and memory storage. When we consider the physicality of reading, typing on a keyboard is the cognitive equivalent of reading virtual text.

A recent Pew survey identifying global attitudes and trends shows that print books remain much more popular than books in digital formats. This presents a powerful counter-narrative to the techno-belief that we live in a world constantly improving through our use of digital technology. Sax tells us digital experiences cannot provide us with the same kind of real-world pleasure through human interaction and tactile interface with our experiences (2016).

Using Technology In Speech Therapy

We may be experts in using technology and apps, and can be tempted to use that knowledge to drive treatment, rather than allowing the client's needs to determine if technology can serve to advance clinical goals (Gosnell, Costello, & Shane, 2011; Munoz, Hoffman, & Brimo, 2013). Screens are purely a delivery mechanism—we still get to control content. The question we must first answer is: are screens the best delivery mechanism for my client?

De Curtis and Ferrer discussed the use of mobile technology as a conduit for learning interactions. They provide *the 7 P's of using mobile technology in speech therapy.* These principles are as follows (DeCurtis & Ferrer, 2011a, 2011b; Sidock, 2012):

1. *Preparation:* What is the rationale for integrating a mobile device with a child, versus traditional toys alone?
2. *Participants:* What is the child's age and developmental level, and should this device be used individually or in a group?
3. *Parameters:* How much time will be spent integrating the device and which environments will yield the best results?
4. *Purpose:* What is the advertised purpose of the technology and how can it meet your client's individual goals? Consider adapting technology and apps to suit your purpose.
5. *Positioning:* What are the effects of sitting side-by- side versus face-to-face?
6. *Playtime:* How will you incorporate the child's preferred style of play with the device and how will you experience shared enjoyment?

7. *Potential:* How will you extend and expand the learning gained from using technology to real-life experiences?

Digital Media Is Not a Replacement

Digital one-dimensional versus real and representative three-dimensional—*nothing replaces the exchanges, the holding, the reciprocal routines, the turn-taking, the eye pointing and physical contact, the manipulation, and the touching.* Dragging and tapping is not as effective as hand rotating, touching different textures or physically moving objects to different locations (Barack, 2014). Digital media should not replace opportunities for real-life exploration with physical activities and creative play (Sauermilch, 2013). We need to find the balance and use technology as a supplemental tool, rather than to have technology be the focus of all learning experiences (Baron, Cayton-Hodges, Copple, Darling-Hammond, & Levine, 2011).

One solution might be to *integrate tangibles with virtual reality*—regular toys and books with interactive toys. When we add a physical manipulative to a digital activity we transform a one dimensional experience to one of multi dimensions. A child's thinking is grounded in touch and movement, which is the essence of traditional Montessori education. Children need to explore and manipulate the world in order to understand it. They need tactile interactivity. Educational technology is in the process of changing to become a more tactile experience for hands-on learning. This is called connected technology, which pairs a physical object that the child can hold with some time of digital interface. Connected technology provides a bridge to the digital world (Murdock, Ganz, & Crittendon, 2013; Rosenburg, 2015; Tynan-Wood, 2016).

REFLECTIVE SUMMATIVE QUESTIONS

1. Make up ten different activities for the same material, and ten different materials for the same activity.
2. Why is it important in our work to understand the difference between a material and an activity?
3. How would you integrate aspects of play with your therapy approach for adolescents and young adults?
4. Identify critical activity features for three speech therapy activities.
5. What thoughts do you have about the use of "communication enhancers"?
6. How do we balance our use of digital media and technology with three-dimensional manipulatives?

REFERENCES

Balluerka, N. (1995). The influence of instructions, outlines, and illustrations on the comprehension and recall of scientific texts. *Contemporary Educational Psychology, 20*(3), 369–375.

Barack, L. (2014, May). *Weaving together touch and digital into early childhood play.* Retrieved June 13, 2016, from http://www.thedigitalshift.com

Barron, B., Bofferding, L., Cayton-Hodges, Copple, C., Darling-Hammond, L., & Levine, M. (2011). *Take a giant step: A blueprint for teaching young children in a digital age.* New York, NY: Joan Ganz Cooney Center.

Barthakur, R (2013). Computer vision syndrome. *Internet Journal of Medical Update, 8*(2), 1–2.

Bateson, P. (2005). The role of play in the evolution of great apes and humans. In A. D. Pellegrini & P. K. Smith (Eds.), *The nature of play: Great apes and humans.* (pp. 13–24). New York, NY: Guilford Press.

Bell, D., & Pross, E. L. (1952). A medicine bag for the speech correctionist. *Journal of Speech and Hearing Disorders, 17,* 397–400.

Benedetto, S., Drai-Zerbib, V., Pedrotti, M., Tissier, G., & Baccino, T. (2013). E-readers and visual fatigue. *PLoS ONE 8*(12). http://dx.doi.org/10.1371/journal.pone.0083676

Bongiorno, L. (2004). How process art experiences support preschoolers. *Teaching Young Children, 7*(3), 18–19.

Brackenbury, T., Folkins, J. W., & Ginsberg, S. M. (2014). Examining educational challenges in communication sciences and disorders from the perspectives of signature pedagogy and reflective practice. *Contemporary Issues in Communication Sciences and Disorders, 41,* 70–82.

Bradley, S. (2015, June). *Design principles: Compositional, symmetrical and asymmetrical balance.* Retrieved from https://www.smashingmagazine.com/2015/06/design-principles-compositional-balance-symmetry-asymmetry/

Brown, S., & Vaughan, C. (2009). *Play: How it shapes the brain, opens the imagination, and invigorates the soul.* New York, NY: Penguin Group.

Burghardt, G. M. (2005). *The genesis of animal play: Testing the limits.* Cambridge, MA: MIT Press.

Conlon, E., & Sanders, M. (2011). The reading rate and comprehension of adults with impaired reading skills or visual discomfort. *Journal of Research in Reading 34*(2), 205–209.

Csikszentmihalyi, M. (1990). *Flow: The psychology of optimal experience.* New York, NY: Harper & Row.

Csikszentmihalyi, M. (1996). *Creativity.* New York, NY: HarperCollins.

DeCurtis, L. L., & Ferrer, D. (2011a). *Maximizing mobile technology with toddlers and preschoolers.* Retrieved from http://pampclub.org/site/2011/07/01/maximizing-mobile-technology-with-toddlers-preschoolers/

DeCurtis, L. L., & Ferrer, D. (2011b). Toddlers and technology: Teaching the techniques. *The ASHA Leader, 16*(11). Retrieved from, http://leader.puts.asha.org/article.aspx?articleid=2280052

Drake, M. (2009, November). *Infection control.* Presented at ASHA Convention, New Orleans, LA.

Dunchan, J. F., Hewitt, L. E., & Sonnenmeier, R. M. (1994). *Pragmatics: From theory to practice.* Englewood Cliffs, NY: Prentice Hall

Edwards, L. (2010). *The creative arts: A process approach for teachers.* Hoboken, NJ: Pearson.

Eisenberg, R. (2014). Using comic strips in speech intervention. *The ASHA Leader Blog.* Retrieved July 7, 2016, from http://www.blog.asha.org

Eisenberg, R. (2015a). Using menus as a treatment tool. *The ASHA Leader Blog.* Retrieved July 7, 2016, from http://www.blog.asha.org

Eisenberg, R. (2015b). 10 low-cost, low-tech tools for SLPs treating teens and adults. *The ASHA Leader Blog.* Retrieved July 7, 2016, from http://www.blog.asha.org

Elkind, D. (2007). *The power of play: Learning what comes naturally.* Philadelphia, PA: Perseus Books Group.

Entertainment Software Association. (2014). *Industry facts.* Retrieved June 13, 2016, from http://www.theesa.com/facts/gameplayer.asp

Florsheim, M. J., & Herr, J. J. (1990). Family counseling with elders. Special issue: Counseling and therapy for elders. *Generations, 14*(1), 40–42.

Folkins, J. W., Brackenbury, T., Krause, M., & Haviland, A. (2016). Enhancing the therapy experience using principles of video game design. *American Journal of Speech-Language Pathology, 25,* 111–121.

Frazier, A. M., & Hooper, C. R. (2012, November). *How to create a perfectly difficult CSD course.* Presented at ASHA Convention, Atlanta, GA.

Frost, L., & Bondy, A. (2002). *The Picture Exchange Communication System training manual (PECS).* New Castle, DE: Pyramid Educational Consultants.

Gerlach, J., & Buxman, P. (2011). Investigating the acceptance of electronic books—The impact of haptic dissonance on innovation adoption. *European Conference on Information Systems 2011 Proceedings,* Paper 141. Retrieved from http://www.aisel.aisnet.org/ecis2011/141/

Goldberg, S. (1997). *Clinical skills for speech-language pathologists.* San Diego, CA: Singular.

Goossens', C., Crain, S., & Elder, P. (1992). *Engineering the preschool environment for interactive symbolic communication.* Birmingham, AL:

Southeast Augmentative Communication Conference Publications—Clinician Series.

Gopnik, A. (2002). What children will teach scientists. In J. Brockman (Ed.), *The next fifty years: Science in the first half of the twenty-first century* (pp. 62–73). New York, NY: Vintage.

Gopnik, A. (2016). *The gardener and the carpenter: What the new science of child development tells us about the relationship.* New York, NY: Farrar, Straus and Giroux.

Gosnell, J., Costello, J., & Shane, H. (2011). There isn't always an app for that. *Perspectives on Augmentative and Alternative Communication, 20,* 7–8.

Gray, C. (2015). *The new social storybook.* Arlington, TX: Future Horizons.

Gray, C., & Garand, J. (1993). Social stories: Improving responses of students with autism with accurate social information. *Focus on Autistic Behavior, 8*(1), 1–10.

Grube, M., & Nunley, R. (1995). Current infection control practices in speech-language pathology. *American Journal of Speech-Language Pathology, 4,* 14–23.

Horn, E., & Banerjee, R. (2009). Understanding curriculum modifications and embedded learning opportunities in the context of supporting all children's success. *Language, Speech, and Hearing Services in Schools, 40,* 406–415.

Howard, J., Jenvey, V., & Hill, C. (2006). Children's categorization of play and learning based on social context. *Early Child Development and Care, 176,* 379–393.

Hsin-Yuan Huang, W., & Soman, D. (2013). *A practitioner's guide to gamification education.* University of Toronto, Rotman School of Management. Retrieved June 23, 2016, from http://inside.rotman.utoronto.ca/behavioural economicsinaction/files/2013/09/GuideGami ficationEducationDec2013.pdf

IconTalk. (n.d.) Retrieved from http://www.icon talk.com/downloads/Resource_Guide.pdf

Jabr, F. (2013, April). The reading brain: The science of paper versus screens. *Scientific American.* Retrieved from http://www.scientificamerican.com /article/reading-paper-screens/

Kapp, K. M. (2012). *The gamification of learning and instruction: Game-based methods and strategies for training and education.* San Francisco, CA: Wiley.

Knewton Infographics. (2016). *The gamification of education.* Retrieved June 23, 2016, from https://www.knewton.com/infographics/gami fication-education/

Konnikova, M. (2014, June). What's lost as handwriting fades. *The New York Times.* Retrieved from http://www.nytimes.com/2014/06/03/science/whats-lost-as-handwriting-fades.html

Kuhaneck, H. M., Spitzer, S. L., & Miller, E. (2010). *Activity analysis, creativity, and playfulness in pediatric occupational therapy.* Boston, MA: Jones and Bartlett.

Lubinski, L. (2007). Infection prevention. In R. Lubinski, L. C. Golper, & C. M. Frattali, (Eds.), *Professional issues in speech-language pathology and audiology* (pp. 444–460). Clifton Park, NY: Thomson Delmar Learning.

Mangen, A., Walgermo, B. R., & Brønnick, K. (2013). Reading linear texts on paper versus computer screen: Effects on reading comprehension. *International Journal of Educational Research 58,* 61–68,

Margolin, S. J., Driscoll, C., Toland, M. J., & Kegler, J. L. (2013). E-readers, computer screens, or paper: Does reading comprehension change across media platforms? *Wiley Online Library.* http://dx.doi.org/10.1002/acp.2930

Mayer-Johnson. (n.d.). *Writing with symbols.* Retrieved July 10, 2016, from http://www.mayer-johnson.com

Meister, J. C. (2013). How Deloitte made learning a game. Retrieved from, *Harvard Business Review* Blog Network: http://blogs.hbr.org/cs/2013/01/how_deloitte_made_learning_a_g.html

Mesibov, G., Shea, V., & Schopler, E. (2010). *The TEACCH approach to autism spectrum disorders.* New York, NY: Springer Science & Business Media.

Meyer, A., Rose, D. H., & Gordon, D. (2014). *Universal design for learning: Theory and practice.* Wakefield, MA: CAST Professional.

Milliot, J. (2014, April). Print, digital book sales settle down. *Publishers Weekly.* Retrieved from http://www.publishersweekly.com/pw/by-topic/industry-news/publisher-news/article/62031-print-digital-settle-down.html

Mueller, P. A., & Oppenheimer, D. M. (2014). The pen is mightier than the keyboard. *Psychological Science, 25*(6), 1159–1168.

Munoz, M. L., Hoffman, L. M., & Brimo, D. (2013, Fall). Be smarter than your phone: A framework for using apps in clinical practice. *Contemporary Issues in Communication Sciences and Disorders, 40*, 138–150.

Murdock, L. C., Ganz, J., & Crittendon, J. (2013). Use of an iPad play story to increase play dialogue of preschoolers with autism spectrum disorders. *Journal of Autism and Developmental Disorders, 43(9)*, 2174–2189.

Myrberg, C., & Wiberg, N., (2015). Screen vs. paper: What is the difference for reading and learning? *Insights. 28*(2), 49–54.

National Center on Universal Design for Learning (UDL). (n.d.). Retrieved from http://www.udlcenter.org

National Institute for Play. (n.d.). *Pattern of play.* Retrieved from http://www.nifplay.org/science/pattern-play/

Oregon Department of Education (ODE). (1995). Retrieved July 2, 2016, from http://www.eed.state.ak.us/tls/frameworks/wrldlang/wlinstr3.html#Early

Pan, S. C. (2015, August). *The interleaving effect: Mixing it up boosts learning.* Retrieved from http://www.scientificamerican.com/article/the-interleaving-effect-mixing-it-up-boosts-learning/

Papir-Bernstein, W. (Ed.). (1987). *Donation resource guide.* NYCDOE Citywide Speech Services, D.75, New York, NY.

Papir-Bernstein, W. (Ed.). (1992) *Activity-based language experiences (ABLE).* NYCDOE Citywide Speech Services, D.75, New York, NY.

Papir-Bernstein, W. (2002, March). *Developing AAC super-vision: Essential components of speech/language therapy programs.* Presented at LIU/UCP AAC Conference, Brooklyn, NY.

Papir-Bernstein, W. (2012). The artistry of practice-based evidence (PBE): One practitioner's path —Part I. In R. Goldfarb (Ed.), *Translational speech-language pathology and audiology* (pp. 51–57). San Diego, CA: Plural.

Parham, L. D., & Fazio, L. S. (Eds.). (2007). *Play in occupational therapy for children.* St. Louis, MO: Mosby Elsevier.

Piaget, J. (1972). *Psychology of the child.* New York, NY: Basic Books.

Popp, T. (2006, November). *Lovise: A visual, logically sequenced language program using graphic organizers.* Paper presented at ASHA Convention, Miami Beach, FL.

Price, P. (2009). The therapeutic relationship. In E. B. Crepeau, E. S. Cohn, & B. A. Boyt Shell (Eds.), *Occupational therapy.* Philadelphia, PA: Lippincott Williams & Wilkins.

Richards, J. C. (2015). *Key issues in language teaching.* Cambridge, MA: Cambridge University Press.

Robb, D. (2012). Let the games begin. *HR Magazine, 57*(9), 93–97.

Rohrer, D., & Taylor, K. (2007). The shuffling of mathematics problems improves learning. *Instructional Science, 35*, 481–498.

Rose, D. H., & Meyer, A. (Eds.). (2006). *A practical reader in Universal Design for Learning.* Cambridge, MA: Harvard Education Press

Rosenburg, A. (2015, October). *What connected technology and Maria Montessori have in common.* Retrieved June 14, 2016, from http://www.tiggly.com and www.edsurge.com

Rouse, C., & Murphy, K. (1999). *Quick and easy ideas for using classroom materials to teach academics to nonverbal children and more.* Solana Beach, CA: Mayer-Johnson.

Runco, M. A. (2007). *Creativity theories and themes: Research, development and practice.* San Diego, CA: Elsevier Academic Press.

Sauermilch, W. (2013, November). *Designing 21st century therapy programs that integrate evidence-based practices, apps, and multimedia sources.* Presented at ASHA Convention, Atlanta, GA.

Sax, D. (2016). *The revenge of analog: Real things and why they matter.* New York, NY: Public Affairs.

Schwarz, S., & Miller, J. H. (1996). *The new language of toys: Teaching communication skills to children with special needs.* Bethesda, MD: Woodbine House.

Sidock, J. (2012). *Critical review: Is the integration of mobile device apps' into speech therapy effective clinical practice?* Retrieved from https://www.uwo.ca/fhs/lwm/Sidock.pdf

Skard, G., & Bundy, A. C. (2008). Test of playfulness. In L. D. Parham & L. S. Fazio (Eds.), *Play in occupational therapy for children* (pp. 71–93). St. Louis, MO: Mosby Elsevier.

Snapp, J. C., & Glover, J. A. (1990). Advance organizers and study questions. *Journal of Educational Research, 83*(5), 266–271.

Sutton-Smith, B. (1997). *The ambiguity of play.* Cambridge, MA: Harvard University Press.

Tanner, M. J. (2014). Digital vs. print: Reading comprehension and the future of the book. *SJSU School of Information Student Research Journal, 4*(2). Retrieved from, http://scholar works.sjsu.edu/slissrj/vol4/iss2/6

Taylor, R. R. (2008). *The intentional relationship: Occupational therapy and use of self.* Philadelphia, PA: F. A. Davis.

Tynan-Wood, C. (2016, March). *iPads in the classroom: The promise and the problems.* Retrieved June 16, 2016, from http://www.greatschools.org/gk/articles/ipad-technology-in-the-classroom/

Wang, R. (2011, December). *Demystifying enterprise gamification for business.* Retrieved June 26, 2016, from http://www.constellationr.com

Wertheimer, M. (1959). *Productive thinking.* New York, NY: Harper & Row.

Wetherby, A., & Prizant, B. (1989). The expression of communicative intent: Assessment issues. *Seminars in Speech and Language, 10,* 77–91

Wilson, J. (2007). *The performance of practice: Enhancing the repertoire of therapy with children and families.* London, UK: Karnac Books.

Wolf, M. (2007). *Proust and the squid: The story and science of the reading brain.* New York, NY: Harper Perennial.

Zarbatany, L., Ghesquiere, K., & Mohr, K. (1992). A context perspective on early adolescents' friendship expectations. *Journal of Early Adolescence, 12*(1), 111–126.

CHAPTER 11

Measuring Progress

1. THE PROCESS OF ASSESSMENT

What Is Assessment?

Assessment serves many different purposes including screening, diagnosing, placement, and program planning (Westby, Stevens-Dominguez, & Oetter, 1996). One last purpose, determining progress and effectiveness of intervention, is our focus in this chapter.

The terms assessment and evaluation are sometimes used interchangeably, but refer to very different types of events (Todd, 2012). *Assessment* is a constant process rather than a one-time happening, and can be defined as the systematic collection, review, and use of information for the purpose of improving outcomes. *The assessment process* begins with the evaluation and continues through the writing of *goals, objectives, target behaviors, and the clinical intervention plan.* Assessment is *formative and ongoing* for the purpose of fostering improvement. Evaluation is *summative and final* for the purpose of measuring performance. Assessment is *process-oriented* and answers the question "How is it going?" Evaluation is *product-oriented* and answers the question, "What has been accomplished?" Assessment is *reflective* based on internally defined goals, and evaluation is *prescriptive* based on externally imposed standards.

Be SMART

A.R.T.: SMART

One day while sitting in a doctor's office in early 2013, I picked up a fishing magazine for lack of much of anything else to read. The article was about catching fish, and the importance of planning and implementing goals within the fishing process. There was an acronym used that really caught my eye, SMART, which stood for specific, measureable, attainable, relevant, and timely. I read the entire article and was struck at how applicable this concept was for our work. I Googled it, talked about it in my classes, and in September of that year was happy to discover that other professionals were paying attention to "interdisciplinary" messages.

When we construct an Individualized Education Program/Plan (IEP) for students with special education needs, we will generally include annual goals and short-term objectives or benchmarks (Moore & Montgomery, 2008). The terms *goal and objective* are used relative to the *assessment jargon* of your state and local work setting. Goals are sometimes called annual, treatment, or long-term goals. Objectives have been called short-term, behavioral, or instructional. The *SMART* acronym can apply to either that addresses the variables contained within (Todd, 2012; Torres, 2013a, 2013b):

- *Specific:* to what needs to be addressed. Consider strengths and weaknesses, deficient skills, compensatory skills, order of acquisition, and supports.
- *Measureable:* outcome changes must be documented either quantitatively or qualitatively.
- *Appropriate/attainable:* must be feasible to accomplish with the period of time and appropriate to the environmental conditions.
- *Realistic/relevant:* must be related to functional life skills and academics. Will it serve a purpose in the child's life and assist with academic, social-emotional, and vocational success?
- *Timed:* must include target dates for completion, interim steps, and a monitoring plan.

In IEP lingo, what is the difference between a goal and an objective? A goal is a more generalized and wider description, whereas an objective is more detailed and answers "the who, what, where, why, when, and how." One of the terms in vogue over the last several years is "benchmark." A *benchmark* is a description of performance that serves as a *standard of comparison* for evaluation or judging quality (Todd, 2012).

Task Analysis

A.R.T.: Task Analysis

As I think about *task analysis,* I remember a staff development idea I presented to the speech supervisors, and subsequently to the speech practitioners throughout our organization. Their assignment was to come up with an activity, completely unrelated to their work in speech therapy, and task analyze it into performable and discrete steps. The assortment of activities ranged from pouring orange juice into a glass to looking for missing keys. We had a lot of fun explaining the activities and providing rationales for step inclusions.

In my classes, I demonstrate this same concept with a student who is wearing sneakers. I ask for a volunteer to sit on my desk, untie their sneaker, and then have other students describe the first thing that needs to be taught in order to tie the laces. Of course, initially students provide steps much later in the sequence, but this is demonstrated as we purposefully make errors by trying to follow a direction we cannot yet accomplish. It is much easier to learn this skill by removing it from our professional content and out of the purview of *subject matter experts* (SME). The complex sometimes overshadows the simple.

A task analysis is a well-organized list of sequential steps or target behaviors, leading to the accomplishment of a larger outcome. The validity of small, manageable steps relates to a philosophical stance of living in the present as opposed to the future. Eckhart Tolle describes the tension and inner conflict that exists for us between the present and the future (2004). The more we wait for action to take place in the future, the more we are expressing discontent with the present. Positive psychologist Joseph Haidt refers to this same phenomenon as "the progress principle" (2006). Pleasure comes from making progress towards a goal rather than knowing you will be achieving it some time in the future. This is a great rationale for structuring targets into very small achievable steps via a task analysis.

The Clinical Intervention Process

There are many variables within the clinical intervention process; however, one constant remains. It will be reassuring to know that these components do not change, regardless of the setting, the population, or the years of experience. Every therapy session has five components, and each one must be addressed on an ongoing basis: the student's motivation and content rationale, specific target behaviors, materials and activities, clinical strategies (procedures, methodologies, or techniques), and session evaluation (Citywide Speech Services, 1993).

New and seasoned practitioners alike will need to spend time in their planning and evaluative processes on each one of these variables. The five clinical variables form a natural linear hierarchy, which makes implementation proceed in a natural progression. When addressed, nothing will be haphazard as these variables provide meaning and direction for all you do in every therapy session (Citywide Speech Services, 1993):

1. *Student motivation and content rationale* can be addressed by asking the clinical question, "*Where is the student now?*" It focuses us on thinking about current levels of performance as well as attitudes and interests of the student as they relate to the appropriateness of our content choice.
2. *Specific target behaviors* are an outgrowth of task analyzing your short-term objective into discrete and more manageable steps. The smaller the step, the easier it will be for us (and our clients) to notice and track progress. This can be accomplished in answer to the question, "*Where do I want the student to be by the end of the next session or two?*"
3. *Materials and activities* were discussed in more detail in an earlier chapter, and answers the question: "*What will I use to help him or her get there?*"
4. *Clinical procedures, strategies, methodologies, and techniques* are all of the clinical tools you acquire in your disorder-specific

coursework and textbooks. The question is, "*How will I use the materials and activities?*"
5. *Session evaluation* answers the question, "*How did it go, where do I go next and what needs to be changed?*" This component allows for feedback about the session as part of our reflection-on-action and reflection-about-action for later sessions.

Another way of thinking about the terminology for tracking each therapy session is the tried and true SOAP format that is used in clinics and universities for keeping therapy notes (Heifferon, 2005; Moore, 2010). SOAP notes are used in the medical and allied medical communities as well. The SOAP format includes: *subjective* notes about your opinion regarding relevant client behavior or current status; *objective* collection and recording of behaviors observed; *assessment,* which includes recording of data for tasks and targets during each therapy session as well as interpretation of data relative to level of performance; and *plan,* which includes an projection of targets for the following therapy session.

2. THE POWER OF OBSERVATION

A.R.T.: Participant Observer

It was not uncommon for me, as a speech supervisor, to be observing the practitioners under my supervision. Because there were no "two-way" clinical setups in the schools, my two choices were to sit in the back of the space and "observe," or sit with the participants and become part of the group. Either situation worked best when the therapist introduced me and explained that I was "their boss" and that it was my job to watch how he or she worked, and offer suggestions. (Otherwise, the situation becomes even more artificial because the students think you are there to evaluate them.) We made it into the game, and sometimes the students became part of the "supervisory experience" as well, as they offered their own suggestions for improvement.

The Observer and the Observed

When we observe, we become part of the observed "clinical universe." McTaggart describes the relationship between the observer and the observed when she talks about observation from the perspective of classical physics and quantum physics (2008). There is always a relationship between the observer and the thing being observed. In classical, or Newtonian physics, the scientist was thought of as a silent observer (behind glass). The universe carried on doing whatever it was doing, unaffected by whether or not it was being observed.

Quantum physics, however, explains a relationship between the observer and observed, and the consciousness of the observer changes the observed. Every minute of each day, we are creating and changing our world by our presence, even if only watching. It suggested that the universe, at its most basic, exists as a complex web of interdependent relationships. Everything influences everything else, and once connections are made, they exist forever (McTaggart, 2008). Therefore, it is important to remember that when you are an observer, you are part of the context and, therefore, a participant in the observational process (Stone-Goldman & Olswang, 2003).

Visual Skill Building

Since the practice of diagnostic medicine is in part a visual science, medical schools have begun to use fine arts training to enhance their curriculum for developing visual thinking, interpretative skills, and observational strategies (Klugman, Peel, & Beckmann-Mendez, 2011; Perry, Maffulli, & Willson, 2011). From a clinical perspective, *visual literacy* can be described as skill in observation, description, and interpretation. Research has indicated that *visual literacy* improves from careful and unbiased observation and detailed description of photographs, representational paintings, and sculpture (Bardes, Gillers, & Herman, 2001; Naghshineh et al., 2008).

This relatively new role for the integration of art within medical education helps practitioners learn how to use their eyes to connect with patients and enhance their practice. A museum experience is incorporated into training and staff development programs, and art becomes the catalyst to strengthen clinical skills and enhance team building. When patients are surveyed for satisfaction of services, very few complain about knowledge base of doctors. What they complain about is that they are ineffective in seeing the patients, sharing their perspective, and directly communicating with them (Gaufberg & Williams, 2011).

A program such as this takes everyone out of their comfort zone. It is used for training in integrated teaching units, and as participants focus on things other than people. It takes personal aspects out and students are better able to solve problems and appreciate the perspectives of others. Successful observation includes the identification of key pieces of data, pattern recognition and interpretation of items relaying significance and meaning (Shapiro, Rucker, & Beck, 2006). Art captures a multitude of meanings and help us see the world in different ways.

One systematic approach, called *Visual Thinking Strategies* (VTS), was codeveloped by a cognitive psychologist and an art educator (Housen, 2002). Housen's original research focused on the thinking strategies people use to find meaning when looking at a work of art. The VTS is now used by medical schools, and facilitate the learning of critical thinking, visual literacy, and collaborative teamwork.

The Physical Environment

As we observe, we learn about the role that physical environments play on expectations for and outcomes of student communicative behaviors. The physical environment includes lighting, temperature, organization, and furniture. By limiting distractions and increasing seating comfort, you can facilitate enhanced outcomes. It is important for furniture to be matched for tables to chairs, and size of body to overall height of chairs.

A.R.T.: Mismatched Furniture

As a staff developer, I was involved with developing a training session on diversity consciousness for the speech practitioners. One part of the seminar that I was not involved with putting together, assessment practices, was presented via a DVD of a therapy session for a 4-year-old. I was seeing this for the first time, and as I watched I sank lower and lower into my chair. Unfortunately, this young girl was seated on a very high seat with her little body trying to accommodate the mismatch through a slouched posture, and her legs swinging because they had no platform. To make things worse, the table was so high that her elbows were on the table at the level of her ears. The worst part of this entire experience for me was the acknowledgment that none of the seasoned professionals making the DVD had picked up the mismatch, and I wondered if practitioners sitting in the audience even noticed.

Our space becomes relevant because it *sets the stage* for therapy. Sometimes, we get few choices—other times, none. Stage setting involves heat, lighting, furniture, storage, and arrangements. Think about minimal needs. Space should be arranged in such a way that the students can accomplish what is expected. The ideal environment is orderly yet stimulating. It is inviting and feels safe. The physical stage has a more significant effect on what happens during the session than is generally assumed (Rubin, 1984).

A.R.T.: Observing Space

When discussing perspectives in Chapter 6, I used the phrase *standing outside the circle*. This phrase has large implications when observing space. One very talented practitioner under my supervision had no recognition of the impact that mismanagement of her therapy space was having on some of her students (and her supervisor) until it was brought to her attention by asking her to "step outside the circle." What she saw was intense disorganization, overcrowded shelves looking like they were ready to tumble, mystery boxes from years ago covered with dust, and overall ineffective use of limited space. The environment was unhealthy, distracting, and felt unsafe. As soon as it reached her level of awareness, it was rectified.

Observational Snapshots

It has been suggested that observations be conducted as would a series of snapshots using a variety of different lenses: microclose-up, close-up, regular, and wide angle (Silliman & Wilkinson, 1991; Westby et al., 1996). *The microclose-up lens* focuses on a particular child and what that child can or cannot do when trying to accomplish a specific task or during a particular activity. *The close-up lens* explores the social interactions that impact the child's performance during a particular task or activity. *The regular lens* focuses on the nature of the activity, including its components and the child's familiarity with it. The *wide angle lens* focuses on the context within which the activity takes place.

There are three global elements to consider for developing and practicing observation skills (Hedge, 2002; Stone-Goldman & Olswang, 2003).

- *The context:* It is a good idea to practice with both live and recorded contexts because they provide you with different elements. For example, a live session connects you with the emotions and sensory experiences, whereas a prerecorded session allows you to observe and write without having to think about your perceived role.
- *The expectations:* Watch broadly rather than narrowing your perspective and possibly limiting or biasing your observation with predrawn hypotheses or conclusions. The observer is not looking for anything in particular, and not making judgments about the validity of observed behaviors.
- *The focus:* Stay alert to what you see and hear (objective notes) as well as to your thoughts, feelings, and reactions (subjective notes).

---

3. DATA COLLECTION

Reminder About Our Relationship With Evidence

In Chapter 1, we talked about evidence-based practice (EBP). An EBP is not only about the research base, it is also about the way we ask questions and train ourselves to think. It is about theory as well as data. It provides the basis for our knowledge about theoretical foundations of science research, understanding treatment efficacy research, and the importance of documenting ongoing progress (Stone-Goldman, 2009, 2012). An EBP informs us about the science behind our practices.

Because of EBP, we can use some treatment programs and techniques routinely and with greater confidence. As for others, we may use them more cautiously knowing that evidence has not yet been generated. We integrate the other two legs of the EBP triangle to support our decision; the expertise of ourselves and that of other practitioners, as well as the preferences and values of our clients and their caregivers (Hegde, 2002). In those cases, our responsibility to document progress by collecting data becomes even more important. As practitioners, school-based or otherwise, we have a responsibility to document the benefits of our treatment implementations by collecting data. The collection of data will provide direction in the following areas (Stone-Goldman, 2012):

- Best treatment for a particular client
- Effectiveness of treatment under specific circumstances
- Implementing treatment under different conditions to different clients
- Acknowledging what is working and modifying what is not

Clinical Activities Are Similar to Scientific Activities

Hegde gives one of most compelling descriptions of similarities between *activities of the scientist and the practitioner* (2002). Both begin with a phenomenon, problem, question, event, or situation that needs to be analyzed and ultimately answered. Both, then, gather whatever information is available to assist with their quest, including research, assessment, and description of behaviors. Both the scientist and the practitioner will specify a dependent variable; the scientist will specify the phenomenon he or she wants to explain, and the practitioner will specify the communication disorder he or she wishes to treat.

The *scientist* will then conduct the experiment to discover what causes the event, by arranging an experimental situation under controlled conditions and manipulating independent variables to see if something changes. Scientists try to gain control over the event being studied. In scientific research, when causes of an event have been isolated under controlled situations and can be replicated by other scientists, the event has been controlled.

The *practitioner*, on the other hand, will begin to treat the client and will also be manipulating independent variables to see what facilitates positive changes in the communicative behaviors. In clinical practice, when the effectiveness of the same treatment variables can be replicated by different practitioners for different clients, it can be stated that the disorder has being manipulated or controlled. This chain of *control and prediction* is one of the goals of both scientific and clinical activity.

We collect and analyze data to further understand the phenomenon under investigation. In the social sciences, including the field of communication disorders, research confirms the belief that we are providing the best possible services for our clients. Practitioners and scientists alike are researchers who allow our field of study to flourish and grow (Keegan, 2012).

The Importance of Data Collection

Data collection is a routine component of our therapy program. It allows us to monitor progress and know when changes need to be made. The collection of data does not replace the importance of clinical intuition within the decision making process, but rather supplements it (Olswang & Bain, 1994). Because data are a necessary part of making informed decisions about the client's management, ongoing questions need to be asked and answered (Bain & Dollaghan, 1991; Olswang & Bain, 1994):

- Is the client responding to the therapy program?
- If change is occurring, is the change significant and important enough to impact the client's well being?
- Would that change be occurring anyway, or is the therapy responsible for the change? In research, we use the term "threats to validity" (such as maturation) to explain any force that could be responsible for the change of behavior other than the treatment itself.

A.R.T.: Threats to Validity

In my private practice, I often worked with young children. There were times that parents felt I was a "miracle worker," and I know I got credit for changes due to the normal developmental critical growth periods the child was passing through. I also know that had I not been there capitalizing on those linguistic growth periods, the results would not have been as dramatic. So most of the time, and in response to the parent's praise, I simply reminded them that we are all working well together and the proof is in the outcomes.

Types of Data

Clinical data can be viewed as of three different types: *treatment data, generalization probe data, and control data* (Denzin & Lincoln, 2011; Olswang & Bain, 1994). *Treatment data* are gathered during therapy, and is descriptive of the child's performance in response to what is done before (antecedents) and after the response (consequences). *Treatment data* measure behaviors that have been selected as treatment targets. This type of quantitative data would contain notes about attending behaviors, participation, types of cues and prompts, and reinforcements (Franklin, 2012; Olswang & Bain, 1994).

Generalization probe data are collected outside of the usual therapy framework, when the child's generalization performance is examined. *Generalization data* measure behaviors that are related to the treatment targets are expected to change through generalization as a result of treatment (Olswang & Bain, 1994). This is done in two ways, using stimulus generalization probes or response generalization probes. *Stimulus generalization probes* examine performance on trained items with new material, people or contexts. *Response generalization probes* examine performance on untrained items with the same stimulus materials, people, or contexts (Lindlof & Taylor, 2002).

Control data reflect behaviors that might change but would not be directly related to treatment effects. *Control behaviors* are unrelated to the treatment targets, and are not expected to change with treatment. If we select behaviors for purpose of having control data, those behaviors might be chosen because there are developmental expectations due to maturational influences (Olswang & Bain, 1994).

Data Distinctions

One distinction we must consider is between *quantitative and qualitative* (Stone-Goldman, 2012). *Quantitative* data come from counting behaviors using a specific measurement sys-tem. Qualitative data come from observations and other descriptive measures, and are often collected using ethnographic methodology (Stone-Goldman & Olswang, 2003). Quantitative assessments are used to determine how children compare to others of similar age or experience. They tend to be discrete point assessments that tell us what a child can or cannot do, but provide little useful information for guiding intervention (Westby et al., 1996).

When we use *quantitative data*, behaviors are operationally defined for the purpose of observation and measurement. Quantitative data are objective, whereas *qualitative data* have a subjective element. Qualitative data refer to what is observed in a particular context, and often bear the mark of the data collector (Olswang & Bain, 1994). Data from observations, interviews, written documents such as surveys, and diaries are considered of qualitative in nature.

In order to collect *qualitative data*, one needs to have defined and established a *taxonomy of behaviors* before the collection begins. The data will consist of behavioral descriptions and interpretation based upon the taxonomy or framework and the data collector. Both quantitative and qualitative data contribute to our decisions and judgments about the course of clinical treatment and practice.

For intervention and progress decisions, we need to consider combinations of qualitative assessments that are judgment-based, ecological and dynamic. Most of these types of assessments will be performed as we observe the child's performance in structured and unstructured settings (Hayes, 1990; Westby, 1990). Ecological assessments include judgment-based portions, focusing on insights and impressions of the professionals, teachers, and caregivers that best know the child. Dynamic assessments are usually conducted using a series of tasks to observe how the child learns and the strategies that are being used (Lidz, 1991).

Quantitative behaviors have two categories of focus: behaviors you are *directly treating*, and behaviors you are *not directly treating*. Behaviors you are treating will be your treatment targets, but sometimes other non-treated behaviors will change by virtue of their *shared relationship* with the treated targets. Some relationships will be closely related, and others will be less related. Theories and developmental guidelines will help us recognize those patterns for analysis. Changes in untreated behaviors help us predict generalization patterns (Stone-Goldman, 2012).

What to Measure: Quantitative Data

The term *quantitative* infers objective, overt, countable, and measurable behaviors. Quantitative data are used for documenting change, and has its roots in the fact-gathering and hypothesis proving stages of clinical research (Olswang & Bain, 1994). When using quantitative data, you must decide which area of behaviors you will be measuring: treatment outcomes, generalization behaviors or control behaviors. Once that decision is made, be certain to *operationalize your definition* of the behavior so that the characteristics of behaviors are clearly identified and all clinical variables are isolated. Olswang and Bain suggest the following questions can be used as guidelines for observing behavioral characteristics (1994):

- Is the behavior a *discrete event*, such as a sound production?
- Is the behavior *sustained over time*, such as joint attention?
- Can the behavior be judged as *correct or incorrect*, such as use of verb forms?
- Is the behavior *occurring or not occurring*, such as use of regular plurals?

- Is the behavior *appropriate or inappropriate*, such as requesting information?

When we understand the behavioral characteristics, it becomes easier to choose appropriate types of measurement techniques. There are many ways of measuring behaviors, and ultimately some aspect needs to be counted if the data is to be considered quantitative. Some of the most common measures are (Olswang & Bain, 1994; Papir-Bernstein, 2000): frequency of occurrence of desired target, latency (time it takes for initiation of desired target), duration of desired target during session, response rate, percent accuracy of desired target, degree of independence, and number of peer interactions (during group sessions).

What to Measure: Qualitative Data

Qualitative measures describe client behaviors in specific contexts from someone's point of view (the practitioner, the client, the teacher, the parent, etc.). The data are subjective, reflect interpretations, inform how contextual variables influence communicative performance, and can contribute vital feedback for evaluating client progress (Olswang & Bain, 1994). As professionals, we often use qualitative data when it is inappropriate or insufficient to simply quantify target behaviors. Although *accountability demands* press us to operationally define and quantify isolated communication behaviors, practitioners sometimes feel at odds with this solo method of data collection and supplement with interviews, protocols, questionnaires, and field-notes.

There are many sources of qualitative information: (Papir-Bernstein, 2000): informal and formal observations, record of conversations with students, interviews with parents and teachers, anecdotal records, ecological inventories, recordings of student work, criterion-referenced assessments, checklists, interest inventories, work portfolios, progress logs, field-notes, and narratives and attitude surveys. Qualitative measures, especially observations and field-notes, have two components: *descriptive and reflective*. The *descriptive component* includes everything that is occurring, with as many details as possible. The *reflective component* includes personal observations, thoughts, ideas, and interpretations of what is occurring (Bogdan & Biklen, 1992; Olswang & Bain, 1994).

A.R.T.: Narrative Observations

As a supervisor, I had opportunity to observe the practitioners at the beginning of the school year when they were collecting assessment information about their students. One of their tools was a *classroom observation protocol*, developed by our team of staff developers. The process of observing the student and completing the form left a huge gap: were they mindful of what they were observing? How were they interpreting the information? Can you be both descriptive and reflective at the same time?

I began to use "narratives" as an exercise, and modeled the process of narrating everything that the student was doing. As soon as the practitioners heard the descriptions, they were better able to interpret them. We then switched roles back, and they were able to experience the power of spoken narratives as a bridge between description and reflection.

How to Measure

Data collection methodologies range from *naturalistic to highly structured*, and can best be thought of on a continuum (Lund & Duchan, 1993). In a naturalistic environment, little if any structure is imposed when observing the child. The environment is familiar to the child, and direction imposes structure (which changes the nature of the environment). Although this is an ideal environment for collecting qualitative date, such may not be the case when needing large numbers of target behavior exemplars for quantitative data collection (Olswang & Bain, 1994).

We can collect both quantitative and qualitative data in structured settings. Protocols and checklists are used for qualitative information, and elicited probes are used for quantitative information. As we move to a structured collection setting, the activity and context can be purposefully manipulated. Elicited probes help us operationalize target behaviors and allow us to collect data in a time efficient manner.

Using Probes

One way of collecting data using nonstandardized measures is to construct *probes*. Probes are an effective way of collecting *quantitative information. A probe* is a measure that we have created to sample behaviors. There are several factors we need to consider when we construct probes (Stone-Goldman, 2009, 2012):

- *Specific behavior:* This is the treatment target, and the more specific you are the better able you will be to probe that behavior and measure change.
- *Linguistic level:* This is the response level you are expecting, or the complexity of the unit in which the behavior occurs (syllable, word, sentence, connected speech, etc.).
- *Type of communicative event:* This is the type of materials and activities you are including, from drill to game to naturalistic events.

- *Number of opportunities:* This is the chance to use the target response. As a general guideline, we can choose 10 opportunities as a maximum and five as a minimum.

An example of a probe for comprehension of prepositions (locatives) might be: Have a toy animal, another object, and several types of container that allow placement of the animal in, under, on, in front of, and so forth. Elicit the target by asking the student to place the animal some place relative (in, on, next to, etc.) to the other object or container. Probes can be used at different stages of the treatment process. At the beginning, they serve as a baseline. During treatment and to document treatment efficacy, they can serve as pre- and postcomparisons when you begin a new target behavior. Ultimately, probes serve the purpose of documenting the benefits of treatment, so they become extremely important as an accountability measure.

Probes are effective to use for the research construct called *single-subject design* (SS). In SS design, you are examining the individuals' responses at different points in time, so that the individual is being compared to himself or herself rather than to others (control subjects). Probes allow for the systematic and repeated measurement of behavior so that *performance trends* can be identified. When a probe is administered, the results are summarized by a number (or a percentage), and this summary becomes a *data point* (Hedge, 2002; Stone & Stoel-Gammon, 1994; Stone-Goldman, 2012). Trends reflect multiple data points (at least three) being flat, increasing, or decreasing in frequency.

As we become more skilled and comfortable with the process of collecting date, whether quantitative or qualitative, our eyes and our ears become better trained and more highly tuned to make clinical judgments. In addition to better serving our clients, our credibility and accountability both increase.

4. QUALITATIVE STRATEGIES OF INQUIRY

The Choice of Qualitative Methodology

In school-based practices, qualitative methodologies are sometimes the research of choice. Qualitative research as a research methodology in our field is sometimes referred to as phenomenological, descriptive, grounded, interpretive, or ethnographic. There are a number of factors that may influence the choice of qualitative research methods: the nature of the research problem, the researcher's theoretical lens, the researcher's skills, and the academic politics (Rowlands, 2005; Trauth, 2001). You will see commonalities and lots of crossover throughout these descriptions. There are many strategies of inquire that are used in qualitative methods, including narrative studies, content analysis, life histories, historical research, biographical studies, and discourse analysis (Irwin, Pannbacker, & Lass, 2008; Keegan, 2012). Qualitative methods are interpretative, and data sources can assume a variety of forms such as observations, interviews, recordings, surveys, protocols, and checklists.

Qualitative research seeks answers to questions regarding naturalistic, social and real-world experiences, and the types of inquiry used can have a dramatic influence on our therapy methodologies (Damico, Simmons-Mackie, Oelschlaeger, Elman, & Armstrong, 1999). It focuses on the participants' perspectives and incorporates authentic methods of analyzing data from social situations. Researcher bias can sometimes influence the results, and sample sizes tend to be smaller which makes generalization of results more difficult. However, validity and reliability can and should be checked in the following ways (Creswell, 2009; Keegan, 2012). *Validity* can be ensured through accuracy checks, providing rich descriptions, clarification of researcher bias, and the possible use of an external auditor. *Reliability* can be ensured through checking for transcription mistakes, consistency in theme assignment, and accuracy of code designations.

Interpretative Practice

Developing expertise of practice should be part of core training for SLPs. Expert practitioners who are skilled in *interpretative practice* need training in both *principles or values* and *practice or skills*. We already know that qualitative research tends to work with words rather than numbers, and includes diverse techniques in order to describe and translate the meaning, rather than the frequency, of phenomena in the social world (Rowlands, 2005; Schwandt, 2001). Interpretative research and practice, a type of qualitative research, is one way of doing just that.

Interpretive practice allows concepts to emerge from field studies and experiences, as it shows how meaningful practice generates observable outcomes. Interpretive methodologies encompass an experience-near perspective that sees actions as meaningful (Bevir & Kedar, 2008). An interpretive study focuses on human actions as a product of interpretations, interventions and individual decisions (Rowlands, 2005). The actions drive the data, rather that the "a priori–determined" concepts. Interpretive methods include: action research, case study analysis, conversational analysis, discourse analysis, reflective analysis, life history, narrative analysis, oral history, phenomenological research, and storytelling analysis (Lakoff, 1987; Yanow & Schwartz-Shea, 2006). The elements of an interpretative process are reading and listening, responding immediately to what one has seen or heard, and pausing to critically analyze that informa-

tion (Glasziou & Irwig, 1995). The following is true of interpretative research (Klein & Meyers, 1999; Rowlands, 2005):

- It assumes that knowledge is filtered through language and shared meanings.
- It acknowledges the intimate relationship between the research and what is being explored.
- It does not set out to test hypotheses or quantify independent or dependent variables.
- It is conducted through a *theoretical lens*, and collected through a variety of qualitative methods. What do we mean by a *theoretical lens*? For researchers, the starting point is to identify one's philosophical and theoretical assumptions about the nature of knowledge (epistemology), and the nature of ways of studying phenomena (methodology) (Trauth, 2001). In all fields, an interpretive paradigm is based upon the view with which people construct their own organizational realities.

Phenomenological Research

The purpose of the *phenomenological approach* is to identify phenomena through how they are perceived by individuals in a particular situation. This normally translates into gathering deep information and perceptions through qualitative methods such as interviews, discussions, and observations. *Phenomenology* is concerned with the study of experience from the perspective of the individual and is based on personal knowledge (Schutz, 1970). It emphasizes the importance of personal *perspective, interpretation and conventional wisdom*. The analysis of data involves the identification of themes, and often relate to feelings and perceptions on the parts of clients and caregivers about disabilities and lifestyle changes (Smith & Osborn, 2003).

One of the main issues with using this type of research is that professionals may not understand what it is, and tend to expect similar parameters to apply as for quantitative research. Although phenomenological approaches are effective for surfacing deep issues or making voices heard, they are not always comfortable for funders of science because this research can challenge status quo or assumptions that have been taken for granted. They are very appropriately used in our practice when gathering data as part of our practice-based evidence (PBE) philosophy.

Phenomenological approaches can be applied to single cases or to selected samples. Although single-case studies are difficult to use for drawing inferences, they can be used to identify issues that draw attention to discrepancies. However, one of the problems we face when performing or using this type of research is that it generates a large and often unorganized quantity of information that needs to be analyzed (Lester, 1999). One process of organization is through the use of semantic or mind maps or even Post-It notes for identifying key themes and issues in each text (Hycner, 1985). Data entered under different headings can be juxtaposed, compared, and used to identify relationships between different themes and factors.

These types of studies and approaches often include a detailed report highlighting *comments about individual situations*. Reports sometimes contain three sections (Lester, 1999; 2012; Moustakas, 1994):

- A *summary of the findings*, including themes, topics, and key issues. The purpose of this section is to *describe* rather than explain.
- A *discussion section*, containing *interpretations and linkages* to research, personal experience, common-sense opinions, and development of tentative theories.

- A *recommendations section*, containing issues and implications.

Grounded Theory

Another strategy of inquiry, grounded theory, is a methodology for developing theories that are grounded in data. The data are coded based upon the emergence of patterns of behaviors and themes, which then allow theories to be developed (Charmaz, 2003). Grounded theory is a way of thinking about qualitative data, and is a methodology used in the social sciences that involves *construction of a theory through the analysis of data*. It often begins with a clinical question or a collection of qualitative data. Data are reviewed for patterns and repeated ideas, which are tagged with codes, grouped into concepts and categories. It is these categories that become the basis for the promulgation of a new theory. Grounded theory helps *close the gap between theory and research*, and ultimately research and practice (Martin & Turner, 1986).

Through the use of grounded theory, *behaviors are coded, grouped into concepts, and named*. Broad groups of similar concepts are used to generate hypotheses and theories. One of the benefits of grounded theory methodologies is ecological validity, as the research represents real-world settings. It has helped legitimize qualitative research as an analytic type of scientific inquiry across the fields of medicine and social sciences (Bernard & Ryan, 2010).

Grounded theory is an alternative to standard deductive research methods, and uses a system that is widely used as a research method in the social sciences. It often takes an inductive approach, which requires the researcher to be immersed within the data for the purpose of finding themes through which the hypothesis may be assessed and *grounded* (Smith, 2012). A researcher who uses contemporary grounded theory methodology believes that "meaning and truth" can be elicited best through individualized client perspectives, theories and stories as a fluid and dynamic type of knowledge creation (Allen, 2008).

Nonstandardized Measures

Nonstandardized assessment procedures are used for a number of reasons and serve a variety of purposes. Sometimes, there are simply no standardized measures that determine the specific competencies you are investigating, or for that particular population. These types of assessments are often called *informal*, but that does not mean they are casual or haphazard. They are used to highlight strengths, abilities, and difficulties for the purpose of providing a direction within the therapy program. They generally are not used to compare one child to another (normative peers), but rather compare that child's performance at different points in time (Coelho, Ylvisaker, & Turkstra, 2005; Turkstra, Coelho, & Ylvisaker, 2005).

Once the student has been diagnosed and is in our speech therapy program, we need to select and target specific communication behaviors and measure progress. To do this, we will use stimulability testing, interviews, language samples, and criterion-referenced probes. One of the most popular types of nonstandardized assessment for measuring learning is a criterion-referenced tool. In essence, it measures the child's performance on the target behavior at different points in time in the treatment process (Stone-Goldman, 2012). As we document that treatment benefit, and expand our evidence base.

There are other reasons we use nonstandardized procedures. Formal testing situations rarely require the individual to initiate behavior on their own, inhibit irrelevant behavior, or self-monitor and evaluate. When we want assessment information about strengths and weaknesses in relation to a variety of contextual variables (settings, people, times of day, activities, materials, communication partner, etc.), we often use a nonstandardized procedure (Coelho et al., 2005).

Ethnographic Research

Ethnographic research is a qualitative methodology used for observing behaviors in context that can be observed, interpreted and described. One of the elements of ethnographic methodology is to use a *thick description* when recording and interpreting your observed behaviors. A thick description refers to a detailed and rich account of everything that is observed, including objective and subjective comments (feelings, reactions, and thoughts) (Stone-Goldman & Olswang, 2003).

Ethnographic interviewing is one qualitative technique used to gather information about the client's and family's perception of the communication disability and its functional impact on life skills (Westby et al., 2003). This type of interview is approached as "client directed" and perceived through the lens of the person being interviewed. Therefore, the questions should begin as broad and open ended to facilitate vivid descriptions of their experiences.

Westby and colleagues offer general question-asking principles and guidelines for types of ethnographic questions to use (2003). The *question-asking principles* include:

- Use *open-ended* questions rather than questions that trigger a yes-no response.
- Try to *restate* what the client said rather than paraphrasing.
- *Summarize* statements and give the client an opportunity to correct.
- Ask questions *one at a time*, and avoid multiple or multipart questions
- *Be supportive* rather than judgmental with your use of questions, so it is better to avoid

the use of "why" questions which can sometimes sound judgmental.

Three general types of questions are commonly used in ethnographic interviews (Westby et al., 2003). *Descriptive questions*: eliciting information about broad experiences, describing activities or events, asking about an experience in a particular setting. *Structural questions*: including inclusion (What kinds of things . . . ?), causality (What causes you to . . . ?), rationale (What are the reasons . . . ?), locations (Where do you . . . ?), means-end (In what way do you . . . ?), and sequence (Tell me the steps you . . .). *Social questions:* including people involved, places, activities and routines, objects and materials, and feelings.

---

5. MEASURING OUTCOMES

The New Accountability

The most obvious reason that data are vital pertains to the nature of funding and the need for *accountability*. Accountability is necessary for evaluating productivity, documenting efficacy, and justifying treatment decisions (Olswang & Bain, 1994). Traditionally, when people examine feelings about their own accountability to the larger organization, they usually view it strictly in terms of individual responsibility (Connors, Smith, & Hickman, 1994). As a result, responsibilities tend to fall through the cracks because they fall outside of the boundaries drawn around independent aspects of their job and the job of others. However, when we view our accountability as something larger, we find ourselves feeling responsible for things beyond the literal interpretation of job descriptions. In other words, by adapting an attitude of "100-100" rather than "50-50," the cracks and boundaries disappear (Papir-Bernstein, 1995).

A.R.T.: How Much Do We Give?

I am reminded of that LifeSpring training, and a lesson learned regarding an expression that most of us heard in our childhood: 50-50 (Hanley, 1990). In fact, 50-50 never works. Nobody other than "the self" can measure effort, or knows who is really giving more of less than their capability. The only formula that facilitates a win-win is 100-100.

Outcome-Based Intervention

Our commitment to the client is to go the extra mile and persist, even when we feel "stuck." Our work demands a commitment to spontaneity within the flow of therapy, and an acknowledgment that every client deserves *a new therapy*. We have to fight the temptation to deliver a uniform, formula-based, cookbook type of approach (Yalom, 2002).

Outcome-based intervention involves systematic collection and reporting of client outcomes as the beginnings of an "evidence base" (Green, Klecan-Aker, & McGehee, 2006). Documentable evidence allows for open-ended or dynamic change. A wide variety of documents can and should be used to represent and celebrate the therapeutic gains a client has made. Equally important is to be aware of our own beliefs, values and attitudes about disability. Our core beliefs can interfere with hearing a person's perspective, so our own ability to be reflective and self-aware is a crucial component of any assessment and treatment approach (Barrow, 2011; Charon, 2006).

Green and colleagues cite a variety of reasons why *it simply makes sense* to collect outcome data (2006). We have the clinical expertise, we are trained to think as scientists, we know our clients well, we are familiar with data collection and we look for outcomes on a regular basis.

What Does Measurable Mean?

Most interpretations refer to measurable having the following components (Blosser & Neidecker, 2002; Eger, 1997; Ehren, 1999):

- Measurable is observable
- Measurable is repeatable
- Measurable is functional
- Measurable is understandable
- Measurable is achievable

The first step is to *specify a target behavior* with an operational definition that is measurable and observable. The target behavior should have an exact skill, a criterion, and the context (materials, stimuli, setting, etc.). The next step is to take a *baseline measurement* before you begin treatment. *Baseline* is the standard by which things are measured or compared, and becomes the starting point (Todd, 2012). *Treatment data* need to be collected during treatment, and *generalization probes* to assess generalization of treatment.

The next step is to decide upon a *clinical design* before treatment begins. An AB design is composed of two phases: the A phase is the baseline and the B phase is the intervention. Two of the most common AB designs to use as part of the therapy program are ABA designs (test, treat, and test) and ABAB designs (test, treat, test, and treat) (Kazdin, 1982). The final step is to *share results at meetings and conferences* so that other professionals will get the benefit of your research.

Clinically Significant Change

When tests of *statistical significance* were introduced many decades ago, researchers paid little attention to practical significant (Fisher, 1925; Meline & Paridiso, 2003). *Practical significance* relates to the meaningfulness of the results, and impacts the applicability of the evidence. As important as that is, a third type of significance was identified in our field called *clinical significance* (Kazdin, 2001). Kazdin described it as the practical impact and value of the intervention, which makes real, genuine, and noticeable difference in everyday activities and interactions for the client (2001).

How do we decide on the meaningfulness of particular information as it relates to practice (Meline & Paridiso, 2003)? EBP tells us that the answer lies within both practical significance and clinical significance. When our services are valued and truly matter for the students, our work will hopefully result in "clinically significant change." Bain and Dollaghan propose that clinically significant change is a change in communication behavior that is due to intervention and not maturation, real and not random and important and not trivial (1991; Moore & Montgomery, 2008).

Functional Outcomes

Evidence of progress is often referred to as the "functional outcomes" resulting from the intervention that we provide. In order to state that the speech-language pathology services are valuable and necessary for students with communication disorders, we must be able to show that the services have made a meaningful difference in that student's life (Moore & Montgomery, 2008). Functional or performance outcomes always focus on the larger picture for students: easier access to curriculum, social-emotional skills, and vocational/life-skills success. That is why it is so important for our goals and objectives or benchmarks to reflect the outcomes desired for that individual student.

In special education, intervention must be linked to a student's *core curriculum* and proficiency in core subject areas. This concept of functional outcomes is reflected in the Individuals with Disabilities Education Act (IDEA) (2004). According to IDEA, comprehensive annual goals must address curriculum standards in a measurable way. Short-term objectives or benchmarks, discrete points along the larger pathway, may be required by some states or local education agencies (LEAs) in addition to annual goals (Moore & Montgomery, 2008).

Treatment effects refer to a narrow and specifically defined outcome of a treatment procedure. For example, the expected treatment effect of a *production task of adjective + noun* would be increased frequency in use of adjective + noun. *Functional outcome* refers to broader improvement in general, meaningful and natural communication, and extends beyond the effects of treatment. Functional outcomes involve generalization in natural settings so that overall communication is improved. *Functional outcomes* might include enhanced social communication facilitating friendships, improved vocational opportunities, more fulfilling life, increased independent functioning, and better academic performance (Hedge, 2002). We discuss this in more detail in a later chapter, but here are some examples of targeting treatment effects rather than functional outcomes (Lewis, 1987):

- Learning to put pegs in a grid rather than quarters in a vending machine
- Identifying your nose rather than learning to blow it
- Folding paper rather than clothing
- Rolling play-dough rather than dough for baking bread
- Lacing a pattern card rather than shoes
- Putting a cube into a larger box rather than learning to dispose of trash in a receptacle

The Underpinnings of Academic Standards

Specific learning disability, as defined by the IDEA (2004) is as follows: "A disorder in 1 or more of the basic psychological processes involved in understanding or in using language, spoken or written, which disorder may manifest itself in the imperfect ability to listen, think, speak, read, write, spell, or do mathematical calculations" (LDonline, 2015). Of course we must know about curriculum standards, but why?

In fact, literacy has always been part of our field even before it became officially part of our scope of practice. We know that learning is language based, and that school success depends upon a student's communicative competence in the areas of reading, writing, speaking, and listening (Rudebusch, 2014). In addition, remember from Chapter 8 that According to the U.S. Department of Education and the Individuals with Disabilities Education Act of 2004 (IDEA, 2004), speech-language pathology service in the special educational setting is a *related service*. Related services assist a child with a disability to benefit within their primary special educational placement (which is usually considered to be their instructional classroom).

When we hear the word literacy, some of us cringe. I have met seasoned practitioners who resent having to work on literacy—they say they feel like reading teachers. Literacy involves much more than reading and writing. It is the ability to use available symbol systems that are fundamental to learning. Being literate is at the heart of learning in every subject area (Literacy in Learning Exchange, 2012). The meaning has been expanded to include the ability to use not only language, but numbers, images and screens to understand, communicate and gain useful knowledge (UNESCO, 2006).

Reading development involves language underpinnings that we are more than familiar with: awareness of speech sounds (phonology), grammar (syntax), patterns of word formation (morphology), and word meaning (semantics). Literacy problems can result from language problems, and language problems can manifest in literacy issues (Rudebusch, 2012; UNESCO, 2006).

We are clearly doing something right, because data from the American Speech-

Language-Hearing Association's National Outcome Measurement System (NOMS) surveyed classroom teachers about whether they think that our services have an impact on the students' classroom performance. The vast majority (65% to 70%) of those surveyed thought that our services helped students improve their prereading, reading, or reading comprehension skills, as well as listening and writing skills.

Language Demands of the Curriculum

A.R.T.: Language Demands of the Curriculum

Before Common Core Standards, we had something called *curriculum*. When I was a practitioner working in a specialized school for children with language impairments in the mid-1970s (the title predates "disability consciousness"), I became familiar with language curriculum from the inside out. There were few standards, and few special education school programs had formalized curriculum. I, along with a few key classroom teachers, were out to change that. We organized a Language Curriculum Committee, and who better to chair it than I.

We had the support of school administration, and a core group of dedicated professionals who vowed to stay late every Wednesday so that the committee might complete its charge. Of course, that didn't happen until years later (and not because of the committee's dedication), but the process was a tremendous introduction to language demands of the curriculum.

More than ever before, our schools are under federal and state pressure to meet criteria involving mastery of academic standards. Our role becomes even more critical, because we are the professionals who can identify and

address the linguistic, metalinguistic, and literacy issues at the base of academic underachievement (Ehren, 2015). Because of our language expertise, we are able to provide unique contributions to the curriculum. This may not be news to us, but it is to many teachers and school administrators, and we need to get the word out. We need to be certain that our goals, objectives, and target behaviors relate to the underpinnings of academic, social-emotional, and vocational educational standards. Most importantly, we need to be able to document that connection.

It is within the scope of our work to contribute to student achievement, college, and career readiness by supporting student access to curriculum, and thereby enhance opportunities to master academic standards. How does our work accomplish that goal in the following areas of communication disorders (American Speech-Language-Hearing Association, 2006; Nevada Speech-Language-Hearing Association, 2015)?

- *Articulation/phonology:* A disordered phonological system impacts spelling and reading. Differences, delays, or disorders in speech production may have a negative impact on self-confidence, social relationships, and vocational opportunities.
- *Pragmatics: Fluency:* Disorders in fluency such as stuttering can inhibit classroom participation and impact academic performance, peer relationships, and career preparation.
- *Language and literacy:* The relationships here are a bit more explicit. Deficits in the area of *auditory processing* (attention, memory, discrimination, sequencing, etc.) can affect performance in all academic areas that involve processing of curricular material and oral directions. Deficits in *semantic areas* (vocabulary, definitions, concepts, relationships, etc.) may impact all areas of communication (listening, speaking, reading, and writing) and therefore all areas of

curriculum. Deficits in *morphology and syntax* (grammar, sentence construction, etc.) will impact the student's ability to communication through the "language of academics" in all subject areas. Deficits in *pragmatics* (critical thinking, nonverbal communication, inferencing, etc.) can affect listening, comprehension, problem solving, study skills, and social interactions.

Standards (CCSS) become one of the yardsticks against which we evaluate student strengths and areas of need. One of the first steps is to review the content standards in all areas for the student's grade level. Do the same for prior grade levels to identify content that should have already been mastered. The next step is to simply analyze the standards for communication expectations that have been subsumed in the standards. Look specifically for pragmatic, semantic, phonologic, syntactic, morphologic, and metalinguistic skills (Rudebusch, 2014). You will see much that is familiar with your own knowledge base.

Rather than using the CCSS as a listing of skills that will be taught to the students, think of it as a blueprint for speech-language pathology services that will allow the students to participate and progress within the general curriculum (Rudebusch, 2012, 2014; Common Core State Standards Initiative, 2016). Most of what we work on in the language/literacy areas are already embedded within the language and reading standards. Reading and writing is "braided" through language, and are the visual portals of language processing (Rudebusch, 2014).

The Importance of Using Checklists and Measurement Protocols

Our greatest responsibility is to our clients, assuring them that our work together is making a positive difference in their lives. The support we provide assures a higher likelihood of communicative competence as will as academic success. We need to insure that is happening, and if it is not, we need to make the necessary adjustments. As we discussed in Chapter 8, pointing one finger out there points three at ourselves. It is up to us; however, we are all fallible.

In the 1970s, a short essay on human fallibility was written by physicians Gorovitz and Macintyre (1976). They talked about why we fail at what we set out to do, and came up with interesting insights. They referred to "necessary fallibility" due to the fact that much of the world is outside our purview of comprehension and therefore control. But there are aspects that we can control, and, even then, we sometimes fail. Why? One reason is *ignorance* or lack of knowledge. A second reason is *ineptitude,* or failure to correctly apply what we do know. Ineptitude happens because we are overwhelmed by the volume and complexity of our responsibilities. We need a different strategy. We need *checklists* (Gawande, 2010).

Even some of the smartest and best trained doctors make errors. With all of our high technology and medical solutions, Frakt reports some frightening statistics: one in about 100,000 surgeries is on the wrong body part, and for one in 10,000 surgeries, a foreign object is accidentally left inside the surgical area (2014). He says that something as simple as a checklist can reduce such errors. When we use protocols, we can think of them as a means of providing reference points on a continuum to assist with decisions about where to start or where to proceed next. They provide directions for practice (Wilson, 2007).

Checklists provide protection against leaving out necessary steps or considerations. They provide us with *discipline of a higher linear order,* a kind of *cognitive net.* They catch mental flaws of attention, memory, and thoroughness inherent in all of us (Gawande, 2010). They provide procedures that allow us to balance craft with protocol, discipline with routine. Checklists reflect a philosophy about work and our profession. They should be easy to follow and simple to complete, and provide reminders of the most important steps to follow. They increase efficiency and ultimately save time. They become part of our *systems approach* to our professional practice.

Questions for Assessing Effectiveness of an Intervention Strategy

In most cases, we can consider an intervention strategy *ineffective* until there is evidence to the contrary (Hegde, 2002; Silverman, 1998). As we research the effectiveness of the strategies and methodologies we use, it is helpful to consider its impact in a number of points related to space-time (periods of time in given situations) (Silverman, 1998): the impact of the strategy on increasing or decreasing *specific communication behaviors;* the impact of the strategy on *specific attitudes and feelings* that may contribute to the communicative disorder; the impact of the strategy on *attitudes of friends, teachers, and caregivers*; and the impact of the strategy on the *required investment* of clinician, client, support personnel, and home caregivers.

REFLECTIVE SUMMATIVE QUESTIONS

1. How is assessment an important part of our ongoing attempt to document progress?
2. Task-analyze an exercise routine that you do on a weekly basis.
3. Describe how you would set up an observational training session at a museum.

4. How is your role as practitioner similar to that of a scientist?

REFERENCES

Allen, J. (2008). *Psychotherapy: The artful use of science.* Smith College Social Work, *78*, 2–3.

American Speech-Language-Hearing Association. (2006). *Professional performance review process for the school-based speech-language pathologist* [Guidelines]. Retrieved from http://www.asha.org/policy

Bain, B., & Dollaghan, C. (1991). Treatment efficacy: The notion of clinically significant change. *Language, Speech, and Hearing Services in Schools, 22*, 264–270.

Bardes C.L., Gillers D., & Herman A.E. (2001). Learning to look: Developing clinical observational skills at an art museum. *Medical Education, 35*(12), 1157–1161.

Barrow, R. (2011). Shaping practice: The benefits of really attending to the person's story. In R. J. Fourie (Ed.), *Therapeutic processes for communication disorders: A guide for clinicians and students.* New York, NY: Psychology Press.

Bernard, H. R., & Ryan, G. W. (2010). *Analyzing qualitative data: Systematic approaches.* Thousand Oaks, CA: Sage.

Bevir, M., & Kedar, A. (2008). Concept formation in political science: An anti-naturalist critique of qualitative methodology. *Perspectives on Politics, 6*(3), 503–517.

Blosser, J. L., & Neidecker, E. A. (2002). *School programs in speech-language pathology: Organization and service delivery.* Boston, MA: Allyn & Bacon.

Bogdan, R., & Biklen, S. (1992). *Qualitative research for education: An introduction to theory and methods.* Boston, MA: Allyn & Bacon.

Charmaz, K. (2003). Grounded theory. In J. A. Smith (Ed.), *Qualitative psychology.* Thousand Oaks, CA: Sage.

Charon, R. (2006). *Narrative medicine: Honoring the stories of illness.* New York, NY: Oxford University Press.

Citywide Speech Services (CSS) Staff Development Unit. (1993). *The clinical intervention process.* NYCDOE, D. 75.

Coelho, C., Ylvisaker, M., & Turkstra, L. (2005). Nonstandardized assessment approaches for individuals with traumatic brain injury. *Seminars in Speech and Language, 26*(4), 223–241.

Conners, R., Smith T., & Hickman, C. (1994). *The Oz principle: Getting results through individual and organizational accountability.* New Jersey, NJ: Prentice Hall.

Damico, J. S., Simmons-Mackie, N. N., Oelschlaeger, M., Elman, R., & Armstrong, E. (1999). Qualitative methods in aphasia research: Basic issues. *Aphasiology, 13*, 651–666.

Creswell, J. (2009) *Research design* (3rd ed.). Thousand Oaks, CA: Sage.

Denzin, N. K., & Lincoln, Y. S. (2011). *The handbook of qualitative research.* Thousand Oaks, CA: Sage.

Eger, D. L. (1997). Outcomes measurement in the schools. In C. M. Fratteli (Ed.), *Measuring outcomes in speech-language pathology.* New York, NY: Thieme.

Ehren, B. J. (2015). Shout it out: We are critical to students' academic achievement. *The ASHA Leader, 20*, 6–8.

Ehren, T. (1999). *Developing a professional growth plan for speech-language pathologists.* In-service meeting for Broward County School District, Ft. Lauderdale, FL.

Fisher, R. A. (1925). *Statistical methods for research workers.* Edinburgh, UK: Oliver & Boyd.

Frakt, A. (2014). High-tech care can save lives—But it also may create incentives that result in lives lost. *JAMA, 312*(20), 2081–2082.

Franklin, M. I. (2012). *Understanding research: Coping with the quantitative-qualitative divide.* London, UK: Routledge.

Gaufberg, E. G., & Williams, M. R. (2011). Reflection in a museum setting: The personal responses tour. *Journal of Graduate Medical Education, 3*(4), 546–549

Gawande, A. (2010). *The checklist manifesto: How to get things right.* New York, NY: Henry Holt.

Glasziou P. P., & Irwig L. M. (1995). An evidence based approach to individualizing treatment. *British Medical Journal, 311*, 1356–1359.

Gorovitz S., & Macintyre, A. (1976). Toward a theory of medical fallibility. *Journal of Medicine and Philosophy, 1*, 51–71.

Green, L., Klecan-Aker, J., & McGehee, K. (2006). *Outcome-based intervention: Practical ideas for practicing clinicians.* Paper presented at ASHA Convention, Miami, FL.

Haidt, J. (2006). *The happiness hypothesis.* New York, NY: Basic Books.

Hanley, J. (1990). *Lifespring.* New York, NY: Fireside.

Hayes, A. (1990). The context and future of judgment-based assessment. *Topics in Early Childhood Special Education, 10*(3), 1–12.

Hegde, M. N. (2002). *Treatment procedures in communicative disorders.* Austin, TX: Pro-Ed.

Heifferon, B. A. (2005). *Writing in the health professions.* New York, NY: Pearson/Longman.

Housen, A. (2002). Aesthetic thought and critical thinking. *Arts Learning Journal, 18*, 1–2.

Hycner, R. H. (1985). Some guidelines for the phenomenological analysis of interview data. *Human Studies, 8*, 279–303.

Irwin, D., Pannbacker, M., & Lass, N. (2008). *Clinical research methods in speech-language pathology and audiology.* San Diego, CA: Plural.

Kazdin, A. (1982). *Single-case research designs.* New York, NY: Oxford University Press.

Kazdin, A. (2001). Bridging the enormous gaps of theory with therapy research and practice. *Journal of Clinical Child Psychology, 30*, 59–66.

Keegan, L. (2012). Review of research methods in communication disorders. *Contemporary Issues in Communication Science and Disorders, 39*, 98–104

Klein, H., & Myers, M. (1999). A set of principles for conducting and evaluating interpretive field studies in information systems. *MIS Quarterly, 23*(1), 67–94.

Klugman, C., Peel, J., & Beckmann-Mendez, D. (2011). Art rounds: Teaching interprofessional students visual thinking strategies at school. *Academic Medicine, 86*(10), 1266–1271

Lakoff, G. (1987). *Women, fire and dangerous things: What categories reveal about the mind.* Chicago, IL: Chicago University Press.

LDonline: The educators' guide to learning disabilities and ADHD. (2015). Retrieved July 22,

2016, from http://www.ldonline.org/features/idea2004

Lester, S. (1999). *An introduction to phenomenological research.* Taunton, UK: Stan Lester Developments. Retrieved June 3, 2016, from www.sld.demon.co.uk/resmethy.pdf.

Lester, S. (2012). Creating original knowledge in and for the workplace: Evidence from a practitioner doctorate. *Studies in Continuing Education, 34*(3), 267–280.

Lewis, P. (1987). *A case for teaching functional skills.* St. Louis, MO: TASH Newsletter. Retrieved from http://www.geocities.ws/our_super_class/functional.html

Lidz, C. S. (1991). *Practitioner's guide to dynamic assessment.* New York, NY: Guilford Press.

Lindlof, T. R., & Taylor, B. C. (2002) *Qualitative communication research methods* (2nd ed.). Thousand Oaks, CA: Sage.

Literacy in Learning Exchange (LLE). (2012, April). Retrieved July 21, 2016, from http://www.literacyinlearningexchange.org/defining-literacy

Lund, N., & Duchan, J. (1993). *Assessing children's language in naturalistic contexts.* Englewood Cliffs, NJ: Prentice-Hall.

Martin, P. Y., & Turner, B. A. (1986). Grounded theory and organizational research. *Journal of Applied Behavioural Science, 22*(2), 141.

McTaggart, L. (2008). *The field.* New York, NY: HarperCollins.

Meline, T., & Paradiso, T. (2003). Evidence-based practice in schools: Evaluating research and reducing barriers. *Language, Speech, and Hearing Services in Schools, 34,* 273–283.

Moore, B. J. (2010). Ethics: If it's not documented, it didn't happen. *ASHA SIG 11: Perspectives on Administration and Supervision, 20,* 106–112.

Moore, B. J., & Montgomery, J. K. (2008). *Making a difference for America's children: Speech-language pathologists in public schools.* Austin, TX: Pro-Ed.

Moustakas, C. (1994). *Phenomenological research methods.* London, UK: Sage.

Naghshineh S., Hafler J.P., Miller A.R., Blanco M.A., Lipsitz, S. R., Dubroff, R. P., . . . Katz, J. T., (2008). Formal art observation training improves medical students' visual diagnostic skills. *Journal of General Internal Medicine, 23*(7), 991–997.

National Governors Association Council of Chief State School Officers. (2016). *Common Core State Standards Initiative.* Retrieved June 20, 2016, from http://www.corestandards.org

National Outcome Measurement System (NOMS) Fact Sheet. Do SLP services have an impact on students' classroom performance? What teachers think. [PDF] Retrieved June 22, 2016, from http://www.asha.org/topics/literacy/

Nevada Speech-Language-Hearing Association (NSHA/NV) Coalition Leadership Team and SEAL Champions. (2015, May). *I contribute.* Presented at ASHA Convention, Denver, CO.

Olswang, L. B., & Bain, B. (1994). Data collection: Monitoring children's treatment progress. *American Journal of Speech-Language Pathology, 3*(3), 55–66.

Papir-Bernstein, W. (1995). *Supervision for the 21st century: Facilitating self-directed professional growth.* Presented at NYSSLHA Mini-Seminar, New York, NY.

Papir-Bernstein, W. (Ed.). (2000). *Measuring outcomes: Clinical variables to measure.* New York, NY: NYCDOE Citywide Speech Services, D.75.

Perry, M., Maffulli, N., & Willson S. (2011). The effectiveness of arts-based interventions in medical education: A review. *Medical Education, 45*(2), 141–148.

Rowlands B. (2005). Grounded in practice: Using interpretive research to build theory. *Electronic Journal of Business Research Methodology, 3*(1), 81–92.

Rubin, J. A. (1984). *The art of art therapy.* New York, NY: Brunner/Mazel.

Rudebusch, J. (2012, March). From Common Core State Standards to standards-based IEPs: A brief tutorial. *ASHA SIG 16: Perspectives on School-Based Issues, 13,* 17–24.

Rudebusch, J. (2014). *Common Core State Standards and service delivery models: Connecting speech-language services to curriculum.* New York, NY: PESI Rehab.

Schutz, A. (1970). *On phenomenology and social relations.* Chicago, IL: Chicago University Press.

Schwandt, T. (2001). *Dictionary of qualitative inquiry.* Thousand Oaks, CA: Sage.

Shapiro J., Rucker L., & Beck J. (2006). Training the clinical eye and mind: Using the arts. *Medical Education, 40*(3), 263–268.

Silliman, E., & Wilkinson, L. C. (1991). *Communicating for learning: Classroom observation and collaboration.* Gaithersburg, MD: Aspen.

Silverman, F. H. (1998). *Research design and evaluation in speech-language pathology and audiology.* Needham Heights, MA: Allyn & Bacon.

Smith, H. (2012). *The spaces in-between: How the art of intuition informs the science of evidence-based practice in psychotherapy.* Master of Social Work Clinical Research Papers. Paper 93. Retrieved from http://sophia.stkate.edu/msw_papers/93

Smith, J. A., & Osborn, M. (2003). Interpretative phenomenological analysis. In J. A. Smith (Ed.), *Qualitative psychology* (pp. 51–80). Thousand Oaks, CA: Sage.

Stone-Goldman, J. (2009). Choosing where to start. In C. Bowen, *Children's speech sound disorders* (pp. 256–262). Oxford: Wiley-Blackwell.

Stone-Goldman, J. (2012). *Where the personal and professional meet: The lecture circuit.* Retrieved June 7, 2016, from http:// www.judystonegoldman.com

Stone-Goldman, J., & Olswang, L. (2003). Learning to look, learning to see: Using ethnography to develop cultural sensitivity. *The Asha Leader, 8*(8), 6–7, 14–15.

Stone, J., & Stoel-Gammon, C. (1993). Phonological development and disorders in children. In F. Minifie (Ed.). *Introduction to communication disorders* (pp. 149–188). Clifton Park, NY: Delmar Cengage Learning.

Todd, S. (2012). *Assessment jargon: The who, what, where why when and how of writing end of year reports.* Retrieved July 22, 2016, from https://www.canton.edu/.../Assessment_Jargon_Presentation-Academic_ Programs.pptx

Tolle, E. (2004). *The power of now.* Novata, CA: New World Library.

Torres, I. (2013a, September). Tricks to take the pain out of writing treatment goals. *ASHA Leader Blog.* Retrieved June 27, 2016, from http://blog.asha.org/2013/09/10/tricks-to-take-the-pain-out-of-writing-treatment-goals/

Torres, I. (2013b, November). Make it work: Write targeted treatment goals. *The ASHA Leader, 18,* 26–27.

Trauth, E. M. (2001). *Qualitative research: Issues and trends.* Amsterdam, Netherlands: Idea.

Turkstra L, Coelho C, & Ylvisaker M. (2005). The use of standardized tests for individuals with cognitive- communication disorders. *Seminars in Speech and Language, 26*(4), 215–222.

UNESCO. (2006). *Education for all global monitoring report.* Retrieved July 20, 2016, from http://www.unesco.org/education/GMR2006/full/chapt6_eng.pdf

United States Department of Education. (2004). *Individuals with Disabilities Education Act (IDEA).* Retrieved July 5, 2016, from http://idea.ed.gov

Westby, C. E. (1990). Ethnographic interviewing: Asking the right questions to the right people in the right ways. *Journal of Childhood Communication Disorders, 13*(1), 101–111.

Westby, C., Burda, A., & Mehta, Z. (2003). Asking the right questions in the right ways: Strategies for ethnographic interviewing. *The ASHA Leader, 8,* 4–17.

Westby, C. E., StevensDominguez, M., & Oetter, P. (1996). A performance/competence model of observational assessment. *Language, Speech, and Hearing Services in Schools, 27,* 144–156.

Wilson, J. (2007). *The performance of practice: Enhancing the repertoire of therapy with children and families.* London, UK: Karnac Books.

Yalom, I.D. (2002). *The gift of therapy: An open letter to a new generation of therapists and their patients.* New York, NY: HarperCollins.

Yanow, D., & Schwartz-Shea, P. (Eds). (2006). *Interpretation and method: Empirical research methods and the interpretive turn.* Armonk, NY: M. E. Sharpe.

CHAPTER 12

Incorporating Good and Best Practices

1. FROM GOOD TO BEST (AND BACK AGAIN)

Good Practice

When we use the term *good practice*, we are denoting educational or intervention techniques that are research-based, measurable, and effective for students with communication disorders (Moore & Montgomery, 2008). *Good practice* in schools necessitates the acknowledgement of commonalities and differences among all children. Good practice dictates that our decisions and actions will most likely result in progress for the students. Progress in speech, language, and communication has always been the goal for the school-based speech-language pathologist; however, as a result of IDEA (2004), the progress must be linked to educational benefit and achievement (Brannen et al., 2000).

Best Practice

A *best practice* is a method or technique that has consistently shown results superior to those achieved with other means, and that is used as a benchmark. In addition, a "best" practice can evolve to become better as improvements are discovered. Best practice is considered by some as a buzzword, used to describe the process of developing and following a standard way of doing things that multiple organizations can use.

The term *best practice* implies that one technique or model for therapy is better than others, and for that reason is can be a bit misleading. What we use will depend on individual needs of students, the school culture, and the innovation and skill level of the practitioner (Moore & Montgomery, 2008). Best practice methods and techniques are something to aspire to and are what should keep pushing us forward; good practice is the here and now and is a step on the journey toward best practice. If the assumption is that best practice is as good as it can get, then no one would challenge the status quo to improve things and progress would stop (Bogan & English, 1994).

Is the Difference Important?

I have observed that many of us confuse good practice with best practice. The difference may not be all that important. Whenever it is recommended that a practice *should* be followed, it is said to be a best practice. When this practice becomes a part of life, it becomes a good practice. So, a *good practice* is a practice that is usually followed by all concerned professionals. On the other hand, think of best practice as what we strive for, and good practice as the step along the way. *We can say that a best practice, when followed over a period of time, becomes a good practice.*

The terminology used sometimes causes misconceptions around best practice. The term *best practice* indicates that not only is this the best way to do something, but that it will always be the best. What is actually meant by the term is that this is the best way to do something right now. As best practices are adapted and evolved based on new technologies, techniques and ways of thinking it makes sense to call them good practices. Best practice is what we aspire to but good practice is what we work with every day—today we do this activity this way but tomorrow we will adapt it to a new and more effective good practice on our way to a best practice.

Both terms are used. What is determined to be a *best practice in one field* for people with one type of disability or chronologic age may be a good practice when working in other fields of practice or with clients of different disabilities or ages. Our decisions must be informed, but it may never be totally apparent at the start that one choice would be better than another. That is the exciting and creative part of the artistic process—we get to choose.

2. NATURALISTIC

A.R.T.: Naturalistic

We all have "favorites," and one of mine was a young woman Brenda. Brenda was 14 years old, and had just lost her puppy. She was so sad that I asked the principal if I could have a conversational speech session over lunch with Brenda in a neighborhood coffee shop. Off we went, and she was her usual sophisti-

cated self as we got a table and menus were brought over. She had some literacy skills, and I was prepared to help her read from the menu. However, I was astounded with the fact that she had no knowledge of how a menu worked, how the foods were categorized, and how to find things that she may want to eat. Although I was working on vocabulary and categorization, it had never dawned on me to work with real materials that she might come into contact with in her everyday activities. You can be sure I never made that mistake again.

Participation in Everyday Activities

A universal aspect of early childhood intervention is to promote learning opportunities and experiences through participation in everyday activities. These naturalistic activities provide contexts for learning socially situated and culturally meaningful behaviors (Dunst, 2013). There are a number of factors that shape and influence child learning in the naturalistic context of everyday activities. These factors include the child characteristics, caregiver/interventionist characteristics and the activity setting characteristics (Bronfenbrenner, 1993). *Child characteristics* refer to child temperament, personal interests, and type of disability. *Caregiver/interventionist characteristics* refer to cultural values, beliefs, and attitudes, and interactional styles. *Activity setting characteristics* refer to activity locations, types of routines, and interest level of materials and activities.

Everyday activities are defined as naturalistic contexts in which collaborative interactions and assisted performance occur (Dunst, 2013; Tharp & Gallimore, 1988). Through situation-specific experiences, children have opportunity to learn about their own behavior capabilities as well as the behavioral characteristics of others (Dunst et al., 2001). Children's interests (preferences, choices, and likes) play a major role in influencing learning. As we discussed in Chapter 10, materials and activities that are engaging, challenging, of high interest, and well matched to a child's interests are our best bet (Dunst et al., 2001; Dunst, 2013).

In Richter's research review of child-caregiver practices across a variety of countries and cultures, universal features for health child development include *caregiver sensitivity, responsiveness, nurture, and support* (Dunst, 2013; Richter, 2004). These same practitioner characteristics, when integrated within naturalistic language intervention environments, provide opportunities for optimal behavioral and developmental outcomes.

Naturalistic Intervention Strategies

Naturalistic intervention strategies are sometimes referred to as informal methods because they are child-directed rather than adult-directed. Informal strategies include teaching methods that are responsive to a child's attempts (initiations) to communicate (Dunst, Raab, & Trivette, 2011). They promote communication and language development within the context of everyday activities in naturally occurring and socially relevant situations. Several of these methodologies had been developed for use by home caregivers and their young children, and later adapted for instructional use by teachers and speech-language pathologists. Naturalistic intervention approaches include Enhanced Milieu Teaching, Incidental Teaching, Activity-Based Language Experiences (ABLE), and It Takes Two to Talk (Girolametto & Weitzman, 2006; Hart & Risley, 1978; Papir-Bernstein, 1992).

Naturalistic teaching strategies share the following explicit features (Dunst et al., 2011 Horn & Banerjee, 2009):

- The use of *everyday, recognizable, and age-appropriate activities* as contexts for language learning
- The instructional sequence includes *natural consequences* such as desired materials or activities
- *Adult sensitivity* to a child's attempt to communicate
- *Adult responsiveness* to maintain child's attention
- Adult *following the child's lead*
- *Adult modeling* of desired behavior
- Interactions between the child and adult should reflect a *good fit*, indicated by the child's response to prompts and sustained motivation in the activity

---

A.R.T.: Sensemaking

A young, severely language-impaired student was on the receiving end of my routine for eliciting language. I had collected boxes of large pictures, and was in the habit of using the pictures to facilitate conversation. She was motivated and enthusiastic about interacting with me, and thoroughly enjoyed talking about the pictures as I took each one out of the box. I simply had to say, "What's this?" and away she went. After the 4th or 5th picture, she began to change her expression and increase the intensity of how she was looking at me. She finally said, with tears in her eyes (and a pronounced w/l substitution), "Oh, are you blind?" My life changed in that instant, and never again did I use unnaturalistic elicitation questions.

Naturalistic methodologies evolved out of the need for more meaning-based and socially oriented language intervention. That approach is sometimes referred to as *sense-making*. The challenge, however, is to remain naturalistic and interactive while maintaining accountability and organization (Norris & Hoffman, 1990). Naturalistic intervention is consistent with principles of *whole language learning*, which enable the child to use a linguistic code for interacting with the physical and social environment (McLean & Snyder-McLean, 1978; Muma, 1978).

Scaffolding Interactive Strategies

Scaffolding strategies are used to assist the child with communication during naturalistic activities through the provision of prompts, questions, restatements, and other supportive procedures. A naturalistic and activity-based approach to intervention can be motivational, fun, age and developmentally appropriate, and provide natural reinforcement of the language learning process. Activities may be chosen to accommodate a wide variety of interests and values so that they appeal to students from a wide variety of cultural backgrounds. The following are suggested strategies to assist communication during naturalistic activities (Norris & Hoffman, 1990; Papir-Bernstein, 1992; Wiig & Semel, 1976):

- *Cloze procedures* (convergent productions), similar to "filling in the blanks"
- *Gestures and pantomime* provide nonlinguistic cues as prompts
- *Relational words* that indicate more of a certain type of information is needed (and, because, or but)
- *Questions* that prompt for comprehension or additional information
- *Binary choices* that offer alternatives
- *Turn taking cues*
- *Word finding cues*, such as syllabic or phonemic

- *Statements that suggest* the need for non-given information from given information (semantic implications: what would happen if . . .)

---

3. RECIPROCAL

Reciprocity as Joint Partnership

Bronfenbrenner developed an ecological theory of human development, and proposed the idea of "joint activity" as a venue for the development of partnerships between children and adults (1979). In joint activity, a *partnership between the child and adult* will form as long as three variables are present: *balance of power, an affective attachment, and reciprocity.* We have touched upon the first two variables in Chapters 5 and 6, so now we will discuss the importance of *reciprocity*.

Reciprocity is the process by which each person influences the other, rather than the adult controlling everything about the content and direction of the interaction (MacDonald, 1989). The process demands some advance planning and coordination, but the payoff is huge. Reciprocity leads to safe and friendly feedback, which in turn leads to motivation. Because the child feels valued, the reciprocal activities may become self-reinforcing.

A vast field of research in the 1970s and 1980s focused on principles for developing social and communicative partnerships with children. We have learned that as long as adults interact with the child in "productive" ways, the child will have a higher likelihood of being an active participant in his or her own development and growth. Some adult styles are more productive than others. Some come naturally, and others we need to learn. *Productive adult styles* presume a balanced and reciprocal partnership, and include the ability to be behaviorally and cognitively matched, sensitive and responsive, emotionally attached, and child-directed (MacDonald, 1989)

Turn-Taking Exchanges

One popular strategy for building reciprocity is *turn-taking*, or mutual give-and-take, which facilitates the much needed *balance of power* (MacDonald & Gillette, 1989). Turn-taking is like a game of Ping-Pong. Each partner takes one turn at a time, and then waits for the return and tries to keep the game going. It is unlike the game of darts, where one person controls the action with no response, followed by the next person's turn (MacDonald, 1989). Turn-taking creates a type of *interactive loop* that is part of a natural learning process. The loop continues as long as each person maintains the exchange or interaction that helps the other continue to participate.

There are several reasons that account for imbalance during attempted turn-taking routines. They include (MacDonald, 1989):

- Limited give-and-take style, usually accompanied by low expectations of the partner
- Activity domination by one partner
- Interrupted exchange of action
- Lack of sustained contact
- Same actions again and again
- Change from mutual activity (Ping Pong) to parallel activity (darts)

The Golden Rule

Most of us have grown up knowing *the golden rule*: do unto others as you would have others do unto you. Professionally, however, we need to be sure that our idea of "client welfare" is consistent with the client's own ideas. Duchan reminds us that the following strategies would most likely pass *the golden rule test* (2000):

- Focus on what the client *can do.*
- Include *the voice of the client* in anything you write.
- Work on *life-related goals.*
- Select activities and materials that connect with *client interests and preferences.*
- *Solicit input and feedback* from clients and caregivers.

In the last two decades, our field has made multiple strides moving toward *a basic and universal golden rule.* The following are some examples of how we have been doing just that. We have broadened *our understanding of evidence and data* to include ethnographic practices, multiple perspectives, and most importantly, client viewpoint. We include contextual and participatory factors within our intervention approaches, and thus *support inclusionary practices* within a range of educational, social, and life experiences. Finally, we are implementing a *social-medical* model that focuses on *the person rather than the problem* (Frank, 1995; Frattali, 1998; Simmons-Mackie & Damico, 1999; WHO, 1998).

The Social-Medical Model

The social-medical model is supported by the World Health Organization's definition of health as well as by the narrative medicine movement. The World Health Organization's (WHO) definition of health is a *state of physical, mental, and social well-being.* Communication disorders are considered part of the health field, whether the setting for intervention is medical or educational.

The WHO's International Classification of Functioning, Disability and Health (ICF) considers the health condition to be a function of three factors: body function and structural impairment, activity limitations (environmental and personal), and participation restriction (Threats, 2016; WHO, 2008). The WHO supports the removal of contextual barriers to facilitate *greater life participation* for individuals with disabilities.

4. CURRICULUM-RELATED

> ### A.R.T.: Embedded
>
> When I began work in the last few months of the 1960s, our caseloads consisted largely of students with articulation disorders (and a few with fluency disorders). We worked on the disorder, using drill and repetition, vocabulary lists, and sentence constructions. How was the content chosen? No way in particular. It was not particularly based on student preferences, naturalistic activities, curriculum. or parent requests. We knew what we had to remediate, and the rest was up to us.
>
> Consider this: we are fortunate because we work in an area of speech, language and communication that is part of everything we do. Here is the secret: we should be able to embed our clinical targets into curriculum expectations, and then into some larger context—favorite activities, vocational preparation, community experiences, social interactions, life skills, universal/cross cultural themes, and so forth. It is all about *embedding*.

What Is Curriculum?

The world is every changing, and the process of curriculum development and implementation must remain dynamic to keep up with those ongoing changes. Professionals working in the vital field of "childhood learning" rarely agree about the definition of curriculum. We know that curriculum must be purposeful and well defined (Wiles & Bondi, 2007). However, the cornerstone of *belief of and adherence to curriculum* will depend upon your personal and professional philosophies about learning.

At its fullest, curriculum has been defined as the total set of school experiences, much larger than simply the academic subjects (Kelly, 2009). Within this definition, parts of the day, such as lunch, sports, play, and other nonacademic activities, qualify as part of the curriculum experience. The goals and objectives developed from the curriculum direct student learning, and the activities chosen through best practices and student preferences help shape their behaviors (Goodlad, 2004). Wiles & Bondi suggest that curriculum represents a set of values and goals that culminate in successful learning experiences for students by targeting specific knowledge, behavior, and attitudes (2007; Wiles, 2009).

> ### A.R.T.: Curriculum
>
> I know that the word "curriculum" still sends shudders down the spine of many practitioners. I have heard all of the protests, arguments against, and reasons why it shouldn't be. Please remember—by the very definition of our service (speech therapy as a related service), there is no question that our service must relate to "classroom instruction." The only question is will you follow the classroom curriculum and subsequently question your role? Will you conduct your speech therapy only in the classroom, helping your students "read" the class text, and wonder what your service has become? Will you work on directly "teaching your students" the standards and forget about their speech, language, and communication needs?

What Is the Difference Between Curriculum and Standards?

Standards are statements about yearly expectations based upon grade levels. Curriculum is the detailed ongoing day-to-day program created to facilitate student learning about those standards. Decisions about standards are made at the state level, whereas curriculum decisions are locally made and implemented. Curriculum should be (Wiles, 2009):

- Supportive of state standards in all subject areas
- Have clear sequences of objectives
- Be grade and developmentally appropriate
- Include a clear purpose for each standard

The Association of Supervision and Curriculum Development (ASCD) is the largest organization of such in the world, and lists the ten valued learning outcomes for each curriculum as: self-esteem, understanding of others, basic skill, capacity for continuous learning, being a responsible member of society, mental and physical health, creativity, informed participation in the economic world, use of accumulated knowledge to understand the world, and ability to cope with change (Hattie, 2012; Wiles, 2009).

So, in summary, standards are the end, whereas curriculum is the means (EdFly Blog, 2013). Although the terms are sometimes used interchangeably, it is important for us to understand the difference because we will have much more control over developing and implementing curriculum than changing state standards. Every school has access to the state standards; however, you can read about them in detail on the Common Core State Standards (CCSS) website.

How Do We Really Feel About Standards and Curriculum?

By law (IDEA 1997 and 2004), all students with disabilities must be able to access, and participate with and progress in the general curriculum (Horn & Banerjee, 2009). Curriculum provides a roadmap or a blueprint for overall student learning, but school curriculum needs to be adapted and modified to meet the speech, language, and communication needs of students receiving our services in the schools. School curriculum has already been constructed to align with the Common Core State Standards, so they both become resources for us.

Rebecca Visintin, a school-based SLP who moved to the U.S. from Australia, is a contributor on the *ASHA Leader Blog*. She writes about her struggles with understanding the importance of addressing curriculum and standards as an ongoing part of her therapy approach. Some common sense ideas for implementation include (Nippold, 2011; Visintin, 2013a, 2013 b; Wallach, 2014):

- *Collaborate* with classroom teachers about teaching content.
- *Borrow* grade level curriculum handbooks.
- *Become familiar* with the Common Core State Standards, specifically in the area of English Language Arts (speaking, listening, language, writing, and reading). Use them to write IEP goals and objectives and guide informal assessments.
- Integrate *grade-level reading* materials from your school library.
- *Provide in-service* for the teachers, and explain how you will integrate the standards and school curriculum within your therapy approach. Explain about the fundamental role that language plays in the learning process, and how your expertise in language development, language disorders, and language intervention can benefit the students' ability to learn subject content
- Check out the *ASHA resources* for standards and school-based SLPs.
- Be certain that your clinical targets are *relevant to language learning* in general and academic contexts.

> **A.R.T.: Challenging Traditionalism**
>
> Wallach reminds us that this *integrated approach* challenges the long and historical "traditionalism" in speech and

language intervention as a "pullout and isolated" service (2014). Those of us in the field for a while remember the phrase, "I'm going to speech" that our students chanted as they left the classroom for our "mystery room" (assuming we were fortunate enough to have one). The landscape is very different now in what we do, where we do it, and how we accomplish it.

In the mid-1970s, working through curriculum made perfect sense as my early population of students was severely language impaired. I would tip-toe upstairs to the classrooms, because if the teachers heard me coming they would close and lock their doors. We were all friends in that program, and I knew they were kidding when they locked me out—but I also knew there was no uniform curriculum in those days and they knew I was chairing a "language curriculum committee" in the program. My favorite and most productive venue was to work with the students in the classroom, collaborating with the teacher and helping to shape content. We always began with what the teacher was doing because the teacher was the *classroom expert.* The students loved seeing us work together as one interconnected and supportive family, sharing responsibility for academic success.

The relationship between language and learning could not be more clearly stated than by the IDEA 2004 definition of specific learning disability: "a disorder in basic psychological processes involved with understanding or using spoken or written language manifesting in difficulties listening, thinking, speaking, reading, spelling or doing math." Our role is to facilitate the academic success of students with speech and language impairments by integrating the standards and curriculum. Power-

deFur and Flynn describe a no-nonsense process for doing just that (2012):

- *Review the content standards* for the current and prior grades, focusing on the communication expectations underlying the standard (phonologic, morphologic, syntactic, semantic, pragmatic, and metalinguistic).
- *Determine the student's level of functioning* relative to the standards using criterion-referenced assessments and teacher input.
- *Review the student's goals,* objectives, accommodations, and curriculum modifications written on the IEP.
- *Plan on using the classroom materials* so that there will be a natural connection and flow between your services and the classroom.
- *Collaborate with classroom teachers* so that even if services are provided in a setting other than the classroom, content can be coplanned and integrated.

Curriculum Modifications, Adaptations, and Accommodations

In Chapter 10, we discussed the Universal Design for Learning (UDL) as it pertains to materials. However, the use of UDL principles when designing and implementing curriculum does not detract from the importance of making modifications to meet the diverse needs of specific students. *Curriculum modifications or accommodations* cover any category of assisting students to access and progress with the general curriculum. *Accommodation* usually applies to altering an environment or piece of equipment, whereas modification is an individualization of the curriculum (Horn & Banerjee, 2009). The term *adaptation* is more generic and can refer to either modifications or accommodations.

Research conducted largely in early childhood educational programs describes *six types of modification strategies*: environmental support, material adaptations, use of special equipment, implementation of student preferences, activity simplification (task analysis), and personal support (adult, peer, or invisible) (Horn & Banerjee, 2009; Merritt & Culatta, 1998). The first three modification strategies are external to the child and address adapting materials or activities within the instructional environment. The next two focus on matching activities with the student's abilities and preferences. The final strategy focuses on providing personal support.

1. *Environmental support:* This refers to altering the temporal (time sequence for activities), physical or social (interactions) environment to facilitate the student's participation and engagement with the activities.
2. *Material adaptation:* This refers to modifying materials to foster greater independence.
3. *Use of special equipment:* This refers to adapting materials (stabilizing, nonskid backing) using *creative homemade* solutions or commercial adaptations.
4. *Implementation of preferences:* This has been discussed in detail in earlier chapters, and increases both motivation and reinforcement factors.
5. *Activity simplification:* This strategy involves task analyzing activities and perhaps increasing the number of steps or adjusting the pace so that success (successive approximation) is experienced more often.
6. *Adult/peer/invisible support:* We are most familiar with adult support, but peer interaction or support is another powerful variable in the student's environment. Invisible support occurs when aspects

of naturally occurring activities are rearranged to facilitate student involvement (chairs facing a specific direction, materials missing).

Differentiated Instruction

Differentiation, differentiated learning, or *differentiated instruction* (DI) is a philosophy for educating students that involves providing students with individualized avenues for learning (Tomlinson, 1999). It is a type of *personalized instruction* that acknowledges and accounts for differences in readiness levels, beliefs about learning, culture, socioeconomic status, gender, ability/disability, strengths, and personal interests (Inglebret, Banks-Joseph, & CHiXapkaid, 2016; Lawrence-Brown, 2004). Through the process of differentiation, learning methodologies are student-centered and adjusted to accommodate needs and preferences of each learner.

Differentiation is accomplished by differentiating four variables: learning content, learning process, learning product, and learning environment. *Content* can be thought of as what students should understand and be able to accomplish through their content knowledge (Inglebret et al., 2016). One of the most popular ways of differentiating *content* is through the use of *Bloom's taxonomy* of educational learning (Bloom, Engelhart, Furst, Hill, & Krathwohl, 1956). Another is through an educational strategy called *Understanding by Design* (UbD) (Tomlinson & McTighe, 2006). *The Understanding by Design* (UbD) framework focuses on comprehension and learning transfer through authentic performance. According to UbD, comprehension is communicated through the student's ability to explain, interpret, apply, shift perspective, empathize, and self-assess (Tomlinson & McTighe, 2006).

Instructional differentiation is also achieved through distinctions of learning *process*. The process can be defined as learning activities that help students make sense of the content (Tomlinson, 2014). This is where an approach such as *Multiple Intelligences* can be beneficial (Gardner, 1983). When we differentiate by process we are considering learning styles, and how a student best understands and assimilates information. Another such resource for differentiating process can be found in the *Layered Curriculum* approach (Nunley, 2004).

The third type of differentiation is learning *product*, or how mastery of learning is demonstrated (Inglebret et al., 2016). The fourth type is differentiating through *environmental adjustments*, such as space, light, structure, furniture, and classroom management techniques (Pashler, McDaniel, Rohrer, & Bjork, 2008). The DI is a holistic process that includes an assessment component, as well as an extension to home and families.

All components interconnect and communicate with each other. It is in keeping with preferences, values and diverse life experiences of students and their families. The DI is an educational approach that fosters a respect and appreciation for differentiated content (ways of knowing), process (ways of being), and product (ways of doing) (Inglebret et al., 2016). When goals are important and meaningful to the client, they can motivate and empower the client toward more active participation with their therapeutic intervention (Doig, Fleming, Cornwell, & Kuipers, 2009).

5. UNIVERSAL

An Unbroken Golden Thread

There is a component in every behavioral field of knowledge that is based upon experience at its deepest lever. Some of this knowledge cannot develop until the individual activates the *experience mode* with own personal button. Only then does the vast array of professional content come alive and become dynamic, changing with each client, each patient, each student.

There is an unbroken golden thread that weaves through our work. Even the most theoretical genius needs to be grounded in practical realities. Our imagination and ability to integrate our lifelong experiences becomes that grounding (Lesser, 1999). Many of us search for that quality that "lifts the veil between our work and a larger reality" (McTaggart, 2008, p. 27).

Sometimes an overload of information is mistaken for knowledge. To the same extent, we may be uncomfortable to admit that we feel a need for something that we cannot put words to (Lesser, 1999). Admitting that we do not know something is not easy for anyone, as is voicing innocence and a sense of wonder. This essential human condition has changed little over time (McTaggart, 2008). In order to follow and immerse oneself, a change in mentality is required. One must become 'Pharaonic,' and contemplate things and feel them more deeply by means of intuition and intelligence of the heart rather than to study them according to the system advocated by Greek rationalism (Schwaller de Lubicz, 1985). How does this relate to education?

Essentialism and Perennialism as Global Education

The educational philosophy that best mirrors a back to basics approach to education is called *essentialism*. It was popularized in the 1930s but had been the dominant approach to education in our country since the beginnings of American history. Essentialist educations emphasize the importance of facilitating the development of character, social skills, and all that will help students develop effective life-skills (Ruitenberg, 2010).

A second educational philosophy that relates to our topic of discussion is *educational perennialism*. Perennialists believe that the profession of teaching should focus on things of everlasting pertinence and importance, topics and principles for personal development and the most essential elements of humanity at its best (Kneller, 1971). People are always first, and learning how to reason becomes more important than learning the facts—because facts always seem to change. We are people first, and then professionals.

Although essentialism and perennialism seem similar, one basic difference is that the first focuses more on essential skills (doing), whereas the second on personal development (being). Similarities probe us to debate human experiences, such as what it means to be an individual, part of a community, what is worth knowing and why, what are the most productive habits of the mind. The core curriculum becomes about learning how to think, not about accepting specific ideas. One version of it began in 1919 and was developed as the main *transdisciplinary curriculum* used by Columbia University's Columbia College (De Bary, 2007).

Transdisciplinary Themes

Transdisciplinary education simply means that the curriculum is integrated or connected to universal themes. It acknowledges that all teaching and learning should acknowledge human commonality, diversity, and multiple perspectives. Transdisciplinary learning allows students to authentically make connects with information, construct their personal meaning, and thus transfer learning to real-world applications. Transdisciplinary themes provide a basis for discussion and interpretation of local and global perspectives explored in any content. The themes have global significance, and offer students the opportunity to explore commonalities of human experience. All content should be *engaging*, meaning of interest to the students, and involving them actively in their own learning. Content should be *relevant*, and linked to the students' prior knowledge and experience, and current circumstances, and therefore placing learning in a context connected to the lives of the students. It should be *challenging*, and extend the prior knowledge and experience of the students to increase their competencies and understanding. Content should be *significant* as it contributes to an understanding of the transdisciplinary nature of the theme, and therefore to an understanding of commonality of human experiences (Boyer, 1995).

Boyer acknowledged that educating students in a set of isolated subject areas, although necessary, is insufficient. It is also important to explore content that is relevant to students, acquire skills in context, and transcend the boundaries of the traditional subjects. A student must make connections across the disciplines, integrate learnings and relate them to life (1995). He proposed a set of themes or *core commonalities* that represent shared human experiences.

These six transdisciplinary themes provide schools and practitioners the opportunity to incorporate local and global issues into the curriculum and effectively allow students to "step up" beyond the confines of learning within subject areas (Boyer, 1995; Erikson, 2008).

- *Who we are:* Inquiry into the nature of the self; beliefs and values; person, physical, mental, social, and spiritual health; human relationships including families, friends, communities, and cultures; rights and responsibilities; what it means to be human.

- *Where we are in place and time:* Inquiry into orientation in place and time; personal histories; homes and journeys; the discoveries, explorations, and migrations of humankind; the relationship between and the interconnectedness of individuals and civilizations, from local and global perspectives.

- *How we express ourselves:* Inquiry into the ways in which we discover and express ideas, feelings, nature, culture, beliefs, and values; the ways in which we reflect on, extend and enjoy our creativity; our appreciation of the aesthetic.

- *How the world works:* Inquiry into the natural world and its laws, the interaction between the natural world (physical and biological) and human societies; how humans use their understanding of scientific principles; the impact of scientific and technological advances on society and on the environment

- *How we organize ourselves:* Inquiry into the interconnectedness of human-made systems and communities; the structure and function of organizations; societal decision-making; economic activities and their impact on humankind and the environment.

- *Sharing the planet:* Inquiry into rights and responsibilities in the struggle to share finite resources with other people and other living things; communities and the relationship within and between them; access to equal opportunities; peace and conflict resolution.

What We All Have In Common

Some practices are so beautiful that we must adopt them for ourselves. These practices are embedded within and knitted together by events of global and intergenerational significance that occur in our lifetimes. These endur-

ing themes give meaning to art and connect our hearts and minds to those from different times and places (Boyer, 1995; Erickson, 2003). For an overview of such multicultural activities please see Appendix B.

According to this type of universal and transdisciplinary approach, we all do the following: experience life cycles (age: birth, growth, and death); use symbols (use language to express feelings and ideas); know time and place (temporal and spatial concepts: recall the past and anticipate the future); search for a larger purpose (spirituality); have an aesthetic response (interest in art); seek social bonding (members in groups and institutions that shape their lives); connect with nature; need food and water; have a desire to procreate and create families (biological or otherwise); perform labor in exchange for money or favor (work); cloth our bodies; and shelter ourselves (Boyer, 1995; Hall et al., 2012; Levin & Nevo, 2009).

A.R.T.: Universality

During my classes, when I discuss the importance of building universal/cultural components into our therapy programs, I ask the students the following question: what life elements or experiences are the same for people in every culture? It takes a while, but eventually we come up with a list containing things like: everyone eats, sleeps, wears clothing, lives somewhere, has interests, celebrates holidays, has a family, and so forth. That becomes the base for building diversity elements into your intervention program, and we continue our discussion talking about "diversity choices" for materials and activities. For example, make sure your choices of books contain diverse names and people with different skin colors.

---

6. INCLUSIVE

What Is Discrimination?

Abdelal explains the neurobiology of *bias, racial, and ethnic discrimination* (2013). As we remember back to our biology classes, every living organism is the *outward physical manifestation* of *internally coded* and inheritable information. This definition has two parts. The outward physical manifestation of the organism is called the *phenotype*, and consists of the observable structure, function, and behavior of a living organism. The *genotype* is all stored information that serves as the blueprint and genetic code or DNA (Blamire, 2000). Whereas the *genotype* is the set of genes in our DNA that is responsible for a particular trait, the *phenotype* is the physical expression and characteristics of that trait.

Race is defined as the socially constructed reaction to phenotypic characteristics (Abdelal, 2013). Racial differences originated due to geographic isolation, which led to sustained cultural practices as people adapted to their environments. Eventually, genetic adaptations followed suit (Hill & Witherspoon, 2011). Ethnicity, on the other hand, is describes as a common ancestry or history, shared language, beliefs, social rules, and behaviors exhibited in a specific community of members (Abdelal, 2013).

Why Does Discrimination Exist?

Organization is central to how the brain learns. The brain learns through detecting patterns in the environment, and it stores information in a categorical fashion. Categorization facilitates learning by enabling us to make inference about new members of a group that we encounter for the first time (Abdelal, 2016; Quinn et al., 2013). This is called *socially based categorization*, and consists of three levels (Abdelal, 2013):

- Recognizing a difference
- Showing preference toward one social category without assigning social importance
- Showing preference and assigning importance to one social category over another.

According to Kinzler and Spelke, infants as young as 3months old can detect racial differences; however, racially-based social preferences do not emerge until a child is between 2.5 and 5 years of age (2011). At this age most children still have not yet assigned social importance to racial differences. From that point on, the environment takes over by stimulating development of racial and ethnic discrimination (Abdelal, 2013, 2016).

As a result of sensory stimulation, we construct an *inner reality* that is a reflection of the environment. These internal representations become hard-wired by puberty and serve as the lenses through which we will view the world. Those constructs, or lenses, become the standard against which we evaluate people, actions and things (Abdelal, 2013; Wexler, 2006). According to Wexler, conflict is produced when internal constructs contradict with the actual environment (as exemplified with the concept of "alief" in Chapter 4) (2006). This usually occurs after puberty, and conflict will produce the need for either the internal structures or the actual environment to change. To ensure a harmonious state between inner and external reality, people tend to prefer *familiar* people, actions, and things. In fact, familiarity is the primary determiner of preference. Familiarity is predictable and is perceived as safe and pleasurable (Kinzler & Spenkle, 2011).

Research has documented associations in children and adults between racial discrimination and the following outcomes in physical health, cognitive growth, social interactions, and educational success: decreased self-esteem and successful group interactions; increased risk for aggression and violence; early experiences with addiction; decreased academic performance; and sleep and anxiety disorders (Abdelal, 2013, 2016).

It has been suggested that metacognitive skill-building is one our best strategies for lessoning discriminatory practices, by learning to self-analyze thoughts and behaviors and be open to new learning about desensitization and cognitive flexibility (Abdelal, 2013). Familiarity and exposure to other cultures (represented by people, things, and activities) is one of our most valuable tools. Other evidence-based strategies include the improvement of coping and resilience, and programs that foster positive beliefs, self-esteem, and group attitudes (Borders & Hennebry, 2015).

Children notice human differences at a very early age and these distinctions become part of their developing attitudes. These attitudes will be reflected in their early peer interactions, their investment in others, their ability to be in touch with their own emotional experiences, their capacity to empathize with others, and ultimately with their ability to identify with people even though they may look, speak, dress, and act differently than we do (Papir-Bernstein & Rosaly-Santos, 2004). By integrating diversity and multicultural approaches within our therapy program, we are helping our students become independent and socially adept adults.

Cultural Intelligence

Cultural Intelligence (CQ) is a natural evolu-tion from the well-established notions of Intelligence Quotient (IQ) and Emotional Intelligence (EQ). Cultural intelligence is the ability to thrive in and around multiple cultures in our globally complex world. It is something that we can continuously improve and develop during our professional career and over the course of our life (Cheng, 2007; Middleton, 2014; Papir-Bernstein & Rosaly-Santos, 2004). It involves the ability to cross boundaries between cultures and work with people who are different from you.

Middleton describes CQ as the line between *our core and our flex* (2014). Our *core* is the absolutely crucial parts of ourselves that are self-defining, the parts we think we would or could never change. They are our values, and whatever else we consider essential to our lives and to the respect we want from others. Everything else is *flex*. Our flex allows us to adapt and change when necessary. Sometimes we discover aspects of our personality in our cores that create knots, and as we smooth out our knots we can smooth out our relationships. For example, prejudgment is a common knot, and if we work on it we may be able to move that aspect of our personality to our flex.

What is in your core and what is in your flex? Sometimes we have prejudgment or *bias aspects* of our personality in our core. As we work on them, they may be able to move to our flex and allow us to move from intolerance or *ethnocentricity* to *cultural intelligence*. *Ethnocentricity* is a term that describes the use of one's own cultural values as the basis for judging the correctness of the behaviors and values of members of other cultures (Goldberg, 1997). In clinical and educational situations, the conveyance of this attitude often results in the establishment of barriers between the client and the practitioner.

A well-defined and reflected upon core and flex are key to Cultural Intelligence. The balance between the two allows us to experience new situations and adapt to people who are different from ourselves without the fear of losing ourselves or overaccommodating on something that creates discomfort (Earley & Ang, 2003; Middleton, 2014). One useful tool for discovering your knots is ASHA's Cultural Competence Checklists for Personal Reflection and Service Delivery (American Speech-Language-Hearing Association, 2010). For a self-assessment of diversity perspectives, please see Appendix C.

Cultural Competence

Cultural competence involves recognizing differences and respecting those differences. It also involves an understanding that we all have similarities. Medical research has explored the question of whether evidence-based practice and cultural competence (CC) can be complementary goals (Hasnain-Wynia, 2006). Cultural competence in medicine, much like in our own field, begins by understanding cultural diversity in the clinical setting and respecting the beliefs and values of individuals from all cultures. It has evolved into the much broader *patient-centered care* (to be covered in the next chapter) and *narrative practice* (listening to the client's story) (Betancourt, 2003).

Culture of one sort or another infuses and influences every aspect of our identity. Cultural competence is about understanding cultural factors and perspectives that influence everything our clients do and feel (Goldberg, 1997). In order to do that we must first understand how we perceive ourselves relative to our own diversity perspectives (Torres, 2105). Cultural competence implies an appreciation for diverse lenses, world views, and perspectives such as were discussed in Chapter 6. It all begins with self-awareness (Griffer & Perlis, 2007).

Varner and Beamer suggest that the more is known about other cultures, the more important it becomes to make discoveries about one's own (1995). They remind us that many of us may react in these typical ways to unfamiliar cultures (Schraeder, 2013):

- Assumption of *superiority and ethnocentrism*, feeling that their own culture is "right"

- Assumption of *universality*, or that their view of the universe is the only one
- *Bias, discrimination, and prejudice*, all based on preference for comfort and familiarity

Multiperspective Identity Theory (MPIT) has been used to study how individuals perceive the cultural differences and areas of connectedness that exist amongst members of a group. We all have an MPI, and that identity provides a lens that allows us to view the world through specific diversity perspectives (gender, socioeconomics, ability, etc.) One of the strategies for developing an MPI is to dialogue with colleagues about diversity factors and types of differences you have experienced in your personal and professional lives (Griffer & Perlis, 2007). Griffer and Perlis suggest that cultural perspectives can include social class, race, age, religion, ability/disability, gender, sexual orientation, ethnicity, and any other *difference that makes a difference* (2007).

A.R.T.: Diversity Consciousness

As a speech supervisor and staff development coordinator back in the 1980s, one of my responsibilities was to cowrite and implement a series of training sessions for the speech practitioners related to the district-wide bilingual initiatives. This was a wonderful opportunity to talk about diversity perspectives, which was much more global than the linguistic and ethnic differences which were more often the focus during training sessions. Our staff developers constructed an activity whereby each practitioner had to write descriptive phrases for five "cultural" areas that had shaped their life. Culture had a broad interpretation and included interests as well as influences. They were then asked to draw a symbol for each of the five areas, which became a beautiful *diversity mosaic* when they were all pieced together.

Cultural Sensitivity: Macro and Micro Cultures

Culture is a shared way of perceiving, believing, behaving, and evaluating (Goodenough, 1987). Culture has been described as having *macro and micro components* in each country. Macrocultural values are the values that help bind people together within a nation as a whole, but only the microcultural values can explain individual differences (Goldberg, 1997). When we think about cultural differences, we have a tendency to focus solely on micro features such as age, ethnicity, and exceptionality. However, macro values may also be at play. According to Gollnick and Chinn, the following are *macrocultural values* in the United States (1990): status (occupational, educational, and financial); work ethic and achievement (by individual efforts rather than inheritance); cleanliness; rights for self-governance; and health systems.

The terms *multicultural, intercultural, and cross-cultural* have all been used to describe approaches designed to meet the unique needs of students. Cross-cultural special education services is like a puzzle with three pieces: linguistic considerations, cultural considerations, and disability considerations (Echevarria Ratleff, 1989). All three pieces need to be addressed for an approach to be truly considered *cross-cultural*. Although it may be true that it took many years for racial and ethnic diversity issues to become an acknowledged factor in adjusting attitudes and methodologies surrounding clinical treatment, culture is now view from a much larger kaleidoscopic perspective—an experiential mosaic that benefits us all (Papir-Bernstein & Rosaly-Santos, 2004; Screen & Anderson, 1994).

Cultural sensitivity may be one of the most critical factors in establishing a professional relationship when practitioner and client are from differing cultural backgrounds.

One of the primary areas in our field to first emerge in the diversity spectrum was ethnic diversity in the early 1980s (Goldberg, 1997). Diversity is all too often exemplified by differences in gender, ability, race and religion—but we know better. *Collaborative consultation*, by definition, is an interactive process that enables people with diverse expertise to generate creative solutions to mutually defined problems. Therefore, diversity management is the art of discovering new skills, new perspectives, and accessing the greatest resource we have to offer: ourselves (Papir & Legrand, 1994).

REFLECTIVE SUMMATIVE QUESTIONS

1. Think about your *comfort/discomfort level* spending time with a person of a younger/older generation, other faith or race, other sexual orientation, other ability or disability, and different political orientation. What would need to change to enhance your comfort level?

2. What is your core and what is your flex as they relate to *your Cultural Intelligence*? What are the knots that can be shifted from core to flex?

3. Have you ever gone to school or worked with someone who acted in a way or said something that seemed unusual to you, and that you attributed to a *cultural difference*? What was it?

4. Describe the importance of incorporating *universal and transdisciplinary* elements into your speech therapy approach.

5. How would you explain your core values and beliefs as they relate to *curriculum* and its connection to the provision of speech and language therapy for school-aged students?

REFERENCES

Abdelal, A. M. (2013, November). *Neurocognitive seeds of racial and ethnic discrimination: It's all in the mind.* Presented at ASHA Convention, Chicago, IL.

Abdelal, A. (2016). Why the brain discriminates: Neurobiological underpinnings of racial/ethnic discrimination. In *Special Education and Communication Disorders Faculty Publications. Paper 11.* Available from http://vc.bridgew.edu/spec_commdis_fac/11

American Speech-Language-Hearing Association ASHA. (n.d.). *Common Core State Standards: A Resource for SLPs.* Retrieved June 13, 2015, from http://www.asha.org/SLP/schools/Common-Core-State-Standards/

American Speech-Language-Hearing Association ASHA. (n.d.). *School setting resource for SLPs working in the school setting.* Retrieved June 12, 2015, from http://www.asha.org/slp/schools/

American Speech-Language-Hearing Association (ASHA). (2010). Cultural competence checklist: Personal reflection. *Academic Medicine 78*(6), 560–569. Retrieved from http://www.asha.org/uploadedFiles/practice/multicultural/personal reflections.pdf and frameworks for evaluation.

Betancourt, J. R. (2003). Cross-cultural medical education: Conceptual approaches and frameworks for evaluation. *Academic Medicine, 78*(6), 560–569.

Blamire, J. (2000). *Science at a distance: Genotype and phenotype.* Retrieved August 17, 2016, from http://www.brooklyn.cuny.edu/bc/ahp/BioInfo/GP/Definition.html

Bloom, B.S., Engelhart, M. D., Furst, E. J., Hill, W. H., & Krathwohl, D. R (1956). *Taxonomy of educational objectives: The classification of educational goals. Handbook I: Cognitive domain.* New York, NY: David McKay.

Bogan, C.E., & English, M. J. (1994). *Benchmarking for best practices: Winning through innovative adaptation.* New York, NY: McGraw-Hill.

Borders, A., & Hennebry, K. A. (2015). Angry rumination moderates the association between perceived ethnic discrimination and risky behaviors. *Personality and Individual Differences, 79,* 81–86.

Boyer, E. L. (1995). *The basic school: A community for learning.* Princeton, NJ. The Carnegie Foundation for the Advancement of Teaching.

Brannen, S, J., Cooper, E. B., Dellegrotto, J. T., Disney, S. T., Eger, D. L., Ehren, B. J., . . . Secord, W. A. (2000). *Developing educationally relevant IEPs: A technical assistance document for speech-language pathologists.* ASHA Product Sales, 10801 Rockville Pike, Rockville, MD: American Speech-Language-Hearing Association.

Bronfenbrenner, U. (1979). *The ecology of human development.* Cambridge, MA: Harvard University Press.

Bronfenbrenner, U. (1993). The ecology of cognitive development: Research models and fugitive findings. In R. H. Wozniak & K. W. Fisher (Eds.), *Development in context: Acting and thinking in specific environments.* Hillsdale, NJ: Erlbaum.

Cech, M. (1991). *Globalchild: Multicultural resources for young children.* Boston, MA: Addison-Wesley.

Cheng, L. (2007). Cultural intelligence (CQ): A quest for cultural competence. *Communication Disorders Quarterly, 29*(1), 36–42.

Common Core State Standards (CCSS). (2016). Retrieved August 23, 2016 from http://www.corestandards.org

De Bary, W. T. (2007). *Confucian tradition and global education.* New York, NY: Columbia University Press.

Doig, E., Fleming, J., Cornwell, P. L., & Kuipers, P. (2009). Qualitative exploration of a client-centered, goal-directed approach to community-based occupational therapy for adults with traumatic brain injury. *American Journal of Occupational Therapy, 64,* 559–568.

Duchan, J. (2000, May). What would Mrs. Doasyouwouldbedoneby think of speech therapists in America? *Royal College Speech-Language Therapy Bulletin.* London, UK.

Dunst, C. J. (2013, June). *Efficiency of everyday activities as sources of early childhood intervention.* Paper presented at the Efficiency of Early Childhood Intervention Conference, Berlin, Germany.

Dunst, C. J., Bruder, M. B., Trivette, C. M., Hamby, D., Raab, M., & McLean, M. (2001). Characteristics and consequences of everyday natural learning opportunities. *Topics in Early Childhood Special Education, 21*, 68–92.

Dunst, C.J., Raab, M., & Trivette, C. M. (2011). Characteristics of naturalistic language intervention strategies. *Journal of Speech-Language Pathology and Applied Behavior Analysis, 5*(1), 8–16.

Earley, P. C., & Ang, S. (2003). *Cultural intelligence: Individual interactions across cultures.* Stanford, CA: Stanford University Press.

Echevarria Ratleff, J. (1989). *Instructional strategies for cross-cultural students with special education needs.* Sacramento, CA: RiSE.

EdFly Blog. (2013, June). *Common core fact of the day: Standards v. curriculum.* Retrieved September 2, 2016, from http://www.excelined.org/ 2013/06/03/common-core-fact-of-the-day-standards-v-curriculum/

Erickson, H.L. (2003). *Curriculum integration: Major trends and issues. Curriculum handbook.* Alexandria, VA: ASCD.

Erikson, L. (2008). *Stirring the head, heart and soul.* Thousand Oaks, CA: Corwin Press.

Frank, A. (1995). *The wounded storyteller.* Chicago, IL: University of Chicago Press.

Frattali, C. (Ed.) (1998). *Measuring outcomes in speech-language pathology.* New York, NY: Thieme.

Gardner, H. (1983). *Frames of mind: The theory of multiple intelligences.* New York, NY: Basic Books.

Girolametto, L., & Weitzman, E. (2006). It takes two to talk: The Hanen program for parents: Early language intervention through caregiver training. In R. J. McCauley & M. E. Fey (Eds.), *Treatment of language disorders in children* (pp. 77–103). Baltimore, MD: Brookes.

Goldberg, S. (1997). *Clinical skills for speech-language pathologists.* San Diego, CA: Singular.

Gollnick, D., & Chinn, P. (1990). *Multicultural education in a pluralist society.* New York, NY: Merill/Macmillian.

Goodenough, W. (1987). Multi-culturalism as the normal human experience. In E. M. Effy & W. L. Partridge (Eds.), *Applied anthropology in America.* New York, NY: Columbia University Press.

Goodlad, J. (2004). *A place called school.* New York, NY: McGraw-Hill.

Griffer, M. R. & Perlis, S. M. (2007). Developing cultural intelligence in preservice speech-language pathologists and educators. *Communication Disorders Quarterly, 29*(1), 28–35.

Hall, K. L., Vogel, A. L., Stipelman, B. A., Stokols, D., Morgan, G., & Gehlert, S. (2012). A four-phase model of transdisciplinary team-based research: Goals, team processes and strategies. *Translational Behavioral Medicine, 2*(4), 415–430.

Hart, B., & Risley, T. R. (1978). Promoting productive language through incidental teaching. *Education and Urban Society, 10*, 407–429.

Hasnain-Wynia, R. (2006). Is evidence-based medicine patient-centered and is patient centered care evidence-based? *Health Services Research, 41*(1), 1–8

Hattie, J. (2012). *Visible learning for teachers: Maximizing impact on learning.* New York, NY: Routledge.

Hill, N. E., & Witherspoon, D. W. (2011). Race, ethnicity, and social class. In M. Underwood & L. Rosen (Eds.), *Handbook on social development* (pp. 316–346). New York, NY: Guilford.

Horn, E., & Banerjee, R. (2009). Understanding curriculum modifications and embedded learning opportunities in the context of supporting all children's success. *Language, Speech, and Hearing Services in Schools, 40*, 406–415.

Inglebret, E., Banks-Joseph, S. R., & CHiXapkaid, E. (2016). Differentiated instruction: A culturally-congruent practice. *ASHA SIG Perspectives 14 Cultural and Linguistic Diversity, 1*, 43–55.

Kelly, A. V. (2009). *The curriculum: Theory and practice.* Newbury Park, CA: Sage.

Kinzler, K.D., & Spelke, E. (2011). Do infants show social preferences for people differing in race? *Cognition, 119*, 1–9.

Kneller, G. F. (1971). *Introduction to the philosophy of education.* Hoboken, NJ: John Wiley & Sons.

Lawrence-Brown, D (2004). Differentiated instruction: Inclusive strategies for standards-based learning that benefit the whole class. *American Secondary Education, 32*(3), 34–62.

Lesser E. (1999). *The new American spirituality.* New York, NY: Random House.

Levin, T., & Nevo, Y. (2009). Exploring teachers' views on learning and teaching in the context of a trans-disciplinary curriculum. *Journal of Curriculum Studies. 41*(4), 439–465.

MacDonald, J. (1989). *Becoming partners with children: From play to conversation.* San Antonio, TX: Special Press.

MacDonald, J,. & Gillette, Y. (1989). *ECOScales manual.* San Antonio, TX: Special Press.

McLean, J. E., & Snyder-Mclean, L. K. (1978). *A transactional approach to early language training: Derivation of a model system.* Columbus, OH: Charles E. Merrill.

McTaggart, L. (2008). *The field.* New York, NY: HarperCollins.

Merritt, D. D., & Culatta, B. (1998). *Language intervention in the classroom.* San Diego, CA: Singular.

Middleton, J. (2014). *Cultural intelligence (CQ): The competitive edge for leaders crossing borders.* New York, NY: Bloomsbury.

Moore, B. J., & Montgomery, J. K. (2008). *Making a difference for America's children: Speech-language pathologists in public schools.* Austin, TX: Pro-Ed.

Muma, J. R. (1978). *Language handbook: Concepts, assessment and intervention.* Englewood Cliffs, NJ: Prentice-Hall.

Nippold, M. A. (2011). Language intervention in the classroom: What it looks like. *Language, Speech, and Hearing Services in the Schools, 42,* 393–439

Norris, J. A. & Hoffman, P. R. (1990). Language intervention within naturalistic environments. *Language, Speech, and Hearing Services in Schools, 21,* 72–84.

Nunley, K. (2004). *Layered curriculum* (2nd ed.). Amherst, NH: Brains.org.

Papir-Bernstein, W. (Ed., 1992) *Activity-Based Language Experiences (ABLE).* New York, NY: NYCDOE Citywide Speech Services, D.75.

Papir-Bernstein, W., & Legrand, R. (1994, November) *Removing barriers: Creating diversity consciousness through self-regulatory process training.* Presented at ASHA Conference, New Orleans, LA.

Papir-Bernstein, W., & Rosaly-Santos, M. (2004). *Diversity training for providers of speech therapy.* NYC District 75: Citywide Speech Services Staff Development.

Pashler, H., McDaniel, M., Rohrer, D., & Bjork, R. A. (2008). Learning styles: Concepts and evidence. *Psychological Science in the Public Interest. 9*(3), 106–116.

Power-deFur, L., & Flynn, P. (2012). Unpacking the standards for intervention. *Perspectives on School-Based Issues, 13,* 11–16.

Quinn, P. C., Anzures, G., Lee, K., Pascalis, O., Slater, A., & Tanaka, J. W. (2013). On the developmental origins of differential responding to social category information. In M. R. Banaji & S. A. Gelman (Eds.), *Navigating the social world: What infants, children, and other species can teach us* (pp. 286–291). New York, NY: Oxford University Press.

Richter, L. (2004). *The importance of caregiver-child interactions for the survival and healthy development of young children: A review.* Geneva, Switzerland: World Health Organization, Department of Child and Adolescent Health and Development.

Ruitenberg, C. (Ed.). (2010). *What do philosophers of education do? And how do they do it?* New York, NY: Wiley-Blackwell.

Schraeder, T. (2013). *A guide to school services in speech-language pathology.* San Diego, CA: Plural.

Schwaller de Lubicz, R. A. (1985). *The Egyptian miracle: An introduction to the wisdom of the temple.* New York, NY: Inner Traditions.

Screen, R., & Anderson, N. (1994). *Multicultural perspectives in communication disorders.* San Diego, CA: Singular Publishing Group.

Simmons-Mackie, N., & Damico, J. (1999). Qualitative methods in aphasia research: Ethnography. *Aphasiology, 13,* 681–688.

Tharp, R., & Gallimore, R. (1988). *Rousing minds to life: Teaching, learning, and schooling in social context.* Cambridge. UK: Cambridge University Press.

Threats, T. (2016). *Overview of the WHO ICF.* ASHA Ad Hoc Committee on the ICF. Retrieved August 24, 2016, from http://www.asha.org/slp/icf/

Tomlinson, C.A. (1999). Mapping a route toward a differentiated instruction. *Educational Leadership, 57*(1), 12.

Tomlinson, C. A. (2014). *The differentiated classroom: Responding to the needs of all learners.* Alexandria, VA: ASCD.

Tomlinson, C. A., & McTighe, J. (2006). *Integrating differentiated instruction and understanding by design.* Alexandria, VA: ASCD

Torres, I. (2015). How to recognize your cultural competence. *The ASHA Leader, 20,* 6–7.

United States Department of Education. (2004). *Individuals With Disabilities Education Improvement Act (IDEA) of 2004.* Retrieved June 2, 2015, from http://idea.ed.gov

Varner, I., & Beamer, L. (1995). *Intercultural communication in the global workplace.* Chicago, IL: Irwin.

Visintin, R. (2013a, March). *Connecting with the curriculum.* Retrieved August 1, 2016, from http://blog.asha.org/author/rvisintin/

Visintin, R. (2013b, May). *Believe it or not: The Common Core Standards can make your job easier.* Retrieved August 1, 2016, from http://blog.asha.org/author/rvisintin/

Wallach, G. P. (2014). Improving clinical practice: A school-age and school-based perspective. *Language, Speech, and Hearing Services in Schools, 45,* 127–136.

Wexler, B. (2006). *Brain and culture: Neurobiology and social change.* Cambridge, MA: MIT Press.

Wiig, E. H., & Semel, E. M. (1976). *Language disabilities in children and adolescents.* Columbus, OH: Charles E. Merrill.

Wiles, J. (2009). *Leading curriculum development.* Thousand Oaks, CA: Corwin Press.

Wiles, J., & Bondi, J. (2007). *Curriculum development: A guide to practice.* Upper Saddle River, NJ: Prentice Hall.

World Health Organization (WHO): Primary Care. (2008) *Now more than ever.* Geneva, Switzerland: Author. Retrieved from http://www.who.int/whr/2008/whr08_en.pdf

CHAPTER 13

Working in Community

1. PERSON-CENTERED CARE (PCC)

What Comprises Person-Centered Care?

Person-centered care (PCC), far from being a new concept, evolved from the work of Carl Rogers, and values the knowledge, experience, autonomy, and competence of the client with regard to decision-making and problem solving (DiLollo & Favreau, 2010; Rogers, 1942). It is one of the earliest references to the importance of *working in community with the client*. The PCC, used in a variety of fields, has been associated with increased perception of and satisfaction with quality of care. The following behaviors have been described as indicators of the provision of PCC (DiLollo, 2010): indicating interest, expressing approval, giving choices, assessing client comfort, showing empathy, asking permission, maintaining appropriate physical contact, proximity, and eye contact, and treating the client as an equal partner with shared "power."

Over the last few years, reference has been made to the decreased public confidence in the professions disciplines within the educational and health-care industries. DiLollo calls this "crisis of professional confidence" one symptom that calls for the need for greater *person-centered rather than task-centered ther-*

apy (2010). In order to make this shift, we would need to transform our focus from *what we know* to *how we perform*, from "*professional knowledge* to *artistry of practice*" (p. 85). According to the National Academy of Sciences, care is considered "patient-centered" when the following conditions are present: it is respectful of and responsive to individual needs and preferences, it ensures that client values guide clinical decisions, and it encompasses qualities of empathy and compassion (Erdman, 2013).

The Goals of PCC

The goals for this type of care include attitudes of respect of the person with emphasis on empowerment and participation in everyday life. The person is viewed as "the expert" on his or her own condition. The question to ask your client is, "What matters to you?" *Shared decision-making (SDM)* is a component of a client-centered approach. Client participation is encouraged, as we express our appreciation of the client's responsibility to play an active role in decision-making. We offer choices, and discuss the benefits (Erdman, 2013).

PCC relates to *quality of life issues* and functional outcomes. The World Health Organization suggests measuring quality of life using scales, inventories and questionnaires (WHO, 2008). Questions to school-aged children might include the following (Moore & Montgomery, 2008):

1. Are you happy when you come to school?
2. Are you able to get what you need?
3. Do you have friends who you can talk with easily?
4. Do you have hobbies to do when you go home?

Client-Directed Planning

Ultimately, clients (patients and students) must feel empowered to put in the work and get the best outcomes from treatment. Although this means that they need to be drivers in their own treatment, they begin the process looking for us to have the answers. We are simply the guide, and at our best when we become client-directed rather than treatment-directed (Preston, 2015). One of our most important roles is to show our clients how to *assume responsibility* for their own choices and changes (Van Riper, 1978). As client-directed professionals, we must draw on the tenets of counseling, along with all of our other knowledge arenas. A meta-analysis published in the *Journal of Consulting and Clinical Psychology* addressed the importance of the practitioners' ability to create a *supportive, working alliance* with their clients. To do so, we need to consider three core elements: a *positive bond*, a *joint agreement on goals*, and a *team approach* (Martin, Garske, & Davis, 2000; Preston, 2015;).

How is a *positive bond* achieved? One of the first steps is the creation of what Diane Kendall calls "unconditional regard" from the clinician toward the client (Kendall, 2000). This attitude of *unconditional regard* will enable the client to discuss all aspects of the communication issue. It comes from the understanding that the greatest wisdom resides within the clients because they know their communication disorder better than anyone else (Donaher & Richels, 2012). When we listen closely, the client reveals everything that we need to know in order to facilitate change. In order to tap into this wisdom, we need to practice focused listening and withholding judgment (Ciccia, 2011).

The work we do is sometimes referred to as *identity-based* when we take into account what our clients think about themselves, their accomplishments, their abilities, their disabilities, and their future (Duchan, 2003). This type of interaction includes person-centered planning, personal narratives, and work toward social inclusion. *Person-centered planning* is an empowering approach that focuses on people and their needs, rather than the systems that function around them (Simpson, O'Brien, & Towell, 2013). It serves to promote their inclusion in schools, communities, and society during all phases of their lives. The term originated with a social rather than a medical model, and involves a toolbox of methods and resources that enable people to choose their own pathways leading to active participation.

Person-centered planning provides the client with a context for exploring personal identity. The practitioner is responsive, yet low-keyed, whereas the client is empowered and actively engaged. The dialogue is symmetric, and the intervention is connected to the client's identity and personal preferences. The client's voice about life expectations and experiences becomes a primary vehicle for gathering information (Duchan, 2003; Wells & Sheehay, 2012).

We need to critically examine our own perspectives about the role our everyday practices play in therapeutic outcomes. In order to accomplish this, we operate simultaneously on a *macro- and microlevel*, consistently adjusting the scope of our lens to examine our own perspectives and those of our clients as reflected within our work routines.

Ylvisaker's research reminds us to question our belief, philosophy, and involvement with person-centered outcomes and *client collaboration* (O'Brien & Krause, 2014; Ylvisaker et al., 2007). Although much of his research targeted individuals with traumatic brain injury (TBI), the philosophy of his approach is applicable to all clients as it pertains to a core belief in *the competence and agency* of the individuals with whom we work. When we experience a client as "noncompliant," we are actually viewing the difficulty the client is having with that particular intervention approach (Ylvisaker & Feeney, 2000). We need to work in cooperation with our clients.

It is often best to target intervention to the goals of the client within their life's context. Ylvisaker recommends goal identification with a *GOPDR framework*: goal, obstacle, plan, do, and review (O'Brien & Krause, 2014; Ylvisaker, 2006). The framework consists of:

- *Goal:* the clients describe what they want to improve and accomplish
- *Obstacle:* what might be blocking their achievement
- *Plan:* how they will accomplish their goal
- *Do:* practice under controlled and functional conditions
- *Review:* what is working, not working, and what changes need to be implemented

Self-selection of goals can and should be supported by the practitioner. When we involve clients in the selection of their own goals and objectives, meaningfulness and motivation are present and become naturally embedded into the therapeutic continuum (O'Brien & Krause, 2014). This type of approach also improves client's experience of empowerment and decision-making through the power of choice and control (French & Swain, 2001).

Personal and Situational Interests

In Chapter 10, we discussed the importance of choosing materials and activities that match the student's interests. Young children's personal and situational interests have been studied in relationship to language and literacy learning experiences. *Personal interests* include a child's topical likes and preferences, whereas *situational interests* refer to the persons, objects, and activities that evoke prolonged child attention and engagement. Children's interests are one set of factors that have been shown to contribute to literacy and language learning (Dunst, Trivette, & Masiello, 2011; Raab, Dunst, Johnson, & Hamby, 2013).

The most common measures of child interest are parent surveys, practitioner observations, parent interviews, and child interviews (Dunst, Jones, Johnson, Raab, & Hamby, 2011). There are a number of methods and procedures for identifying everyday activities that can be used as sources of interest-based literacy and language learning opportunities. Appendix B is one sample of an Interest Inventory that has been field tested with a variety of school-aged students with varying degrees of disabilities (Papir-Bernstein, 1992). Based on research and practice on everyday interest-based child learning opportunities, optimal benefits can more likely be facilitated when there is a match between children's interests and the activities used as sources of interest-based child learning opportunities (Dunst et al., 2011a, 2011b).

A second set of factors that have been shown to contribute to the language acquisition of young children are characteristics of a responsive interactional style. The style of interaction has been studied in parents, and applied to intervention as part of a naturalistic approach called *responsive teaching*. The six sets of behaviors that have been studied are (Dunst et al., 2011a; Raab et al., 2013; Raab & Dunst, 2009):

1. Sensitivity to a child's behavioral initiations
2. Interpreting a child's behavior as intents to communicate

3. Following a child's lead, shifting focus and engaging in joint attention
4. Responding to a child's behavior promptly, supportively and appropriately
5. Engaging in turn-taking and reciprocal interactions
6. Encouraging child expansions and elaborations by asking questions, repeating what they have said, or adding information

Clinician-Centered Therapy

Although this chapter discusses PCC, it is important to remember that clinician-centered therapy does still occur and continues to serve a purpose and, therefore, be researched. It involves interactions in which the clinician exerts control over therapeutic interactions so that the specific goals of therapy will be addressed. These types of clinician-centered interactions may appear to be characterized by *interactional asymmetry* or therapist dominance, and appear in the following formats (Simmons-Mackie & Damico, 2011):

- Controlling turns
- Requesting known information
- Performance evaluation
- Uneven talk ratios
- Controlling content and topic choices
- Controlling interpretation of meaning
- Choosing materials and activities
- Uneven shared information

This approach to therapy becomes valuable and is used most frequently when creating a learning sequence, described as *request-response-evaluation (RRE)*, or *stimulus-response-contingency (SRC)*. An RRE focuses on the discourse, involving the therapist's request for some performance, client compliance with the request, and the evaluation of the performance by the therapist (Simmons-Mackie & Damico, 2011). A SRC is similar, but focuses more on

the behavioral aspects of the sequence. It is easiest to understand by starting with the R, the response or behavior we are attempting to elicit from the client. The S is everything that comes before the R, all that we are, do, and use to facilitate the response. And the C is everything that happens after the response that ensures that response will continue or be corrected.

The Whole Person

Person-centered care is an approach that focuses on the *whole person*. In the introduction to Galland's book about integrated medicine and as he begins to describe the best use of conventional and alternative approaches, he juxtapositions art restoration with medical care (1997). *Restauro* is an art restoration studio in Florence that models best practices in the following way. The senior member of the restoration team has knowledge about the "whole patient," or the work to be restored. This knowledge includes unique attributes of each work as it has changed over time, and science is a tool that helps the team uncover these unique attributes. Florentine restorers rely on scientific techniques to gather information about the patient's state of health, with the knowledge that every fresco is different, with different problems that require different solutions.

The UK Royal College of General Practitioners report (McWhinney & Freeman, 2009) defines *whole-istic care* as seeing the person as a whole in context and using this perspective as part of one's therapeutic approach. The therapeutic approach is defined by the principle of person-centered decision making which recognizes that health is a resource for living and not an end in itself (Reeve, Irving, & Dowrick, 2011). It emphasizes the importance of integrating multiple sources of knowledge in a dynamic exploration of the individual's experience (Reeve et al., 2013). The patient is viewed as an *active partner rather than a passive recipient* of the treatment. The practitioner monitors the treatment through personal reflections that support an analysis of judgments and decisions. This type of clinical approach is sometimes called *integrative practice*, whereby integration is the process of bringing parts together into a renewed whole. *Integrative practice* addresses the whole person within an environment—mind, body, spirit, heart, and soul. It emphasizes the therapeutic relationship, whereby the client and practitioner are partners in the process (Finley, 2015).

In psychotherapy, reference has been made to qualities that support the co-creative aspects of therapy as "performance of practice" (Wilson, 2007). The term does not infer something false or inauthentic, but rather the recognition that we alter our performance to best fit with our clients' needs. It is a *dynamic play*, much the same way that no two performances of the same show will ever be the same. We all have complex roles, must attend to, and reflect upon features of our practice that keep it alive and flowing.

Medical generalism, or expertise in whole person medicine, is a professional philosophy of practice rather than an evidence-based model of care, and thus calls for implementation of practice-based procedures (McWhinney & Freeman, 2009). The importance of generalist practice is seen as one solution and provides a robust alternative to managing the current problems facing education, as well as health care. Doing more of the same and trying harder is not always the answer; sometimes we need to consider concept redesign and think differently when we ponder models of care (Reeve et al., 2013). The World Health Organization (WHO) has refocused health care and changed the focus of clinical practice from condition to individual, in line with the People First initiative (World Health Organization, 2008).

People First

This renewed focus on the person rather than the disability was reflected in the name change of laws governing education. In 1975, the Education for All Handicapped Children Act (EAHCA) was put into place, initiating the special education system that is still operational. The 1990 revisions to this original act came with a new name, the Individuals with Disabilities Education Act (IDEA), and reflected a new awareness of "people first" (Moore & Montgomery, 2008).

The guiding principle for *people first language* is to maintain the integrity of individuals as human beings (American Psychological Association, 2001). We are to try to avoid using language that has negative overtones (such as a "stroke victim"), sounds judgmental or like a slur (such as "a cripple"), or that equates a person with their condition (such as "the disabled" or "the stutterer"). Descriptions should remain neutral, such as, "a person with . . . ," "a child who has . . . ," or "a woman who uses . . . " (Moore & Montgomery, 2008). That is an important principle when implementing PCC.

2. THE THERAPEUTIC ALLIANCE

The Therapeutic Relationship

One of the aspects of humanity throughout the ages that has guaranteed our survival in harsh evolutionary environments is our desire to cooperate, be with, and look after each other (Fourie, 2011). Fundamental to human survival is to connect and be in relationship with others. A cooperative therapeutic alliance is the underpinning of all effective helping (Clarkson, 2003).

Research supports the claim that central to effective therapy is the importance of relational dimensions. Therapeutic factors about relationships in speech and language therapy have been studied and framed from psycholinguistic, behavioral, and neurological perspectives (Finlay, 2015; Fourie, 2009). The following three components facilitate a therapeutic alliance: agreement about goals, consensus about the content and processes of therapy, and a positive bond (Markin, 2014). There must be a mutual understanding about the nature of therapy, as well as a shared motivation to build and nurture the relationship.

An important aspect of counseling within any field is the development of an effective therapeutic relationship. A client-centered therapeutic focus is more easily facilitated when the SLP follows and reflects clients' emotional responses. We know how tempting it is for the SLP and/or the client to fall into the position of thinking of the SLP as always the "expert"; however, research and experience both teach us differently. Research from *humanistic theory* (Maslow, 1962; Rogers, 1951) suggests that clients' self-discovery and self-actualization is best accomplished when clinicians *listen rather than prescribe* (Luterman, 2008).

A relational approach to therapy reinforces the presence of the practitioner, the client, and something that Finlay calls the *"between"*—that mysterious, sacred space that is impacted in often unseen ways (2015). The relationship is a collaborative partnership and both people contribute to this joint enterprise. In the therapeutic relationship, we are present as a human being first and a practitioner second, as we move fluently between the three spaces (Finlay, 2015; Spinelli, 2015).

It has been proposed that concepts from *systems theory* may present some illumination when used as analytical tools for understanding relationships with family members and other professionals as well as with clients (Stone, 1992). Systems theory was discussed

in Chapter 9, but let us see how it can be applied to relationships within our work setting. Stone describes some basic concepts that can be applied to our work:

1. All participants in the relationship are *interdependent*. What affects one will affect the other, but not necessarily in the same way.

2. Interactions are *shaped and maintained* by all participants in the relationship, and should be viewed as circular (reflecting multiple sources of influence) rather than linear (cause and effect).

3. Relationships have *expectations or rules* based upon roles and patterns of behavior. Rules are not necessarily explicit.

4. Familiarity and routines are comfortable, whereas *rule violation and change* are perceived as stressful.

5. Relationships are components of and affected by larger systems

According to systems theory, well-functioning relationships support the growth of the participants, are characterized by a respect for diverse feelings and beliefs, and contain clear and appropriate roles and rules. The types of relationships that speech-language pathologists found helpful for clinical intervention and service delivery were described as those that stayed within boundaries. *Boundaries* create an empowering and supportive context for the clients and practitioner through mutual respect and shared power base, which is discussed a bit later in this chapter (Stone, 1992; Stone & Olswang, 1989).

Becoming a "systems thinker" does not happen overnight, but systems concepts can be helpful tools for analyzing and resolving relationship problems. It is a process that challenges how we think about ourselves and about our relationships with others. That is not an easy road, but one well worth exploring.

What Is the Therapeutic Alliance?

Psychotherapy researchers and practitioners have postulated that the "therapeutic alliance," defined as the collaborative and affective bond between therapist and patient, is an essential component of the therapeutic process. Theorists and practitioners have used various terms to describe different aspects of the relationship between a therapist and a patient, such as *therapeutic alliance, working alliance, therapeutic bond,* and *helping alliance* (Martin et al., 2000). Although there may be differences among the various alliance conceptualizations, most theoretical definitions of the alliance have three themes in common: (a) the collaborative nature of the relationship, (b) the affective bond between patient and therapist, and (c) the patient and therapist's ability to agree on treatment goals and tasks (Horvath & Symonds, 1991). The therapeutic alliance affirms the presence of community.

One of the reasons that the alliance has grown in significance is a consistent finding that the quality of the alliance is related to subsequent therapeutic outcome (Horvath & Symonds, 1991). Some researchers have looked for common factors across therapies that can explain therapeutic outcomes and several have begun to conceptualize that alliance as a common factor across therapeutic disciplines; some have even begun to argue that the quality of the alliance is more important than the type of treatment in predicting positive therapeutic outcomes (Safran & Muran, 1995).

What is evident from this review is that the strength of the alliance is predictive of outcomes. The implications of this finding are clear: because patients tend to view the alliance consistently throughout treatment, they are more likely to view the alliance as positive at termination if their initial assessment was positive. Thus, therapists must be effective at establishing positive alliances with their patients early in the therapy process (Martin et al., 2000).

There is little question that components of a therapeutic alliance are both valued by clients and experienced as essential for facilitating positive outcomes of speech and language therapy programs. The personal meanings and experiences within the therapeutic relationship have been shown to be impacted by therapeutic attitudes and qualities such as being understanding, gracious, and inspiring, as well as by therapeutic behaviors and actions such as being confident, soothing, practical, and empowering (Fourie, 2009). How do we cultivate meaningful relationships and working alliances we form with our clients, and how are these relationships perceived by our clients? The methodology most often used to research questions involves qualitative interviews and a methodology called grounded theory (Charmaz, 2006). These systems of measurement were discussed more fully in Chapter 11.

As practitioners, our treatment procedures must focus on two issues: the impairment or disability itself, and its impact on the life of our client (Fourie, 2009). The level of participation in specific activities may be restricted, or the client's perception of need for restriction in general life situations may be a function of subjective and existential overlays, resulting from the communication disorder (Fourie, 2009; WHO, 2002). Therefore, the measureable aspects of the impairment may not necessary match how the individual responds and adjusts to a communication disorder within their life. That is where we come in, to help a client adjust and construct personal meaning in response to these challenges (Luterman, 2003, 2008; Spillers, 2007).

The term *rapport* is often used as an alternative for therapeutic alliance, defined as a collaborative and trusting relationship between client and clinician (Frank & Frank, 1993; Terell, Rentschler, & Osborne, 2013). In a survey taken from the field of psychotherapy, clients rated *the working alliance* within the therapeutic relationship as the largest contributor to their own clinical outcomes (Levitt, 2011). Similar research in our own field found that clients who stuttered highly valued a caring therapeutic alliance that facilitated "client participation and agency" (Plexico, Manning, & DiLollo, 2010). *Client agency* was discussed in greater detail in Chapter 7's section on *understanding change*.

One of the biggest obstacles to the establishment of therapeutic alliance is *value imposition*, often related to cultural differences and imposed by the clinician unknowingly. In Levitt's 2011 study, she talks about principles for "wise" clinical practice, and includes:

- Approaching each client with curiosity and humility
- Accepting your own uncertainty about treatment
- Deferring to client values, unless those values were thought to impede productive change
- Helping clients become "agentic" by learning to value their own needs over the needs of the clinician

A Therapeutic Presence

The therapeutic relationship is essential to positive outcomes. *Therapeutic presence* is defined as the state of having one's whole self in the encounter with a client by being completely in the moment on a multiplicity of levels: physically, cognitively, emotionally, and spiritually. Therapeutic presence is not a replacement for anything, but rather a foundational stance that supports deep reflective listening to and understanding of the client (Geller & Greenberg, 2012)

When we use the term therapeutic presence, we tend to focus on the *importance of empathy* and the general tone of relationship with clients and caregivers. As we relate more empathically, we become more attuned to the extent that our presence leads to satisfying and successful clinical service that increases our potential to help others live more meaningful and joyous lives (Silverman, 2008). In addition, we feel a greater sense of professional utility and value, and reduce the likelihood of professional fatigue and burnout.

A therapeutic presence that is welcoming and healing can be communicated through grooming, posture, attire, use of personal space, eye contact, attention, physical touch, rate of speech, tone, and intensity of voice and silence (Silverman, 2008). It is also expressed through whole communication.

Sacred Moments

In the fields of psychology and psychiatry, *the therapeutic alliance* is one of the best-researched and most helpful dimensions of the therapeutic relationship. The term *sacred* has been used to describe moments of intense connection between practitioner and client that may facilitate powerful transformation for the practitioner, for the client, and within the therapeutic relationship (Allen, 2014; Pargament, Lomax, McGee, & Qijuan, 2014). These types of moments have been described as involving authenticity, representing a shared experience, containing spontaneity, and carrying the personal signature of the practitioner that extends beyond the everyday routines (Allen, 2014; Stern, 2004).

A.R.T.: Sacred Moments

The first time I heard the word *sacred* used to describe an aspect of our work

was with regard to rapport, and the impact it has on our relationships. It happened to be during a fluency presentation many years ago, and the name of the presenter is a bit fuzzy. I do however remember my goose bumps when he spoke of *the sacred space* with invisible boundaries that existed between the clinician and the client. He described it as something almost magical—but once violated, would disappear quickly.

Sacred moments have been an ongoing part of my work experiences. They are embedded in my cognitive library of tacit knowledge, and have been shared with practitioners I have supervised and students I have taught. They comprise the A.R.T. *narratives* of this textbook.

Pargament and colleagues suggest that one key element of an effective *therapeutic alliance* may involve the *spiritual character* of the relationship between the practitioner and client (2014). In Chapter 3, we discussed spirituality, and the fact that it is more commonly attributed to describing dimensions of individuality rather that to helping us understand and experience relationships. For the purpose of discussions of spirituality in the helping professions, we focus on the universality rather than the religiosity of the term. The same is true of the term *sacred*, which is used in the psychological rather than a theological sense.

There is, however, a growing body of evidence linking *spirituality* to the practitioners capacity to be interpersonally *attuned* to the client, *mindful* of the client's needs, and *reflective* about ones own beliefs and actions (Hernandez & Mahoney, 2012; Spillers, 2011). *Sacred* refers to human perceptions of qualities (such as interconnectedness and boundlessness) and emotions (such as awe, humility, and serenity) that reflect on human character

and may include the following types of experiences (Pergament et al., 2014):

- *Transcendence:* experiences that are perceived to be set apart for the everyday and ordinary
- *Ultimacy:* experiences of deep truth, perceived to be "really real"
- *Boundlessness:* experiences perceived as beyond the limits or ordinary time and space
- *Interconnectedness:* perceptions of deep mutual understanding and caring
- *Emotions:* such as uplift, awe, humility, mystery, joy, and serenity

Sacred moments can occur in all kinds of relationships, including helping relationships, and are not limited to extraordinary encounters (Hernandez & Mahoney, 2012). Sacred experiences can serve as a vast resource for people by fostering the capacity to sooth, empower, and inspire. Perceptions of sacredness can add to feelings of connectedness with a larger community (Pargament et al., 2014).

Whole Communication

Therapeutic presence expressed through communication involves entering the experience of others as if we were the other person, if only for the moment. This is a type of *experiential intimacy*, which requires perspective shifting (Shapiro & Moses, 2005). When ideas are exchanged or instruction is offered, there is a flow from person to person and a *shared reality*.

As we all work with people, our work must also intersect with social change, community, empowerment, and the integration of the mind, body and spirit of individuals (Slattery, 2013). In his preface, Slattery talks about Thich Nhat Hanh and his movement, known as engaged Buddhism, which reviews precepts about the process of *mindfulness*, discussed in Chapter 5 (2013). Nhat Hanh is a global spiritual leader, poet, and peace activist, and one of the best known and most respected Zen masters in the world today. His percepts are as follows:

- All systems of thought are guidelines, not absolutes.
- Your knowledge is always changing, so avoid being absolute and narrow-minded.
- Learn and practice non-attachment from views in order to be open to receive others' viewpoints.
- Truth is found in life and not just conceptual knowledge.
- Learn through your entire life by observing in yourself and in the world at all times (Nhat Hanh, 2013).

Through communication we represent our best selves. Effective communication is as important to our well-being and happiness as food and water is to our bodies (Nhat Hanh, 2013). One of our tools for effective communication is mindfulness, which requires letting go of judgment and bringing your full attention to what is in you and around you. *Mindfulness* was discussed as a principle of practice in Chapter 5 when we reviewed counsel and care.

Strength Perspectives

Researchers have explored *client strengths* as they affect therapeutic change and increase motivation, cooperative efforts, and acceptance of the need for change. This *strength perspective* has been used in counseling to promote human growth and maximize potential and is supported by the positive psychology movement in the pursuit of optimal human functioning (Lopez, 2008).

Strength-based therapeutic approaches always begin with creating the therapeutic alliance. They then proceed to identifying strengths, facilitating empowerment, and instilling resilience (Scheel, Davis, & Henderson, 2012).

One model described consists of four phases of promoting character strengths and virtues as an important component of the therapeutic process (Wong, 2006). The four phases included *making explicit* or the identification of existing client strengths; *envisioning* or the identification of areas for future development so that goals and objectives can be achieved (goal-setting); *empowering* or the encouragement of positive efforts and amplification of strengths; and *evolving* or the summarization and feedback of gains and outcomes, and generalization to contexts outside of therapy.

Therapeutic Qualities and Actions

In research that studied adults with acquired communication disorders, grounded theory was used to code and group the qualitative interview data collected (to be discussed more fully in Chapter 15) (Fourie, 2009). *Therapeutic qualities and therapeutic actions were described*, and the relationship between the two formed a theory of *Restorative (actions) Poise (qualities)*. *Therapeutic qualities* refer to *values and cognitive/emotional states*, whereas *therapeutic actions* refer to the manner in which therapy was conducted. Of course, this information was collected from client response to questions, and therefore it is all with reference to *client perception*.

Therapeutic qualities (TQ) included (Fourie, 2009):

1. *Being understanding* was represented as having patience, interest, compassion, and really listening. This quality was especially important for addressing alienation, loneliness and other existential issues talked about in Chapter 5.
2. *Being gracious* was represented as being courteous, nice, respectful, kind, and

benevolent. Graciousness was especially related to giving clients enough time.

3. *Being erudite* was represented as being knowledgeable, resourceful, facilitative of reflection, giving feedback, and self-reflective and evaluative. One important factor in this category was the ease of knowledge transfer.

4. *Being inspiring* was represented as being enthusiastic, motivational, relevant, and stimulating. This quality also helped steer clients away from their existential sense of alienation and isolation.

Therapeutic Actions (TA) included (Fourie, 2009):

1. *Being confident* was represented as taking charge, self-assured, truthful, committed, energetic, and enthusiastic. Confidence helped create a sense of safety for the clients.

2. *Being soothing* was represented as being relaxed, calming, peaceful, non-punitive, effective, and non-defensive. This action helped clients feel at ease.

3. *Being practical* was represented as being pragmatic, relevant, efficient, flexible, and on the right level. Practicality facilitated resourceful and creative actions.

4. *Being empowering* was represented as facilitating autonomy, independence, confidence, rebalancing power dynamics, providing choices. Empowerment re-establishes client control and personal power.

As practitioners, we must consider how we can best contribute to a therapeutic relationship and thus reflect upon how therapy is conducted. Fourie's descriptors in the areas of TQ and TA provide for us an exploratory framework for reflecting on principles of practice as well as the importance of cultivating specific clinical behaviors and therapeutic attitudes.

3. COLLABORATIONS AND TEAMWORK

Social Learning

One of the central ideas in Buddhism is that all things exist only in relationship to each other, as a vast *flow of events* that are linked together and participate with one another. This is sometimes referred to as *mutual causality* (Ricard & Thuan, 2001). It infers another concept, that of *interdependence*, meaning that all things and relationships have a type of continuity, coexistence, and contain elements that are mutually dependent. That helps us understand the power of collaboration, and the fact that something changes only when something else changes.

Social learning focuses on learning in social settings through relationship to others, practice settings, and actual situations of practice through observation and authentic participation in communities of practice (Harris, 2011). Major sources of learning evolve from socializing experiences, social role models, collaboration with peers, and direct engagement with the beliefs, roles, and culture of the environment (Wilkerson & Irby, 1998). These experiences allow us as learners to self-regulate, self-assess, self-reflect, and begin to develop perceptions about self-efficacy.

Social learning was described by Vygotsky through his description of the zone of proximal development (ZPD) (1978). The ZPD is a space where aspiring professionals observe and interact with more experienced practitioners. It is a place where they practice, receive feedback, and reflect on their performance (Harris, 2011). Through this type of learning, we develop knowledge and skills about the context, processes and values of professional practice through controlled observation, coaching, practice, and feedback.

As we discussed in Chapter 7, self-efficacy will impact what we choose to do, how much effort, and for how long we invest in our activities (Harris, 2011). Bandura (1986) emphasized that there are four sources of information that contribute to perceptions of self-efficacy:

1. Vicarious experiences of observing others they perceive to be like themselves and who perform effectively;
2. Perceptions of performance achievement during observations of master practitioners;
3. Authentic feedback that is received;
4. Physiological state, specifically their level of tension.

Kaufman and Mann recommend the following strategies for maximizing social learning (2007): develop clear objectives and desired outcomes, provide opportunities for vicarious experiences through modeling and demonstrations, provide opportunities for guided practice with feedback, and provide opportunities to reflect on development of new strategies and approaches to problem solving.

Why Do We Need to Collaborate?

With the implementation of state standards, we are now integrated into the classroom culture as we provide speech therapy services that are academically relevant. We are working as a collaborative team with the student, teachers, and families. This facilitates a diversity of perspectives for creating supports and accommodations (Zurawski, 2015).

In our last chapter, we talked about how collaboration with classroom staff drives the team of professionals to determine appropriate strategies and accommodations for students, keeping in mind what would best match specific needs of students with educational impact for our services (Mount, 2014). Moving out of

our professional "silos" provides opportunities to improve *interprofessional practice outcomes* as we coordinate services and learn from one another (Pickering & Embry, 2013).

Collaboration and collaborative service delivery allows us to implement our services within the more "naturalistic" classroom environment, and take advantage of the expertise that we can only do by crossing through the boundaries of individual perspectives and lines of professional disciplines. Service delivery now demands that we partner with other professionals and engage in interprofessional collaborations for more integrated intervention formats. The issue to ponder is how we can enhance the scope of those collaborations as we strengthen the relationships within.

Challenges of Collaborative Classroom Practices

Collaborative service delivery, although having many benefits, does come with its challenges. One area of challenge concerns training and implementation. Coursework tends to be discipline specific (as does our thinking), and there is limited opportunity for interprofessional collaborations during our training. Team-based service delivery is far from a new concept within our educational speech therapy programs, however we need our mentors, administrators, and supervisors to model, enable, and support it by (Pickering & Embry, 2013):

- Learning from one another and sharing skills
- Not functioning within a knowledge-based or political hierarchy
- Understanding that student needs are not always discipline-specific
- Emphasizing consensus-building within team interactions
- Being willing to respect yet blur professional boundaries for the sake of teamwork

A second pervasive *area of challenge* concerns comfort zones, egos, and belief systems on the part of all players: students, practitioners, paraprofessionals, teachers, administrators and parents (Kaufman, Braswell, Cohen, & Papir-Bernstein, 1995; Mount, 2014; Papir-Bernstein, Braswell, Kaufman, & Magnante, 1995). *Students* may be more accustomed to being pulled out for services, and *practitioners* may be outside of their "sole expert" comfort zones. They are also working in somebody else's space, and may feel "intrusive" or uncertain of classroom procedures. *Teachers* are used to feeling a sense of knowledge and control within their classrooms, and may not want to share resources and teaching techniques for fear of criticism or lack of confidence. *Parents* are uncertain or skeptical about the benefits, and may only be familiar with the more traditional pull-out model of service delivery. They sometimes see isolated services as "more and better." *Paraprofessionals* have been known to take a back seat in the classroom routines, as they may view your role as "teacher's helper" replacing the necessity of their presence. Some *administrators* are more comfortable viewing collaboration as an "all of nothing" process, and thus try to mandate that all services take that format rather than pulling students out of the classroom. We all tend to fear the unknown, and take comfort in the familiar. And so it goes . . .

A.R.T.: Classroom Collaboration Is Not "Push-In"

When we talk about models of service delivery, the traditional model was termed "pull-out," so it seemed logical to coin the term "push-in" for the *other predominant type* of service delivery (collaborative and classroom-based). If we want the service to succeed, we cannot refer to it as "push-in" because that terminology defines the service at it worst—is there any one who would choose to be pushy and intrusive, or be pushed in on? Would any professional think of those as favorable characteristics of a person or an activity? Pushback on using push-in . . .

A third area of challenge is our ongoing preoccupation with individualization, individual efforts, and rewarding individual as opposed to group achievement sometimes to the exclusion of adult collaborations and group activity. Perhaps we are finally ready to move from the *age of the individual to the era of community* and focus on shared work, partnerships of knowledge, dynamics of mutuality, and communities of common thought (John-Steiner, 2006).

Key Principles of Social Influence

Ultimately, the success of our collaborative efforts will depend largely on our persuasive abilities to "sell" the idea of working together. Not everyone will be open to that idea, and we can learn about *theories of influence* as researched within the fields of psychology and marketing. Cialdini identified six *key principles of social influence* to consider when working with other professionals (Cialdini, 2001; Livingston, 2010):

1. *Reciprocity:* Everyone likes to receive a "favor," and when one is given the other person often feels that something is "owed" in return.
2. *Commitment and consistency:* Although our efforts may be unrecognized initially, our diligence will usually pay off as we stand behind our beliefs.
3. *Social proof:* People need to see evidence or hear testimonials that a technique

actually works before they buy into it. If somebody speaks highly about our collaborations, it makes it easier to "buy into."

4. *Authority:* Administrative support is essential, and provides "the permission" or gently persuasion needed to engage with and support new practices.

5. *Liking:* People are more easily influenced by people their "friends" as people they like.

6. *Scarcity:* When an activity or material is limited in time, or amount, that creates demand.

Collaborative Practices

Collaboration is a process that takes time and effort. It is well worth the effort, as positive outcomes emerge from the joint thinking, emotional connections, and the passionately shared struggles that evolve from collaborative relationships (Pickering & Embry, 2013). Implicit in the process is the acknowledgment that each time member has a different personality, area of expertise, world-view, and belief system. The following key components have been suggested as absolutely necessary in order for collaboration attempts to have successful outcomes (Mount, 2014; Papir-Bernstein et al., 1995; Pickering & Embry, 2013):

- *Commitment:* Each team member must let their ego go at the door, and focus on one thing and one thing only—the student.
- *Cooperation:* If we remain focused on the team outcomes, we can agree to disagree as we continue to work open-mindedly with one another.
- *Time for regular communications:* Especially at the beginning of the process, time is needed for meetings and collegial exchanges.
- *Support from parents and administrators:* Input and feedback can make or break

the process, so consider support a major ally.

- *Willingness to share:* Team members need to be open with each other regarding materials and techniques. Your collaborative outcomes become opportunities for constructing a "presentation team" and sharing your practice-based evidence at meetings and conferences.

A.R.T.: Administrative Input

As a result of my involvement with a pilot "classroom collaborative" speech therapy approach in the mind 1990s, I got to experience first-hand what a difference administrative input makes. The speech practitioners in NYC Department of Education had both speech therapy supervisors and building level administrators. In one particular program, the building principal wanted to choose and assign specific classroom teachers to be a part of our collaborations. Although we had experienced greater success with an alternative approach, letting the speech providers decide with classroom staff, the principal was quite insistent on controlling the personnel. Needless to say, the pilot was unsuccessful in his school.

A second more positive area of support concerned another principal, who called me one day with questions about materials and collaborative practices. It seems that the speech personnel were coming into the classroom with all of their materials, working with the teachers and students, and then leaving with their same materials. The principal, through her perspective and feedback, raised issues that I had never considered. As a result, we worked with the classroom teachers to help them generate the same types of materials we were using in our highly effective collaborations.

We will continue with our discussion about collaborations, communities of practice, and professional learning communities in when we discuss *leadership practices*.

4. BOUNDARIES

Power Differentials

Implicit to our work is a complex network of diverse relationships that are dynamically evolving or devolving. In most fields such as ours, there are times when boundary lines get fuzzy and our personal lives, professional lives, and that of the client may cross over (Herd, Waide, & Cohn., 2010). Questions arise calling for our careful assessment of boundaries, decisions about potential crossings, and avoidance of boundary violations. Should I accept a gift, an invitation, or share personal information when they share theirs (Herd & Cohen, 2009)? We must consider related ethical issues, professional ramifications, and potential *triangulation* with our clients.

As was discussed in earlier chapters, the very nature of the *power differential* that exists between a clinician and a client puts us in the position of "expert" and the client in the position of being a "vulnerable." This asymmetry and imbalance creates a different set of boundaries than we experience in our personal relationships. Professional boundaries provide the foundation for growth, by fostering a sense of safety and belief on the part of the client (Herd et al., 2010).

The Use of Peer Tutors

One of the problems we encounter with teaching about client-centeredness is that the same power inequity is at its core, as is with the teacher-student relationship in universities (Beecham, 2004). In other words, certain people speak and tell others what to do (teachers, practitioners and parents), while other people listen and are supposed to do what they are told (students, clients and children). The architectural underpinnings of homes, training programs, and universities all embrace that assumption (Beecham & Dunley, 2004).

There is a widening theoretical separation between the communicative tasks believed to constitute therapeutic intervention and the nature of human relationships as therapeutic (Beecham, 2004). This is not unlike the same research-practice gap that exists in our field, and shows up repeatedly in many of these chapters. The speech therapy training programs at Charles Sturt University in Australia developed an innovative approach in the preparation of their students for client-centered practice (Beecham, 2004; Beecham & Dunley, 2004). They hired client-tutors to help prepare the students for power-sharing negotiations. Client-tutors talked about what it is like living with their disorder, their experiences with therapy, its efficacy, their unmet needs in a variety of domains, and the strategies they use to cope and compensate for their difficulties. As a result of the communication exchanges, the client tutors expressed the following perceptual themes about reasons for their communication improvements: *human connectedness* or hearing them as a human being rather than a disorder; *feeling needed and valued* as a result of what they could teach to the students; *a sense of empowerment* as a result of their influence through student listening; and *increased feeling of autonomy* or choice in guiding their own destiny.

It certainly appears as if caring human relationships is a fundamental and foregrounded building block for improving communication, rather that the less vital position it is often delegated to as a result of our traditional training programs. We are trained to believe that the only way to prove that "what we do works" is to empirically measure tasks and activities. Unfortunately, this counters the recognition and celebration that the *quality of relationships* is fundamental to communicative improvement (Beecham & Clark, 2004).

Triangulation

In the social sciences, *triangulation* is a powerful technique that facilitates credibility and validation of research by combining and converging perspectives, diverse viewpoints, and sources of information. It provides a way of mapping out the richness and complexity of human behavior by studying it from more than one viewpoint, thus deepening our understanding of a topic (O'Donoghue & Punch, 2003).

The theory of triangulation evolved from *family systems theory*, and introduced the concept of the three-person configuration as the building block of the emotional system im-plicit in relationships (Bowen, 1976; Herd et al., 2010). A relationship between two people is subject to instability when one of both individuals in the dyad feels threatened, and that instability creates felt tension. When that occurs, the process of self-care for the practitioner becomes important for maintenance and growth of the therapeutic relationship (Herd et al., 2010). One suggestion in this type of situation that has been offered is to redirect the emotional response of tension back to the client, which is a type of acknowledgment. Acknowledge becomes a first step in avoiding entrapment in the triangle and the potential for violating boundaries (Herd & Cohn, 2009).

Boundary Issues

The word boundary has been defined as, "something that fixes a limit or extent." (Mirriam-Webster, 2017). *Professional boundaries* can be thought of as parameters or lines of division that create and define space between two or more people. They set limits and expectations for what should and should not occur, and define the manner in which professionals are expected to relate and grow within their therapeutic relationships (Baker, 2003; Davis, 1994). Boundaries help us determine restraints and responsibilities, and are meant to protect both the clients and the practitioners. They set guidelines for ethical behavior as well as the use of good clinical judgment (ASHA, 2016). It has been suggested that *optimal distance* is not a specific point on a spectrum, but rather arrived at through a process of ongoing self-regulation through the capacity to observe, listen, and reflect (Geller, 2013).

Boundary issues can result in a practitioner's lose of objectivity in his professional relationships and cloud judgment. In the worst-case scenario, they can lead to clinician hostility, burnout, or use of unethical practices (Baker, 2003; Reamer, 1991). All health care professions have established standards for ethical conduct, which explicitly address professional relationships and boundary statements. Ours is no exception, and offers us guidance to what we should or shouldn't do in given circumstances (ASHA, 2016).

Although the establishment of boundaries helps us maintain compliance with our professional standards, there are additional reasons we need to establish them related to sustaining and growing healthy relationships with clients such as shared therapeutic leverage, maximized trust and confidentiality, sense of safety, and self-care (Baker, 2003; Reamer, 1991).

Potential Boundary Crossings

Whether or not a boundary crossing becomes a *boundary violation* will depend upon the potential or actualized level of harm inflicted on the client. Just as a crossing can undermine or disrupt the therapeutic alliance, it can also serve to enrich intervention and enhance the clinician-client relationship (Pope & Keith-Spiegel, 2008). Our clinical philosophies and beliefs will impact the decisions we make relative to the boundaries within our clinical relationships, which in turn will impact the growth and development of said relationships.

How can we avoid the slippery slope of blurred boundaries? Two types of awareness are called for, awareness of ethics and awareness of self (Pope & Keith-Spiegel, 2008). We need to turn both inward and outward, as we reflect on roles, micro and macro systems, emotional and social biases, and personal triggers (Herd et al., 2010). As we enter a caring and therapeutic relationship, we know this relationship does not exist in an emotional vacuum.

The following behaviors may be considered "yellow lights" or warning signs for potential boundary crossings: spending time with clients beyond what is needed to meet therapeutic needs; establishing personal relationships with clients or caregivers; sharing personal problems with clients; choosing clients based on personal factors such as age or looks; becoming defensive when questioned about your interactions with a client; or maintaining a client in treatment longer than is required (College of Physiotherapists of Ontario, 2005).

If you are uncertain about whether or not a boundary has been crossed, ask yourself the following questions: Would another practitioner have a problem with my behavior? Could my actions with the client be misunderstood? Would I tell a colleague about this? Will my actions bias my clinical decision-making (College of Speech and Hearing Health Professionals British Columbia, 2011)?

Warning Lights

Listed below are some red flags, indicative of unprofessional behavior with clients, and indicating that we are experiencing boundary lapses and not looking after ourselves within the relationship (Baker, 2003; Morrissey & Reddy, 2006; National Council of State Boards of Nursing, 2007):

1. *Excessive self-disclosure:* the practitioner discusses personal or intimate aspects of his or her life with the client.
2. *Secretive behavior:* the practitioner keeps secrets with the client and becomes defensive when questioned about the interaction.
3. *Superman/superwoman syndrome:* the practitioner believes he or she is immune to fostering a non-therapeutic relationship and is convinced nobody else would understand the client's needs.
4. *Singled-out client treatment:* the practitioner spends inappropriate amounts of time or attention with a particular client.
5. *Flirtations:* the practitioner communicates with off-color or offensive language.
6. *You and me against the world:* the practitioner views the client in an overly-protective manner.

Therapeutic relationships are at the core of professional practice in any setting, and the client's needs are first and foremost. The essential components of therapeutic relationships—power, trust, respect, and closeness—must never be violated. Professional boundaries are intended to set limits while facilitating safe therapeutic connections between clients and their practitioners. This is a difficult task, as boundaries are dynamic and change between people, situations and over time (CSHHPBC, 2011).

REFLECTIVE SUMMATIVE QUESTIONS

1. What is there to learn from other fields about the process of *building client's agency* and ability to focus on their own needs?

2. What does *problem-focused* in the context of therapeutic intervention mean to you? How is it different from a "strength" perspective and might you incorporate student strengths within the therapeutic process?

3. How can *sacred moments* be identified and cultivated in practice?

4. What are the greatest *challenges to accomplishing collaborative classroom* therapeutic activities?

5. How can the *key principles of social influence* be utilized in classroom collaborations?

6. What types of situations might activate warning lights for *potential boundary crossings*?

REFERENCES

Allen, J. G. (2014). Beyond the therapeutic alliance. *Spirituality in Clinical Practice, 1*(4), 263–265.

American Psychological Association (APA). (2001). *Publication manual of the American Psychological Association.* Washington, DC: Author.

American Speech-Language-Hearing Association. (2016). *Code of ethics.* Retrieved April 25, 2016, from http://www.asha.org/Code-of-Ethics/

Baker, E. K. (2003). *Caring for ourselves—A therapist's guide to personal and professional well-being.* Washington, DC: American Psychological Association.

Bandura, A. (1986). *Social foundations of thought and action: A social cognitive theory.* Englewood Cliffs, NJ: Prentice-Hall.

Beecham, R. (2004). Power and practice: A critique of evidence-based practice for the profession of speech-language pathology. *Advances in Speech-Language Pathology, 6*(2), 123–125.

Beecham, R., & Clark, E. (2004). Averting the professional gaze from science: "Connecting with Care" as a model of educational development. In B. Murdoch (Ed.), *26th IALP 2004 World Congress of the International Association of Logopedics and Phoniatrics*, Melbourne, Australia: Speech Pathology Australia.

Beecham, R., & Dunley, D. (2004). *Clients as teachers: Innovations within the speech therapy curriculum at Charles Sturt University.* Presented at the National SARRAH Conference, Sydney, Australia.

Bowen, M. (1976). Theory in the practice of psychotherapy. In P. Geurin (Ed.), *Family therapy: Theory and practice* (pp. 42–90). New York, NY: Gardner.

Charmez, K. (2006). *Constructing grounded theory: A practical guide through qualitative analysis.* London, UK: Sage.

Cialdini, R. B. (2001). *Influence: Science and practice.* Boston, MA: Allyn & Bacon.

Ciccia, A. (2011). Pragmatic communication. In J. Kreutzer, J. DeLuca, & B. Kaplan (Eds.), *Encyclopedia of clinical neuropsychology.* New York, NY: Springer Shop.

Clarkson, P. (2003). *The therapeutic relationship,* (2nd ed.). London, UK: Whurr.

College of Physiotherapists of Ontario (CPO). (2005). *Guide to the standard for establishing and maintaining therapeutic relationships.* Retrieved November 18, 2008, from http://www.collegept.org

College of Speech and Hearing Health Professionals British Columbia (CSHHPBC). (2011). *Where's the line? Professional boundaries in a therapeutic relationship.* Retrieved September 9, 2016, from http://www.cshhpbc.org

Davis, C. M. (1994). *Patient practitioner interaction—An experiential manual for developing the art of healthcare* (2nd ed.). Thorofare, NJ: Slack.

DiLollo, A. (2010). Business: The crisis of confidence in professional knowledge: Implications for clinical education in speech-language pathology. *ASHA SIG 11 Perspectives on Administration and Supervision, 20*, 85–91.

DiLollo, A., & Favreau, C. (2010). Person-centered care and speech and language therapy. *Seminars in Speech and Language, 31*(2), 90–97.

Donaher, J. G., & Richels, C. (2012). Traits of attention deficit/hyperactivity disorder in school-age children who stutter. *Journal of Fluency Disorders, 37*(4), 242–252.

Duchan, J. (2003, November). *Identity-based therapies.* Presented at ASHA Convention, Chicago, IL.

Dunst, C. J., Jones, T., Johnson, M., Raab, M., & Hamby, D. W. (2011a). Role of children's interests in early literacy and language development. *CELL Reviews, 4*(5), 1–18. Retrieved August 16, 2016, from http://www.earlyliteracylearning.org/cellreviews/cellreviews_v4_n5.pdf

Dunst, C. J., Trivette, C. M., & Masiello, T. (2011b). Exploratory investigation of the effects of interest-based learning on the development of young children with autism. *Autism: International Journal of Research and Practice, 15,* 295–305.

Erdman, S. (2013, November). *Patient-centered care: Enhancing patient satisfaction and treatment outcomes in audiology.* Presented at ASHA Convention, Atlanta, GA.

Finlay, L. (2015). *Relational integrative psychotherapy: Engaging process and theory in practice.* Chichester, E. Sussex, UK: Wiley.

Fourie, R. (2009). Qualitative study of relationship in speech and language therapy: Perspectives of adults with communication and swallowing disorders. *International Journal of Language and Communication Disorders, 44*(6), 979–999.

Fourie, R. J. (2011). From alienation to therapeutic dialogue. In R. J. Fourie (Ed.), *Therapeutic processes for communication disorders: A guide for clinicians and students.* New York, NY: Psychology Press.

Frank, J. D., & Frank, J. B. (1993). *Persuasion and healing: A comparative study of psychotherapy.* Baltimore, MD: The John Hopkins University Press.

French, S., & Swain, J. (2001). The relationship between disabled people and health and welfare professionals. In G. L. Albrecht, K. D. Seelman, & M Bury (Eds.), *Handbook of disability studies.* Thousand Oaks, CA: Sage.

Galland, L. (1997). *The four pillars of healing.* New York, NY: Random House.

Geller, E. (2013, November). *Broadening the "ports of entry" for speech-language pathologists: A reflective model of clinical supervision.* Presented at ASHA Convention, Chicago, IL.

Geller, S. M., & Greenberg, L. S. (2012). *Therapeutic presence: A mindful approach to effective therapy.* Washington, DC: American Psychological Association.

Harris, I. B. (2011). Conceptions and theories of learning for workplace education. In J. P. Hafler (Ed.), *Extraordinary learning in the workplace.* New York, NY : Springer.

Herd, C., & Cohn, T. (2009). Constructing and maintaining appropriate boundaries within clinical supervision relationships. *Perspectives on Supervision and Administration, 19,* 30–35.

Herd, C., Waide, M., & Cohn, T. (2010). Audiology: Remediating boundary issues: Triangulation and self-care. *Perspectives on Supervision and Administration, 20,* 40–44.

Hernandez, K. M., & Mahoney, A. (2012). Balancing sacred callings in career and family life. In P. Hill & B. Dik (Eds.), *Advances in workplace spirituality: Theory, research, and application* (pp. 135–136). Charlotte, NC: Information Age.

Horvath, A. O., & Symonds, B. D. (1991). Relation between working alliance and outcome in psychotherapy: A meta-analysis. *Journal of Counseling Psychology, 38,* 139–149. Retrieved from http://www.encarta.msn.com/encnet/ref pages/search.=boundary

John-Steiner, V. (2006). *Creative collaboration.* New York, NY: Oxford University Press.

Kaufman, D. M., & Mann, K. V. (2007). *Teaching and learning in medical education: How theory informs practice.* Edinburgh, UK: Association for Study of Medical Education (ASME).

Kaufman, H., Braswell, Y., Cohen, M, & Papir-Bernstein, W. (1995). Citywide speech services collaborative consultation pilot project. *Journal of the New York State Association of Supervision and Curriculum Development (NYSASCD), 10,* 30–34.

Kendall, D. L. (2000). Counseling in communication disorders. *Contemporary Issues in Communication Science and Disorders, 27,* 96–103.

Levitt, H. M. (2011, November). *Principles of change used by expert therapists.* Presented at ASHA Convention, San Diego, CA.

Livingston, A. (2010). Supervision: Essentials of collaboration. *ASHA SIG 11 Perspectives on Administration and Supervision, 20,* 35–39.

Lopez, S. J. (2008). The interface of counseling psychology and positive psychology: Assessing and promoting strengths. In S. D. Brown & R. W.

Lent (Eds.), *Handbook of counseling psychology* (4th ed.). Hoboken, NJ: John Wiley & Sons.

Luterman, D. (2003). Helping the helper. *SIG 4 Perspectives on Fluency and Fluency Disorders, 13*, 19–20.

Luterman, D. M. (2008). *Counseling persons with communication disorders and their families.* Austin, TX: Pro-Ed.

Markin, R. D. (2014). Toward a common identity for relationally oriented clinicians: A place to hang one's hat. *Psychotherapy, 51*(3), 327–333.

Martin, D., Garske, J., & Davis, K. (2000). Relation of the therapeutic alliance: A meta-analytic review. *Journal of Consulting and Clinical Psychology, 68*(3), 438–450

Maslow, A. H. (1962). *Towards a psychology of being.* Trenton, NJ: van Nordstrand.

McWhinney I. R., & Freeman T. (2009). *Textbook of family medicine.* Oxford, UK: Oxford University Press.

Mirriam-Webster. (2017). *Boundary.* Retrieved from https://www.merriam-webster.com/dictionary/boundary

Moore, B. J., & Montgomery, J. K. (2008). *Making a difference for America's children: Speech-language pathologists in public schools.* Austin, TX: Pro-Ed.

Morrissey, S., & Reddy, P. (2006). *Ethics and professional practice for psychologists.* Victoria, Australia: Thomson.

Mount, M. (2014). Facilitating cohesive service delivery through collaboration. *SIG 16 Perspectives on School-Based Issues, 15*, 15–25.

National Council of State Boards of Nursing. (2007). *Professional boundaries: A nurse's guide to the importance of appropriate professional boundaries.* Retrieved from http://www.ncsbn.org/Professional_Boundaries_2007_Web.pdf

Nhat Hanh, T. (2013). *The art of communicating.* New York, NY: Harper One.

O'Brien, K. H., & Krause, M. O. (2014). Fundamentally innovative: The continuing contributions of Mark Ylvisaker. *ASHA SIG 2 Perspectives on Neurophysiology and Neurogenic Speech and Language Disorders, 14*, 10–17.

O'Donoghue, T., & Punch, K. (2003). *Qualitative educational research in action: Doing and reflecting.* New York, NY: Routledge.

Papir-Bernstein, W. (Ed.) (1992) *Activity-Based Language Experiences (ABLE).* New York, NY: NYCDOE, D.75.

Papir-Bernstein, W., Bernstein, S. W., Braswell, Y., Kaufman, H., & Magnante, P. (1995). *Collaborative consultation: An adventure with alternative service delivery models.* New York, NY: New York State Speech-Language-Hearing Association (NYSSLHA).

Pargament, K. I., Lomax, J. W., McGee, J. S., & Qijuan, F. (2014). Sacred moments in psychotherapy from the perspectives of mental health providers and clients: Prevalence, predictors, and consequences. *Spirituality in Clinical Practice, 1*(4), 248–262.

Pickering, J., & Embry, E. (2013). So long, silos. *The ASHA Leader, 18*, 38–45.

Plexico, L., Manning, W., & DiLollo, A. (2010). Client perceptions of effective and ineffective therapeutic alliances. *Journal of Fluency Disorders, 35*(4), 333–354.

Pope, K. S., & Keith-Spiegel, P. (2008). A practical approach to boundaries in psychotherapy: Making decisions, bypassing blunders, and mending fences. *Journal of Clinical Psychology: In Session, 64*(5), 638–652.

Preston, K. (2015) Hands on the wheel. *The ASHA Leader, 20*, 38–43.

Raab, M., & Dunst, C. J. (2009). *Magic seven steps to responsive teaching: Revised and updated.* Asheville, NC: Winterberry Press.

Raab, M., Dunst, C. J., Johnson, M., & Hamby, D. W. (2013). Influences of a responsive interactional style on young children's language acquisition. *Everyday Child Language Learning Reports, 4*, 1–23. Retrieved August 16, 2016, from http://www.cecll.org/download/ECLLReport_4_Responsive.pdf

Reamer, F. G. (1991). *Tangled relationships—Managing boundary issues in the human services.* New York, NY: Columbia University Press.

Reeve, J., Blakeman, T., Freeman, G. K., Green, L. A., James, P. A., Lucassen, P., . . . van Weel, C. (2013). Generalist solutions to complex problems: Generating practice-based evidence. *BMC Family Practice, 14*(112), 1–8. Retrieved from http://www.biomedcentral.com/1471-2296/14/112

Reeve, J., Irving, G., & Dowrick, C. (2011). Can generalism help revive the primary healthcare vision? *Journal of the Royal Society of Medicine, 14*, 395–400.

Ricard, M., & Thuan, T. X. (2001). *The quantum and the lotus: A journey to the frontiers where science and Buddhism meet.* New York, NY: Three Rivers Press.

Rogers, C. R. (1942). *Counseling and psychotherapy.* Boston, MA: Houghton Mifflin

Rogers, C. (1951). *Client-centered therapy.* Boston, MA: Houghton Mifflin.

Safran, J. D., & Muran, J. C. (Eds.). (1995). The therapeutic alliance [Special issue]. *In Session: Psychotherapy in Practice, 1*(1).

Scheel, M. J., Davis, C. K., & Henderson, J. D. (2012). Therapist use of client strengths: A qualitative study of positive processes. *The Counseling Psychologist, 41*(3), 1–36.

Shapiro, D., & Moses, N. (2005). Clinicians' questioning behavior: Achieving intellectual intimacy in a postmodern professional era. *Contemporary Issues in Communication Science and Disorders, 32*, 64–76.

Silverman, E. (2008). Ongoing self-reflection. *American Journal of Speech-Language Pathology, 17*(92). Retrieved from http://ajslp.pubs.asha.org/article.aspx?articleid=1769291

Simmons-Mackie, N., & Damico, J. (2011). Exploring clinical interaction in speech-language therapy: Narrative, discourse and relationships. In R. J. Fourie (Ed.). *Therapeutic processes for communication disorders: A guide for clinicians and students* (pp. 35–52). New York, NY: Psychology Press.

Simpson, J., O'Brien, J., & Towell, D. (2013). Person-centered planning in its strategic context: Towards a framework for reflection-in-action. *The Australian Magazine on Intellectual Disability, 27*(2), 10–30.

Slattery, P. A. (2013). *Curriculum development in the postmodern era.* New York, NY: Routledge.

Spillers, C. S. (2007). An existential framework for understanding the counseling needs of clients. *American Journal of Speech-Language Pathology, 16*, 191–197.

Spillers, C. (2011). Spiritual dimensions of the clinical relationship. In R. F. Fourie (Ed.), *Ther-apeutic processes for communication disorders: A guide for students and clinicians* (pp. 229–243). New York, NY: Psychology Press.

Spinelli, E. (2015). *Practicing existential therapy: The relational world.* London, UK: Sage.

Stern, D. N. (2004). *The present moment in psychotherapy and everyday life.* New York, NY: Norton.

Stone, J. R. (1992). Resolving relationship problems in communication disorders treatment: A systems approach. *Language, Speech, and Hearing Services in Schools, 23*, 300–307.

Stone, J. R., & Olswang, L. (1989). The hidden challenge in counseling. *ASHA, 31*(6–7), 27–31.

Terell, P., Rentschler, G., & Osborne, C. (2013, November). *The supervisor-student-client triad: Fostering intellectual intimacy and therapeutic alliance.* Presented at ASHA Convention, Atlanta, GA.

Van Riper, C. (1978). *Speech correction: Principles and methods* (6th ed.). Englewood Cliffs, NJ: Prentice-Hall.

Vygotsky, L. S. (1978). In C. Michael (Ed.), *Mind in society: The development of higher psychological processes.* Cambridge, MA: Harvard University Press.

Wells, J., & Sheehey, P. (2012). Person-centered planning: Strategies to encourage participation and facilitate communication. *Teaching Exceptional Children, 44*(3), 32–39.

Wilkerson, L., & Irby, D. (1998). Strategies for improving teaching practice: A comprehensive approach to faculty development. *Academic Medicine, 73*, 387–396.

Wilson, J. (2007). *The performance of practice: Enhancing the repertoire of therapy with children and families.* London, UK: Karnac Books.

Wong, Y. J. (2006). Strength-centered therapy: A social virtues-based psychotherapy. *Psychotherapy: Theory, Research, Practice, Training, 43*(2), 133–146.

World Health Organization (WHO). (2002). *Towards a common language for functioning, disability, and health: ICF—The International Classification of Functioning, Disability, and Health (ICF).* Geneva, Switzerland: Author.

World Health Organization (WHO): Primary Care. (2008) *Now more than ever.* Geneva, Swit-

zerland: Author. Retrieved from http://www
.who.int/whr/2008/whr08_en.pdf

Ylvisaker, M. (2006). Self-coaching: A context-sensitive, person-centred approach to social communication after traumatic brain injury. *Brain Impairment, 7*(3), 246–258.

Ylvisaker, M., & Feeney, T. (2000) Reflections on Dobermans, poodles, and social rehabilitation for difficult-to-serve individuals with traumatic brain injury. *Aphasiology, 14*(4), 407–431.

Ylvisaker, M., Turkstra, L., Coehlo, C., Yorkston, K., Kennedy, M., Sohlberg, M. M., & Avery, J. (2007) Behavioural interventions for children and adults with behavior disorders after TBI: A systematic review of the evidence. *Brain Injury, 21*(8), 769–805.

Zurawski, L. (2015). Utilizing behavioral interventions to reinforce therapeutic practices in the schools. *ASHA Perspectives on School-Based Issues, 16*, 4–10.

PART IV

Becoming Our Path:
Leadership Practices

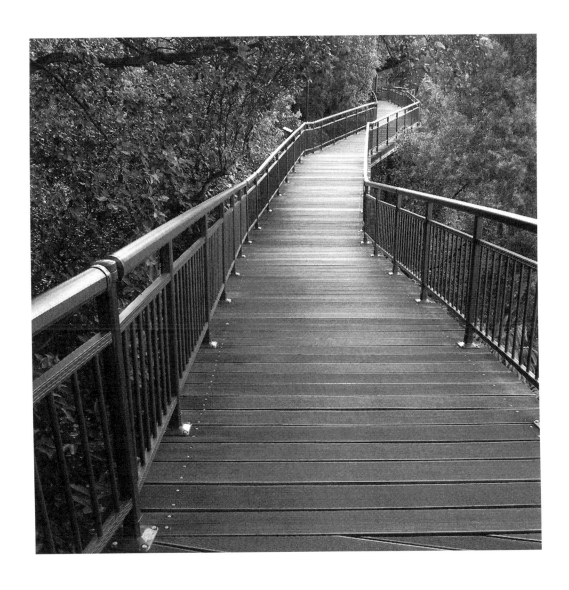

INTRODUCTION

Part IV contains four chapters, and discussing the ownership process, the creation, and implementation of a learning organization, leadership within teaching and learning, and the development of leadership practices in speech-language pathology within a practice-based educational arena. As in other parts of the book, narratives and explanations from my own work experiences are presented.

How do you know if you are a leader? If any of these apply to you, trust me—you are a leader (Hawley, 1993; Palmer, 2000; Vaill, 1996):

- You understand the importance of vision and mission statements.
- You enjoy working with others, sometimes as part of teams or committees.
- You truly enjoy learning and research topics unrelated to assignments.
- Others seem to follow your lead, or ask for your opinions or direction.
- You let others know that they motivate or inspire you, and encourage others to express the same.
- You take pride in expressing your ideas to others.
- You enjoy role modeling, assisting, and influencing others.
- You attend to emotional and political contexts.
- You are self-reflective and operate with transparency.
- You think about "process" or system, and have a big-picture perspective.
- You enjoy assuming responsibility.
- You feel passionate about your studies or work, and have experienced flashes, sparks of ignition, "aha or goosebumps" moments.
- You recognize innovation when you encounter it.
- You do not stay stuck, and believe "love it, change it, or leave it."
- You treat others in a polite, caring, and respectful way.

The leadership journey sometimes begins with not wanting to do something because you feel that you do not have the skills. As we begin to develop confidence and motivation, we try it and then realize that we can in fact accomplish what we once saw as impossible (Robinson et al., 2015). Leadership begins with self-care, and an appreciation of the impact that stress has on our attitudes and performance. It involves the ability to create a learning environment, and then transforms learning and teaching by facilitating opportunities for valued and engaged scholarship. Ultimately, leadership allows us to "become" the practitioner's path, as we model practices for others and contribute to the sustenance of our profession.

REFERENCES

Hawley, J. (1993). *Reawakening the spirit in work.* New York, NY: Simon & Shuster.

Palmer, P. (2000). *Let your life speak: Listening for the voice of vocation.* San Francisco, CA: Jossey-Bass.

Robinson, T., Prelock, P., McCrea, L., Diefendorf, A., Chabon, S., & Papir-Bernstein, W. (2015, November). *Pathways to ASHA leadership: ASHA Committee on Leadership Cultivation (CLC).* Presented at ASHA Convention, Denver, CO.

Vaill, P. B. (1996). *Learning as a way of being: Strategies for survival in a world of permanent white water.* San Francisco, CA: Jossey-Bass.

CHAPTER 14

The Ownership Process

1. SELF-CARE

Well-Being

Even back in the 1970s, research in the fields of medicine and other health professions showed us that when practitioners are able to be friendly and caring, their clients exhibited a greater probability of recovery and rehabilitation (Scott & Hawk, 1986; Traux & Mitchell, 1971). Our attitudes provide the framework and the context for what happens within the clinical and educational process for our clients, and thus we are the most critical "instrument" in the profession (Traux & Mitchell, 1971). Prescriptions for our own self-care and well-being must be at least as important as care for our clients and students.

A.R.T.: Self-Care

So many of us think of ourselves as consummate caregivers. That is certainly true for me. In my work, as well as in my home, my needs would usually come second simply because everyone else came first. That is how I was brought up, and this *culture of self-sacrifice* was naturally carried over into my work setting. I remember the moment many years ago when I first thought about the possible consequences. I was on a plane, traveling out of the country. So many times before, the flight attendants

spoke about safety regulations, demonstrated oxygen masks, and I thought I knew the drill well. This time, however, I really heard it for the first time. When they explained how important it was for you to put on your own oxygen face-mask first—before helping anyone else with theirs—I understood and I took it to heart. After I returned to work, I made some immediate changes with priorities and strategies for my own self-care.

Well being is intangible, difficult to define, and even more difficult to measure (Dodge, Daly, Huyton, & Sanders,, 2012; Thomas, 2009). It is described as a multi-dimensional construct that involves maintenance of balance and equilibrium easily affected and offset by life events or challenges (Cummins, 2010). It helps us understand how people, both children and adults, deal with change. Subjective well being consists of three components: life satisfaction, positive affect, and negative affect. *Life satisfaction* is a cognitive sense, while *affect* refers more to mood and emotions. Dimensions of wellbeing include ability to achieve goals, autonomy, positive relationships, personal growth, and self-acceptance (Diener & Suh, 1997; Dodge et al., 2012).

Psychological well being is sometimes referred to as *happiness*, and has been linked to Aristotle's idea of *Eudaimonia*. Aristotle believed this was the overarching goal of all human actions, and is influenced by the degree that positive affect predominates over negative affect (Bradburn, 1969). Well-being has been compared to *quality of life*, which is defined by The World Health Organization (WHO) as in individual's perception of their position in life in the context of the culture and value systems in which they live in relation to their goals, expectations, standards and concerns (WHO, 1997).

Another term linked to well being is *flourish*, which has now become synonymous with the *positive psychology movement* as a scientific concept rather than as a philosophical ideal (Haidt, 2006). Martin Seligman is a pioneer and leader in the positive psychology movement, and strove to identify those *enabling rather than disabling* conditions that facilitate our ability to flourish (2011). His theory of wellbeing focuses on the building blocks for a flourishing life, which he coined as PERMA: positive emotion, engagement, relationships, meaning, and accomplishment.

We each have a *set point for well being* on a kind of seesaw, with a resource pool that adds to our positive affect and challenges that add to our negative affect. In our work setting, our clinical relationships become an important component of our experience of *positive sense of self*. Our relationships are demanding of time and energy, and self-care begins with the effective use of time management and downtime (Bourne, 2002). When elements affect the fluctuating state of our well being equilibrium and create an imbalance, we need to adapt our resources to meet the challenge (Cummins, 2010; Dodge et al., 2012).

Change facilitates challenge, and resources must be called upon. One resource of self-care is the ability to use perspective and reframe events. The notion of giving may need to be reframed. We all need self-care, especially those of us who are therapists, clinicians, counselors—in fact, everyone who works with people. If you feel depleted rather than fulfilled, consider changing your attitude. There

is nothing more ennobling than helping people, but be sure to take care of your own needs first (Kabat-Zinn, 1994; Luterman, 2003).

The Internal Metric

One could think of *success* as measured by how we contribute to the quality of the lives of others, as well as our own. How do we measure such success? We are familiar with the measures used for client outcomes, but how do we measure our own contributions, which enhance our lives as well as the lives of our clients? Arianna Huffington talks about using a third "metric," one that extends beyond money and power. She calls it *meaning* (Huffington, 2015). The meaning metric *shifts the measurement* from external to internal. When we use meaning as a metric of success, we create opportunity for reflection and self-direction (Tam, 2013).

One method of invoking the "third metric" is to assume ownership and become a *stakeholder*. The term stakeholder has two possible derivations. One source is the holder of the money or stakes when a bit is placed. The other possible source comes from mining and potential land ownership. When you find a property that you want to claim, you drive stakes into the four corners of the property (Mason & Mitroff, 1981).

A.R.T.: Stakeholder

This concept has always been near and dear to my heart, and very much related to our work. I have a strong connection to that word, because it was the early 1990s, and I had just watched a movie called *Far and Away* with Tom Cruise and Nicole Kidman. It was the 1890s in Ireland, and there was a very moving scene where the couple drove a stake into a piece of land to claim it and begin their married life.

> The next week, I attended an IEP training, and it was the first time I thought about the fact that every member of the educational team is a stakeholder who must assume responsibility and ownership for the outcomes.

5. *Cover your tail:* allows us to craft elaborate stories as to why we couldn't possibly be blamed for something that might go wrong.
6. *Wait and see:* is what we do when we choose to wait and see if things will get better.

Above the Line or Below the Line

The *meaning metric* comes alive when we incorporate the importance of *owning it*. When we do that, we honor ourselves as we acknowledge our uniqueness, talents, tendencies, and fears (Heyman & Lieberman, 2014). When we do not, we *become victim* of circumstance, victim of personalities, and victim of bureaucracy. What happens when we play victim (Conners, Smith, & Hickman, 1994; Papir-Bernstein, 2001)? We are captive, and have little control over our circumstances. We blame others and point fingers. We focus more on what we cannot do rather than the "cans." We feel treated unfairly and feel powerless to do anything to change it. We get defensive, view the world with a pessimistic attitude, and say negative things about others.

The victim cycle runs through many states, but six basic ones are common to most people and organizations (Conners et al., 1994):

1. *Ignore/deny:* is a typical beginning point.
2. *It's not my job:* is used to excuse inaction, to redirect blame, and to avoid responsibility.
3. *Finger pointing:* is used when people not only deny their own responsibility for poor results but seek to shift the blame to others.
4. *Confusion/tell me what to do:* is often an excuse to relieve themselves of their accountability. It's easier to not do anything about a situation if we insist that we cite confusion.

Accountability

A thin line separates feeling victimized from feeling accountable. The importance of accountability has woven its way through the fabric of several chapters. In Chapter 6, when discussing balance and harmony, we discussed it relative to science and practice. In Chapter 11, when discussing measuring progress, we discussed it relative to student outcomes. Now, we talk about accountability as it relates to "owning it"—rising above circumstances and doing whatever it takes to get the job done. It's about wondering what else you can do rather than thinking it's not your job. It is a perspective that embraces current and future efforts rather than reactive and historical excuses (Conners et al., 1994; Papir-Bernstein, 2001).

This type of accountability demands that we be proactive in the design of our own self-directed professional development maps. Our program effectiveness is now being judged by additional standards, not only by standards related to our knowledge of professional content and our ability to facilitate improved student communication. It is being judged by competencies related largely to programmatic accountability issues. The better we are able to handle those issues, the more comfortable we feel on a daily basis in our work. This newer definition of accountability tells us that we need to consider the effectiveness of our speech therapy program from the perspective of the larger school organization.

Although we do want to assume responsibility for our programs, it becomes tempting to feel victimized by the system and its bureaucratic barriers and roadblocks that prevent our programs from being the best that they can be. When we get hooked into the victim cycle, we neither feel nor act at our best. In fact, our attitudes of victimization actually can prevent us from obtaining what we personally and organizationally want (Papir-Bernstein, 1995). We feel captive to the system, and tend to blame other people or circumstances for how we are feeling. Perhaps we spend time talking about what other people have done to us, or we simply get defensive and say negative things about others. We know why this happens, but what can we do to change it?

This newer definition of accountability tells us that we need to consider the larger organizational context and ask ourselves,

"How well is our speech therapy program actually running?" In other words, how effective is our program from the perspective of the larger school organization?

We can facilitate real change through the development of a kind of "super-vision" as a process that keeps us focused on our own professional development and personal growth. In this land of emerging roles and shifting priorities, how do we remain focused on self-growth? How can we be constant and true to our own beliefs and stay afloat? How do we stay happy and content with our work, and comply with bureaucratic pressures. How do we not burn out?

In the context of business communities, much has been written about the impact of organizational climate or culture on worker

---

A.R.T.: Accountability

Accountability translates into increased pressure and administrative demands. We know it by many other names: IEPs, standards reform, classroom-based services, authentic assessments, and LRE, just to name a few, but the list of these accountability induced bureaucratic pressures seems to go on forever. We feel accountable to ourselves, our peers, our supervisors, principals, parents, teachers, paraprofessionals, and of course to the students. We feel responsible for the success of our programs. In addition, we work really hard, and sometimes this is the result of our efforts. Do any of these scenarios sound familiar? They all came from programs I have supervised.

1. You prepare a wonderful thematic, curriculum-based lesson, arrive at the class at the designated time. The teacher tells you she is in the middle of something important and asks that you come back later.
2. The Assistant Principal requests that

you to go on a school trip because teachers are absent and he needs an "extra pair of hands." You agree, thinking you can rearrange your sessions and conduct community-based intervention. Once out of the building, you are "assigned" to stay with one student all day and guard his safety.
3. You are attempting to move students along the therapeutic continuum of service, and worked up a great rationale for changing some individual sessions to small groups but the parents don't buy it, because they still believe individual is more and more is better.
4. You have all intentions of using an integrated classroom-based therapy approach, but the teachers want you to take the students out of the room because your presence is "too distracting."
5. Have you ever been conducting a beautifully planned phonemic awareness segment in the classroom, and had a teacher ask you why you are not helping the students with their speech?

productivity, accountability demands, and work satisfaction. The most successful organizations are value driven, with an overriding philosophy, a mission, and a clear basis for decision-making. Most service delivery settings can be enhanced if we consider organizational issues and values that affect productivity and job satisfaction. They include motivation and continuous process improvement.

Motivation

Let's take a quick look at *motivation*. Much of what we know about motivation stems from Maslow's work from the 1940s and 1950s. He presented a five-tiered hierarchy of human needs (Lawler, 1973):

1. *Physiological:* including need for water, food, sleep, and so forth
2. *Safety:* including need for security, absence of threat, and so forth
3. *Love:* including need for affection, belonging, and so forth
4. *Esteem:* including need for recognition and respect
5. *Self-actualization:* including need for self-fulfillment and realization of one's potential

The lower level needs must be achieved before the higher ones can be considered. The lowest level related to physical survival needs such as hunger, sleep, and so on. The second, safety and security needs, such as absence of physical danger, the third—the need for social inclusion, which means that we want to be part of a group. When these three basic levels have been met, we can concern ourselves with the highest levels, esteem, and self-actualization. According to Maslow, the self-actualizing person strives to achieve his or her potential, is challenged by work, seeks intellectual stimulation, and exhibits creativity. Ultimately, the challenge of everyone working within this field

is to enhance self-esteem and foster efforts toward self-actualization, from supervisor to supervisee, from administration to staff, and from staff to students (Papir-Bernstein, 1995).

It has been suggested that one of the most proactive roads leading to self-actualization is to *own it*—do things out of your comfort zone, things that might frighten you. Be courageous and take risks. Take pride in your work and identify its worth and values. Express your confidence, be clear about your expectations, accept your mistakes, and learn from them. Transition from a state of passivity into taking full responsibility for and power over your professional life (Ranchk & Nutter, 2009).

Renewal

Renewal depends on a combination of motivation, conviction, commitment, values, and meaning (Gardner, 1981). We all recognize when a professional is on her (his) toes and another is in a rut. What are the factors that account for such differences? There are processes involved in the rise and fall of people, much like that of human institutions. The aging process diminishes creativity and replaces flexibility with rigidity. Youth is adaptable and more open to change and growth. So the question is how do we stay young and energetic, innovative, creative, and enthusiastic? Continuity must never interfere with *renewal*, the process of bringing the results of change into line with our purposes.

Gardner uses some descriptive metaphors as he addresses our choices about life in his book about self-renewal (1981). It is not like a *train ride*, where you choose your destination, pay your fare, and settle back in your chair as you take a nap. It is more like a *motorcycle ride* over uncertain terrain, being in the driver's seat, and constantly re-aligning your balance and making adjustments depending upon who else is on the road.

In his research about teaching and burnout, Cain identified qualities that, when present, provide practitioners with resilience, perspective, presence, and *professional renewal.* These types of qualities can be identified best through *self-reflective practices* and exercises (2001; ASHA, 2006):

1. A philosophical framework at the core of your professional beliefs
2. A commitment to students, lifelong learning, and the educational setting
3. An awareness of your presence as integral to the school's optimal state of functioning
4. A sense of personal responsibility
5. A passion for your profession
6. The desire/ability to communicate with everyone as the unique individual that they are
7. A sense of community and collegiality
8. The ability to leave your personal agendas at home
9. A strong and well developed sense of leadership

2. SELF-ADVOCACY

What We Call Ourselves

Kamhi raised the question concerning why some names, titles, and concepts catch on while others do not (2004). The answer does not seem to depend only upon something called "the truth value" and logic of a term or idea, or even upon the science behind the evidence. The appeal and acceptance of an idea lies neither with truth nor logic, but with *memetic theory,* traveling to us from the field of evolution. A *meme* is a unit of imitation involved with genetic and cultural transmission, and in part has transformed and expanded our understanding of why "catch phrases" caught on (Blackmore, 1999; Dawkins, 1976).

Examples of memes are contained in everything our culture has to offer including ceremonies, fad diets, fashion, and types of recipes (Kamhi, 2004). Successful memes care only about their own survival by reduplication, so they must get copied accurately and last a long time (fidelity and longevity). They are easy to remember, easy to understand, and easy to communicate to others—which makes them useful for passing on information (Blackmore, 1999; Kamhi, 2004). As a result, successful memes spread most quickly within professional and nonprofessional communities, while other memes may never disseminate and get utilized by the larger community. It seems that "language" is one of those unsuccessful memes, as indicated by its lack of use in the ASHA acronym as well as our most commonly used title, that of speech therapist or speech pathologist.

Had Kamhi expanded his dialogue to cover memes used in the educational setting, he probably would have concluded that the most commonly used title in the schools is that of "teacher.. That is unfortunate for us because that term does little to explain the complexity of our credentials, our scope of practice. and our expertise (Robinson, 2010). On the bright side, "teacher" does reflect our chosen setting, and the fact that we are working with students in the area of learning and behavioral change.

Some of us prefer to use our full title, speech-language pathologist, as a sign on our desks or certainly under our signature. We feel strongly that the word "language" makes it easier for parents to understand our place within their children's intervention on the continuum of speaking, listening, remembering, reading, writing. and spelling (Kamhi, 2004; Verrico, 2016).

If you are an adult working with children, in all likelihood you will be called a teacher. *Speech teacher* accommodates the child's perspective and seems to be the "friendliest" term for teachers to process (Hanes, 2011). Each one of us must balance our professional identity with our professional culture.

A.R.T.: Our Title

During one chapter of my career, I was supervising the speech therapy component of a high-school program for students with multiple disabilities. There was a staff of five speech therapy related-service providers, all of whom shared a common space. Each one had a desk with a wooden sign containing a name and a title. At our first meeting, I scanned the desks and noted that each title was different: speech-language pathologist, speech therapist, speech provider, speech and language specialist, and speech teacher.

We all had a good laugh, and then began to discuss the pros and cons of each title choice as well as the difficulty created by having different titles. The final decision might not have been the best choice for everyone, and was actually none of the above titles. It came from the preference of our district program that used "related service provider," so the sign was going to say *related service provider: speech and language therapy.*

Constructing an Elevator Speech

We are certainly in the sales business, from what to call ourselves to our abilities to create communicative and educational change for students and their school programs. All of this calls for self-advocacy. *Elevator speeches* are sometime the ideal platform for pitching an idea, selling a solution, or simply raising awareness of an issue. They are generally around 3 minutes, the time it takes for people in an elevator to travel from the top floor to the bottom (Ellis, Gottfred, & Freiberg, 2015).

The term originated in Hollywood, when screenwriters had limited time to pitch ideas

to a producer so they had to be ready at a moment's notice. They often had impromptu encounters, such as when riding in elevators, and so the term came into play (Westfall, 2012). Often, an elevator speech gets the ball rolling with beginning a dialogue that needs to be continued, or introducing an idea that needs to be researched and further considered (Sjodin, 2012). For us, our elevator might be the school cafeteria, the yard, or the gym. It generally takes much longer to craft an effective 3-minute speech, than to speak for an hour.

The first step in organizing and crafting your elevator speech is to consider its purpose. Although it should sound natural and conversational, it should also be carefully structured like any other presentation. Every word is carefully planned and chosen, and the speech should contain four components: an introduction, body, conclusion, and "call to action" (Ellis et al., 2015; Sjodin, 2012).

- The *introduction* captures the attention of the listener and informs the listener of what to expect. One needs to consider *diverse perspectives, frames, and lenses,* such as were discussed in Chapter 6.
- The *body of the speech* should have no more than three talking points, and each point should pass the "so what" test (see A.R.T. Box).
- The *conclusion* should be a summary of the main points, and allude to what discussion needs to be continued in the future.
- The *call to action* is the request you will be making to the listener, such as an email, meeting, or phone call.

A.R.T.: The "So What" and" Stranger" Tests

These were actually introduced to me during a turn-key administrative training session for IEP writing. When you write something and you want to make sure it *serves a purpose,* ask and answer the question "so what?" On another note, when you write something and you want to be sure, it is *understandable*, perform the "stranger test." In the context of IEPs, take your goals and objectives, go into the street, and stop the first stranger you see, read the content, and then ask them to restate what you just said. The *stranger test* is easy enough to perform at home with a family member or friend not particularly familiar with your work setting.

Elevator speeches should contain careful consideration and interaction of personal vocal styles, body language, charisma, authenticity, creativity, and timing. Nine Cs have been proposed as necessary for success. Elevator speeches can be thought of as concise, clear, credible, compelling, concrete, conceptual, consistent, conversational, and customized (Ellis et al., 2015; O'Leary, 2008).

What Do We Value?

We all have productivity standards and a continual onslaught of paperwork if we work in public agencies. Why do we do this work? We didn't enlist to become rich and famous. What contributes to the heart of our aspirations and the soul of our professional identity? Therapists value connecting deeply with their clients and helping them to improve. We also have the desire to continue learning about the profession, and professional growth has been cited as a strong incentive and buffer against burnout (Duncan, Miller, Wampold, & Hubble, 2010; Orlinsky & Ronnestad, 2005).

We like to think that as we learn more, we get better over time. In Chapter 7, we learned about *self-efficacy*, and that the better we think we are at doing something, the more invested we are in doing it (Bandura, 1977; Csikszentmihalyi, 2014). Studies have

shown that when practitioners feel engaged and effective with their work, they are happiest. They can sense their *experienced growth* as a result of the progress their clients make, and this feeling of professional accomplishment is unrelated to workshops and academic research from the field at large. However, as professional growth fosters continual professional reflection, it motivates us to seek out further improvements through professional training and enhanced clinical information. It is as if this experience of our current growth helps repair the abrasions and stressors of our work and minimizes the dangers of disillusionment and burnout (Orlinsky & Ronnestad, 2005). Currently experienced professional growth seems to be one of our greatest allies against the dreaded burnout.

Dealing With Role Ambiguity

The appearance of collaborative models of care has created areas of overlap with regard to professional boundaries and ambiguous situations. The term "encroachment" or the more neutral term *role ambiguity* has been used at times to describe these confusing situations precipitated by the prevalence of expansive roles and team-based models of service. In 2009, a committee was convened by ASHA Board of Directors to examine issues (and make recommendations) about role ambiguity (CCVPSLP).

Concerns have been raised about our perceived loss of professional identity as boundaries get confused and blurred. Although we do have clearly stipulated scopes of practice, we do not "own" areas of practice, nor can we dictate what other professions can or cannot do (CCVPSLP, 2009). Professional boundaries are shared, and may even seem to shift around when working within the areas of expertise held by other team members. This calls for the use of a specialized lens and perspective, because educational teaming and collaboration emphasizes a student-by-student "whole-person" approach, rather than a profession-by profession approach. We have a unique scope of practice, some of which intersects with that of other professions. However, what we do own is our professional identity.

3. PROFESSIONAL IMPAIRMENT AND STRESS

What Is Professional Impairment?

The medical, dental, pharmaceutical, and nursing professions are the fields that have most often expressed concern with the problem of health care professionals who have demonstrated signs of *professional impairment* (Pfifferling, 1986). One of the most complete definitions of professional impairment comes from the American Medical Association (AMA) as a practitioner who is unable to practice with skill and safety due to physical or mental illness, deterioration through the aging process, or motor dysfunction, personal or family problems that interfere with the quality or care and interpersonal communication, or substance abuse (Shortt, 1979). This is a potential issue with all educational personal and health care practitioners.

It is no surprise that when job satisfaction is low, and retention rates of speech-language pathologists dip, two of the major contributors have been found to be stress and burnout (Ross, 2011). There are lots of research studies now about common stressors in our field, and the importance of nurturing the mind, body, spirit, and emotions to both decrease stress and increase productivity and work satisfaction (Langdon & Langdon Starr, 2014). Some of the more common work stressors are paperwork, tension in relationships, attitudes of competitiveness, conflicting values, poor

teaming, overcommitment, lack of physical relaxation, and lack of time to complete work (Felt, 2014; Flasher & Fogle, 2012).

> **A.R.T.: Reasons We Feel Stressed**
>
> In recent years, my fascination with architectural books has grown and I have incorporated architectural references and analogies throughout this book. Frederick, in his own book about life lessons he received from architecture school (2007), reminded me about our role as environmental engineer. We are part architect, engineer, designer, and space planner—and must dance between the four for ourselves and our clients. The architect knows something about everything, and the engineer knows everything about one thing. The space planner creates something functional for the individual; however, an architect must consider the meaning and overall value to society. All designers are fast on their feet, and never afraid to throw away an idea if it does not fit with our overall plan or "parti" (see Preface).

It is critical for both students and practitioners to be aware of the causes and symptoms of stress and burnout, as well as self-care and preventive strategies for ensuring well-being (Ross, 2011). *Stress* is caused by external, as well as internal factors, such as hopes, beliefs, fears, and expectation (Patel, 1989; Ross, 2011). In a demanding situation, a stress response may or may not occur depending upon the balance arising from the interaction of the following components: external demands, internal values, personal coping strategies, and external resources and support (Ross, 2011).

Stress is a natural component of our lives, and we all experience it to some degree. An experience with too little stress may be perceived as boring, and a moderate amount of stress can be stimulating and facilitate positive coping strategies (Germain & Gitterman, 1995). Excessive and extensive periods of stress, in combination with ineffective coping and lack of support, can cause poor health. Burnout has been described as the final stage of stress, and can be defined as emotional exhaustion, depersonalization, and reduced feelings of personal accomplishment (Lubinski & Hudson, 2013).

Symptoms of Burnout

The symptoms of burnout can be categorized as physical, affective-cognitive, and behavioral and include fatigue, aches, insomnia, depression, alienation, depletion, anger, impatience, and abuse (Ross, 2011). The most common symptoms related to the *syndrome of burnout* and reduced physical and psychological wellbeing are emotional exhaustion, depersonalization, and reduced sense of personal accomplishment (Ross, 2011). In the helping professions, burnout has been termed "compassion fatigue" because of the emotional demands of caring for people, along with our inability to copy with environmental demands (Ross, 2011). The four most common reasons we experience our work as inherently stressful are: the complexity of our client base, the difficulty of experiencing outcomes, poor perceptions of relationships, and frustration with the systematic decision-making process (Lubinski & Hudson, 2013).

Burnout has been described as occurring when work becomes more tedious and less rewarding (Felt, 2014). Some of the *signs and symptoms* of burnout that have been reported by speech-language pathologists include frequent irritation or increased moodiness, more frequent illness caused by lowered immunity, difficulty focusing, decreased motivation about engaging in new projects, and little

optimism about work population and setting (Flasher & Fogle, 2012; Langdon & Langdon Starr, 2014).

A.R.T.: Potential Burnout

As a supervisor, I was always on the lookout for signs of potential burnout. In one program new to my supervision, there were four very seasoned SLPs who were clearly headed in that direction—each in their own way. Overall, they were discouraged, bored, felt unappreciated, and were considering leaving the field. During a dialogue with one practitioner, I asked her about herself and what she enjoyed doing on her "off time." She couldn't stop talking about her music. I suggested that she figure out a way to integrate her guitar into her therapy sessions and, of course, she did just that. A second practitioner loved her dogs, chow chows, I believe. The next time I was visiting, she had started a knitting club with some of her students—using the "wool" from her dogs. The third supervisee loved to organize things, and decided to go through all of the materials in their therapy space and donate things they were no longer using. The fourth practitioner decided to work on her professional esteem by organizing a dynamite series of parent workshops with the guidance counselor and school psychologist.

Avoiding Burnout

Strategies for stress management include cognitive, emotional, social, spiritual-philosophical, and physical dimensions (Ross, 2011). *Cognitive, intellectual, and mental strategies* begin with having knowledge about what constitutes burnout, followed by such activities as desensitization, problem-setting, and reframing. *Emotional strategies* include promoting self-awareness, consultations, recalibrating treatment goals, and incorporating time-outs and work breaks. *Social strategies* include reaching out for support from other professionals, friends, and family, engaging in morale building activities, and balancing work and home life. *Spiritual-philosophical strategies* include activities to foster renewal and mindfulness. *Physical strategies* include exercise, rest, and anything you do for relaxation.

How can we avoid burnout? One suggestion is to be sure you are appreciating and nurturing your mind, body, spirit, and emotions. Here are some simple suggestions (Langdon & Langdon Starr, 2014):

- *Nurture your mind* by being reflective and self-aware, taking breaks, creating and developing new methods and materials, and scheduling in fun.
- *Nurture your body* by walking during work breaks, sticking to a healthy diet, and considering brief shoulder and chair massages.
- *Nurture your spirit* by focusing on your strengths, staying away from negative people and gossip, looking for coworkers who share your perspectives, and scheduling in a change of scenery.
- *Nurture your emotions* by facilitating positive relationships, consulting with colleagues, and talking with family members or professionals if you need additional support.

Pfifferling and colleagues specialize in physician stress management at the Center for Professional Well-Being in Durham, North Carolina. Their findings and practices can be applied to other of the helping professions as we attempt to increase our knowledge about potential burn-out (Pfifferling, 1980). As stress increases, we attempt to save time by eliminating things that ordinarily would help

revitalize and refresh us, such as exercise, outside interests, time with family and friends, and self-renewal strategies such as meditation, reflection, and healing modalities (Baron & Sholevar, 2009). The training programs of medical schools, as an example, tend to foster attitudes that value technical and scientific management to the detriment of the human encounter between practitioner and patient. The patient feels lost to the "noise" in the system (Pfifferling, 1986).

Burnout is state of physical, emotional, spiritual, and mental exhaustion resulting from poor coping strategies in conjunction with involvement with people and situations that are emotionally demanding (Pines, 1986). Burnout is prevalent in the helping professions as we are constantly exposed to the problems experienced by others and expected to be both skilled with techniques as well as expressive of personal concern. Pines and colleagues conducted over a decade of research with over 5,000 human service professionals from more than 25 occupations in seven countries. They responded to extensive questionnaires about their work environments, resulting in the publication of two books and over 15 book chapters (Pines, 1986; Pines & Aronson, 1980). The conceptual framework for this research was based upon a social-psychological model that assumes most human service professionals start their careers with high levels of motivation.

It works like this: when we work in a supportive environment and achieve peak performance, our motivation gets reinforced and strengthened and becomes self-sustaining (Pines, 1986). Hale and colleagues (2006) reported a relationship between lower stress levels and the utilization of coping mechanisms such as humor, laughter, and friendships in the workplace for speech-language pathologists. However, when we are faced with stressful situations, and have either the additional presence of negative features (exhaustion) or absence of positive features (support), burnout is often the result (Potter & Rudensey, 1984). Ultimately, the determining factor in deciding whether an individual will reach peak performance or burn out is the balance between personal dispositional characteristics and the work environment (Pines, 1986).

Re-establishing a Cycle of Growth

During times of stress, we become more reactive and less proactive. We resist, blame, compete, justify, suspect, and struggle (Felt, 2014). Transforming a downward spiral into a *cycle of growth* is entirely possible, as long as we reflect and rebalance. Felt identifies a number of steps in this process of rebalancing ourselves (2014):

1. *Stop and reflect:* Ask yourself, "What do I love to do?" What are my gifts?" What are my passions?" What are my beliefs?" What do I really enjoy?"
2. *Look:* Assess where you are in all areas of your life. Are there some other areas that need attention? Consider finances, your home, friends and family, fitness and health, significant others, and leisure.
3. *Choose:* Have you chosen to devote more attention to some areas of your life to the detriment of others? Are you choosing to get drawn into ego and political battles?
4. *Reestablish goals:* Draw a map of where you would like to be, and plan out the steps you need to accomplish. Use the SMART system for your goals: be specific, measurable, attainable, realistic, and on a timetable. Track and measure your progress.
5. *Acknowledge yourself:* Solicit positive feedback, and give it to yourself as well. Celebrate your victories and have fun along the way.

4. WORK ENVIRONMENTS AND STRESS

Work Environments and Their Relation to Burnout

The purpose of this section is to help the practitioner understand that although some work factors are under our influence, others are not. We must learn to recognize the factors that will work for us and those that will not, choose carefully, and exert leadership to navigate changes in our work environment when necessary. A second purpose pertains to our work with our clients, and the importance of implementing factors that will enhance their satisfaction and outcomes.

Pines and colleagues (1980, 1986) identified *dimensions and features* of a supportive work environment as distinguished from a stressful work environment. There are a number of variables that play a role in promoting or preventing burnout, and they can be represented by four dimensions of the environment: psychological, physical, social, and organizational (Pines, 1982). A *supportive work environment* is characterized by having the following positive features: autonomy, variety, actualization, significance, growth, support, and challenge. A *stressful work environment* is characterized by having the following negative features: overload, noise, bureaucratic "red tape," paperwork, and communication problems.

Psychological Dimensions of Our Environment *(Pines, 1982, 1986; Pines & Aronson, 1980)*

Psychological dimensions include *cognitive* and *emotional* variables. The cognitive variables are autonomy, variety, and overload. The emotional variables are significance, actualization, and growth. *Emotional and cognitive factors* at work can play a major impact on our perceived psychological well-being in the work environment.

First, we will discuss the *emotional factors*. A sense of *autonomy* ties in with our need for power and control, all of which mediate against stress as it helps us feel that we can predict and determine what will happen in our immediate environment. Autonomy is a high predictor of job satisfaction. *Variety*, too, has been identified with satisfaction, job performance, and attendance. Most of us actively seek variety and avoid monotonous situations. Variety enhances interest and challenge. *Overload* pertains to the tasks we have to complete. An overload can be quantitative (too many) or qualitative (too difficult).

One of the *cognitive factors* that accounts for job dissatisfaction is the belief that our work has no real *significance*. Some jobs feel inherently more significant than others, but work environments can enhance or diminish an individual's perceived sense of such. In our work, the most significant way to feel our impact is through the outcomes that our clients achieve. *Actualization and growth* is a major theme in the field of humanistic psychologists. According to Maslow, our drive toward actualization of our human potential is the highest need in our "hierarchy of needs" (1968). Actualization, according to humanistic psychology and personality theorists, refers to a person's desire for self-fulfillment, and is a continual process of becoming rather than the perfect static state of reaching one's "happily ever after" place (Hoffman, 1988; Maslow, 1968). The growth of self-actualization refers to the need for personal growth and discovery that remains present throughout life.

A.R.T.: Significance

In my years as a speech supervisor for an organization that provided speech therapy services for students with severe and profound disabilities, I remember a turning point in my own perception of the perceived significance of my role on behalf of the "educational bureaucracy." It was a typical New York winter, and we were getting ready for a huge anticipated snow blizzard. Decisions were being made about who had to show up and where they were to report. Speech supervisors were told that because we were "nonessential," we did not have to show up at all. I remember there was a shout of glee from some of the other supervisors in my office. I, on the other hand, felt sad and disappointed that we were not considered "essential" workers. I believed otherwise . . .

Social and Organizational Dimensions of Our Environment

Social dimensions include *service recipients, coworkers,* and *supervisors or administrators*. The social dimensions of our service recipients include numbers, problems, and relationships. The social dimensions of our *coworkers* include work relationships, sharing, time out, support, and challenge (Pines, 1982, 1986; Pines & Aronson, 1980). The social dimensions of our *supervisors or administrators* include feedback, rewards, support, and challenge. The architect is the conductor of the orchestra. As *practitioners,* we coordinate a team of parents and professionals. We must negotiate and synthesize competing demands, and always honor the needs and values of our client.

Organizational dimensions include *bureaucratic, administrative,* and *organizational role*. The bureaucratic organization dimensions include red tape, paperwork, and communication problems. The administrative dimensions include rules and regulations, policy influence, and participation. The organizational role dimensions include role conflict, role ambiguity, and status imbalance.

Physical Dimensions of Our Environment *(Pines, 1982, 1986; Pines & Aronson, 1980)*

Physical dimensions include architectural structure, space and noise as well as flexibility to change fixed features. There is a growing body of evidence that physical dimensions of our environment can play a major impact on our mental and physical health, and that area of study is now called *environmental psychology*. From that perspective, stress has even been defined as a mismatch between the individual's needs and the environmental attributes (Zimring, 1981).

A.R.T.: Physical Dimensions

So many stories come to mind when I think of our physical environment. Clutter, and the lack of it, has always been a big theme. One practitioner was having a problem procuring a therapy space. I suggested she speak with the custodian, who was privy to hidden storage closets not being utilized. With his help, she found one such area previously used for textbook storage. I suggested to her that if she cover all of the bookshelves with large pieces of fabric remnants (acting as curtains), the space would be perfect.

Another theme is light. One practitioner seemed to be going through a difficult chapter, and was exhibiting symptoms such as unusual pallor, expressed lack of motivation, and decreased affect in her communications. We spoke, and she was very honest about her feelings. I noticed that the lights in her therapy space were fluorescent, with one bulb out and the other one flickering. We

---

talked about the importance of lighting, and whether she experienced these symptoms more in the winter than the summer. When she told me she did, I asked her to research Seasonal Affective Disorder (SAD), and that we would talk again soon. The next time I came out to visit her, she had bought and was using a full spectrum lamp both at work and in her home. Her complete manner was back to where it had usually been, and she said she felt so much better. She even noticed a difference with the work that some of her students were doing.

Maximizing Our Physical Environment

If we are fortunate enough to have our own space, it is probably far from ideal. We can throw up our hands and complain, or be proactive about making it the best space that it can possibly be. Some elements are more obvious than others, like clutter, heat, and light. Others, we can learn about by examining some basic design principles used by *feng shui* practitioners to harmonize people with their surrounding environment (Simons, 1996). Alignment and balance are the essence of this ancient Chinese design art, and the first step is to apply both inner and outer approaches to heighten your awareness to the space around you (Skinner, 2001). There may be some easy fixes incorporating shapes, types of materials, colors, decorative objects and their locations, flowers, mirrors, and orientation of furniture.

---

5. REFLECTIVE PRACTICES

Nurturing Reflective Practices

In Chapter 4, we talked about the incorporation of reflection as one of our *philosophical pillars of practice.* We will now continue our discussion as it relates to *owning it.* Reflective functioning integrates cognitive with affective domains, so that insights emerge regarding our own assumptions, beliefs, motivations, and biases. When we are integrating reflective strategies with our work, we leave our agendas and egos home. We view events through a lens of detachment, and are able to view behaviors in a nonthreatening and impersonal way without shutting down because our feelings are hurt. We need to slow down, step back, and attend to our physiological responses and sensations as possible indications of covert meanings. Reflective practice allows us to shift attention from external behaviors to internal feelings (Geller & Foley, 2009).

Reflection has been described as a recurring cycle of learning that takes place between the people who live in the "territory" and the people who provide the "maps." *Experienced reflection* is a process of continuous interplay between experiences and conceptual ideas and theories, which moves from cognitive classroom to job and back again (Mintzberg, 2003; Sawyer & Villaire, 2007). Reflective practice leads to "a demystification of professional expertise." It encourages us to recognize that for practitioners such as us, *special knowledge* is "embedded in evaluative frames that bear the stamp of human values and interests" (Schön, 1987, p. 345; Wilson, 2007). All we can hope to do is be well prepared to *reflect in action.*

Guiding Principles

Finlay offers two guiding principles to use when facilitating or developing reflective practices (2008). The first principle pertains to the way in which it is introduced, and this must be done in such a way to *facilitate interest and motivation.* One suggestion is to introduce opportunities for reflective exercises as a portal, leading to the development of clini-

cal reasoning. It also helps if experiences are student-centered, and focus on other learners or practitioners as they describe their own philosophical values, reflective tools, reflective experiences, and situational uncertainties. Small group work and self-assessments will reinforce autonomy, self-determination, and other core principles of critical reflection (Hobbs, 2007).

The second principle is to make available the *support, opportunities, and tools* necessary for reflection. Reflective practice can be stressful and challenging, and demands a safe learning environment where positive activities can be modeled and practiced. One should participate in a variety of reflective contexts: thoughtful and solitary reflections, dialogical team reflections, written journal reflections, stream of consciousness verbal reflections, and guided verbal reflections (Quinn, 1998). Some of the methodologies and reflective tools include critical incidents, case studies, reflective dialogical exercises with peers, role, plays, and use of reflective journals and diaries (Griffin, 2003). Reflective practices help us make sense of uncertainties, and give us the courage to develop professional artistry through a process of critical self-awareness and self-assessment.

Reflection and Clinical Reasoning

We began discussing reflection and clinical reasoning in Chapters 4 and 7, and will now continue with that topic as it contributes to clinical decision-making, lifelong learning, and professional growth. Schön's traditional *model of reflective practice* contains four stages (Wainwright, Shepard, Harman, & Stephens, 2010). The first stage is *knowing-in-action (KIA).* The process begins with the knowledge and skills possessed by the practitioner and used within a specific context. The second stage is *surprise and experimentation.* When a novel or unexpected problem is encountered, surprise sets the stage for the experimentation as attempts are made to find new solutions. The next stage is *reflection-in-action (RIA).* This stage is the ongoing and spontaneous metacognition of what is happening, that is fueled by surprise and informs the process of experimentation. The final stage is *reflection-on-action (ROA),* which begins as a practitioner looks back on what has taken place and expands or revises the clinical decisions to guide future action.

There have been three *elements of reflection* identified from Schön's model: active engagement with intellectual processes, exploration of experiences, and the resulting new perspectives or insights. The following five abilities have been isolated as necessary for effective reflection to take place (Boud, Keogh, & Walker, 1985; Schön, 1983; Wainwright et al., 2010):

1. *Self-awareness:* to assess how the situation and the person have affected each other.
2. *Description:* to recognize and recall salient events related to the situation
3. *Critical analysis:* to identify and examine assumptions, and explore alternatives
4. *Synthesis:* to integrate new with existing knowledge for problem solving and predicting
5. *Evaluation:* to make value judgments

Just as effective clinical reasoning is central to the development of professional autonomy, reflection is central to the development of clinical decision-making and reasoning skills consistent with expert practice (Elstein, Shulman, & Sprafka, 1978). *Expert knowledge* seems to be characterized by the development of causal networks of knowledge, types of "scripts" or building blocks, which guide the clinical decision-making process as practitioners gain experiential knowledge (Wainwright et al., 2010).

In a study about the ways that reflection informs clinical decisions, distinctions were found in strategies used by "novice" as compared with "expert" physical therapy practitioners (Wainwright et al., 2010). When *reflection was on specific actions* (ROA), both novice and experienced practitioners used reflection to gather insight about their actions and thoughts.

These reflections included assessment of their own thoughts and performance as well as the performance of the client. There were greater differences, however, between how novice practitioners used *reflection-in-action* (RIA) when compared with more experienced practitioners. As a novice, reflections were specific to themselves and their performance with clients. The experienced practitioners were better able to integrate and use information from a variety of sources (including peers, prior experiences, and continuing education), self-monitor, self-evaluate, and self-correct.

Reflecting About Bottom Line Clinical Judgment

Significant changes that have taken place in laws, policies, practices, and classrooms have forced us to re-evaluate our professional identities. What do we know for certain? First, we know that we must provide support for students so that they can participate to the maximum extent possible in social and academic contexts. Second, we know that clinical success is defined in terms of helping students reach measurable and functional outcomes so they can successfully and independently participate in community, family, work, and learning activities.

However, one of the biggest unknowns is the amount and type of intervention that is needed to facilitate a change in communication behavior. Depending upon our state of practice and local educational agency (LEA), we may or may not have specific guidelines for decision-making. Each one of us must acknowledge the huge responsibility in using clinical judgment based upon good and best practices. We need to believe, and actually experience, that the service we are offering will benefit students.

Bottom line clinical judgment often plays the greatest factor in targeting appropriate clinical decisions. Blosser and Neidecker identify eight key factors that help pave the way to uncluttered clinical judgment about student communication abilities and subsequent clinical/educational needs (2002):

1. *Consistency:* inappropriate communication patterns and the conditions under which they present themselves
2. *Developmental factors:* the student's chronologic age as compared to the expected age for developing the targeted communication skills
3. *Home:* the status of speech and language involvement in the home
4. *Stimulability:* the student's response to stimulation
5. *Interactions:* the ability of the student to interact verbally and non-verbally with others
6. *Learning outcomes:* the effect of the communication problem on school performance (academic, social, and vocational)
7. *Response by people:* the impact of the communication problem on the listener
8. *Meeting needs:* the ability of the student to communicate well enough to satisfy his or her own needs

Transformative Learning

Transformative learning has been described as an extension of reflective practice, because it focuses on the use of reflection for exploring premises and assumptions about existing val-

ues and beliefs in order to achieve a paradigm shift in thinking or action, or a transformation (Harris, 1998). Transformations can occur in any or all of the following areas: assumptions about areas of professional practice, methods or materials, defense of beliefs, examining alternate perspectives, testing new assumptions about practice, and exploring alternative professional roles and relationships (Mezirow, 1991).

Self-assessment and professional development planning are two approaches that support the facilitation of reflective practice, as both encourage thinking about our own learning objectives. Through reflective practice, professionals can develop an increased level of self-awareness about the impact of their work, and thus create openings for previously unseen opportunities for professional growth. We continue this discussion about *clinical expertise and personal mastery* in the chapter that follows.

REFLECTIVE SUMMATIVE QUESTIONS

1. What activities do you do on a regular basis to nurture your mind, spirit, and emotions as well as your body? How can you integrate those into your intervention program?
2. What types of accountability issues have you heard about in school-based practice? Describe some strategies that you can use to counter them.
3. How important is renewal in your personal life? How might you carryover your strategies for diffusing stress into your professional life?
4. What professional titles are you uncomfortable with and why? Write an elevator speech about the title you would want to advocate using.

REFERENCES

American Speech-Language-Hearing Association. (2006). *Professional performance review process for the school-based speech-language pathologist* [Guidelines]. Retrieved from http://www.asha.org/policy.

Bandura, A. (1977). Self-efficacy: Toward a unifying theory of behavioral change. *Psychological Review, 84,* 191–215.

Baron, D., & Sholevar, E. (Eds.). (2009). *Psychiatry and behavioral science: An introduction and study guide for medical students.* Philadelphia, PA: Temple University Press.

Blackmore, S. (1999). *The meme machine.* Oxford, UK: Oxford University Press.

Blosser, J., & Neidecker, E. (2002). *School programs in speech-language pathology: Organization and service delivery.* Boston, MA: Allyn & Bacon.

Boud, D., Keogh, R., & Walker. (1985). *Reflection: Turning experience into learning.* London, UK: Kegan Page.

Bourne, E. J. (2002). *The anxiety and phobia workbook.* Oakland, CA: Harbinger.

Bradburn, N. (1969). *The structure of psychological well-being.* Chicago, IL: Aldine.

Cain, M. S. (2001). Ten qualities of the renewed teacher. *Phi Delta Kappan, 82,* 702–705.

Conners, R., Smith, T., & Hickman, C. (1994). *The Oz principle: Getting results through individual and organizational accountability.* Upper Saddle River, NJ: Prentice Hall.

Coordinating Committee of the Vice President for Speech-Language Pathology Practice (CCVPSLP). (2009). Role ambiguity and speech-language pathology. *ASHA Leader, 14*(16), 12–15.

Csikszentmihalyi, M. (2014). *Applications of flow in human development and education: The collected works of Mihaly Csikszentmihalyi.* Dordrecht, Netherlands: Springer.

Cummins, R. (2010). Subjective wellbeing, homeostatically protected mood and depression: A synthesis. *Journal of Happiness Studies, 11,* 1–17.

Dawkins, R. (1976). *The selfish gene.* Oxford, UK: Oxford University Press.

Diener, E., & Suh, E. (1997). Measuring quality of life: Economic, social, and subjective indicators. *Social Indicators Research, 40*(1–2), 189–216.

Dodge, R., Daly, A., Huyton, J., & Sanders, L. (2012). The challenge of defining well-being. *International Journal of Well-being, 2*(3), 222–235.

Duncan, B., Miller, S., Wampold, B., & Hubble, M. (2010). *The heart and soul of change: Delivering what works in therapy.* Washinton, DC: American Psychological Association.

Ellis, K. C., Gottfred, C., & Freiberg, C. (2015). Minute to win it: Using elevator speeches to advocate in educational speech-language pathology and audiology. *ASHA SIG 16 Perspectives on School-Based Issues, 16,* 99–104.

Elstein, A. S., Shulman, L. A., & Sprafka, S. A. (1978). *Medical problem solving: An analysis of clinical reasoning.* Cambridge, MA: Harvard University Press.

Felt. A. (2014). Battling burnout: Change is possible with insight and effort. *Advance Newsmagazine.* King of Prussia, PA: Merion.

Finlay, L. (2008). *Reflecting on "reflective practice."* PBPL CETL, Paper 52. Retrieved March 1, 2016, from http://www.open.ac.uk/pbpl

Flasher, L. V., & Fogle, P. T. (2012). *Counseling skills for speech-language pathologists and audiologists* (2nd ed.). Clifton Park, NY: Delmar Cengage Learning.

Frederick, M. (2007). *101 things I learned from architecture school.* Cambridge, MA: MIT Press.

Gardner, J. W. (1981). *Self-renewal: The individual and the innovative society.* New York, NY: W.W. Norton.

Geller, E., & Foley, G. M. (2009). Broadening the "ports of entry" for speech-language pathologists: A relational and reflective model for clinical supervision. *American Journal of Speech-Language Pathology, 18,* 22–41.

Germain, A., & Gitterman, C. B. (1995). *The life model of social work practice: Advances in theory and practice.* New York, NY: Columbia University Press.

Griffin, M. (2003). Using critical incidents to promote and assess reflective thinking in pre-service teachers. *Reflective Practice, 4*(2), 207–220.

Haidt, J. (2006). *The happiness hypothesis: Finding modern truth in ancient wisdom.* New York, NY: Basic Books.

Hale, S. T., Kellum, G. D., & Burger, C., (2006, November). *Burnout in speech-language pathologists employed in schools.* Presented at ASHA Convention, Miami Beach, FL.

Hanes, S. (2011). More on SLP titles. *ASHA Leader, 16,* 45. Retrieved from http://leader.pubs.asha.org/article.aspx?articleid=2279038

Harris, A. (1998). Effective teaching: A review of the literature. *School Leadership and Management, 18*(2), 169–183.

Heyman, J., & Lieberman, C. (2014, April). How to "own it." *The Huffington Post.* Retrieved September 13, 2016, from http://www.huffingtonpost.com/joanne-heyman/how-to-own-it_b_5072488.html

Hobbs, V. (2007). Faking it or hating it: Can reflective practice be forced? *Reflective Practice, 8*(3), 405–417.

Hoffman, E. (1988). *The right to be human: A biography of Abraham Maslow.* New York, NY: Jeremy P. Tarcher.

Huffington, A. (2015). *Thrive: The third metric to redefining success and creating a life of well-being, wisdom and success.* New York, NY: Harmony Books.

Kabat-Zinn, J. (1994). *Wherever you go, there you are.* New York, NY: Hyperion.

Kamhi, A. G. (2004). A meme's eye view of speech-language pathology. *Language Speech-Hearing Services in the Schools, 35,* 105–111

Langdon, H., & Langdon Starr, M. (2014, November). *Resting is for more than just your voice: Self-care for SLPs.* Presented at ASHA Convention, Orlando, FL.

Lubinski, R., & Hudson, M. (2013). *Professional issues in speech-language pathology and audiology.* New York, NY: Delmar Cengage Learning.

Luterman, D., (2003). Helping the helper. *SIG 4 Perspectives on Fluency and Fluency Disorders, 13,* 19–20.

Maslow, A. H. (1968). *Toward a psychology of being.* New York, NY: D. Van Nostrand.

Mason, R.O., & Mitroff, I.I. (1981). *Challenging strategic planning assumptions: Theory, cases and techniques.* New York, NY: Wiley.

Mezirow, J. (1991). *Transformative dimensions of adult learning.* San Francisco, CA: Jossey-Bass.

Mintzberg, H. (2003). *Managers not MBAs.* San Francisco, CA: Berrett-Koehler.

O'Leary, C. (2008). *Elevator pitch essentials: How to create an effective elevator pitch.* St. Louis, MO: The Limb Press.

Orlinsky, D. E., & Rønnestad. M. H. (2005). *How psychotherapists develop: A study of work and professional growth.* Washington, DC: American Psychological Association.

Papir-Bernstein, W. (1995, April). *Supervision for the 21st century: Facilitating self-directed professional growth.* Presented at NYSSLHA Convention, New York, NY.

Papir-Bernstein, W. (2001, November). *Creating the perfect fit: Merging personal competence with program effectiveness.* Presented at ASHA Convention, New Orleans, LA.

Patel, C. (1989). *The complete guide to stress management.* London, UK: Mcdonald.

Pfiffering, J. H. (1980). The problem: physician impairment. *Connecticut Medicine, 44,* 587–591.

Pfifferling, J. (1986). Cultural antecedents promoting professional impairment. In C. D. Scott & J. Hawk (Eds.), *Heal thyself: The health of health care professionals.* New York, NY: Brunner/Mazel.

Pines, A. (1982). Changing organizations: Is a work environment without burnout a possible goal? In W. S. Paine (Ed.), *Job stress and burnout.* Beverly Hills, CA: Sage.

Pines, A. M. (1986). Who is to blame for helpers' burnout? Environmental impact. In C. D. Scott & J. Hawk (Eds.), *Heal thyself: The health of health care professionals.* New York, NY: Brunner/Mazel.

Pines, A., & Aronson, E. (1980). *Burnout.* Schiller Park, IL: MTI Teleprograms.

Potter, R. E., & Rudensey, K. (1984). Coping with burnout. *Asha, 26* (11), 35–37.

Quinn, F. M. (1998). Reflection and reflective practice. In F. M. Quinn (Ed.), *Continuing professional development in nursing.* Cheltenham, UK: Stanley Thornes.

Ranchk, C., & Nutter, C. L. (2009). *Ignite the genius within.* New York, NY: Dutton.

Robinson, T. L. (2010). What's in a name? *ASHA Leader, 15,* 23.

Ross, E. (2011). Burnout and self-care in the professions of speech pathology and audiology: An ecological perspective. In R. J. Fourie, (Ed.), *Therapeutic processes for communication disor-*

ders: *A guide for clinicians and students*. New York, NY: Psychology Press.

Sawyer, C., & Villaire, M. (2007, Fall). Recapturing relevance in a graduate leadership program: An experiment in self-directed learning. *Leadership Review, 7*, 111–121.

Schön, D. A. (1983). *The reflective practitioner: How professionals think in action*. New York, NY: Basic Books.

Schön, D. A. (1987). *Educating the reflective practitioner*. San Francisco, CA: Jossey-Bass.

Scott, C. D., & Hawk, J. (Eds.) (1986). *Heal thyself: The health of health care professionals*. New York, NY: Brunner/Mazel.

Seligman, M. E. P. (2011). *Flourish—A new understanding of happiness and well-being—and how to achieve them*. London, UK: Nicholas Brealey.

Shortt, S. E. D. (1979). Psychiatric illness in physicians. *Canadian Medical Association Journal, 121*, 283–288.

Simons, T. R. (1996). *Feng shui: Step by step*. New York, NY: Crown Trade Paperbacks.

Sjodin, T. (2012). *Small message, big impact. The elevator speech effect*. New York, NY: Penguin Group.

Skinner, S. (2001). *Feng shui: Before and after*. Boston, MA: Tuttle.

Tam, M. (2013). *The happiness choice: The five decisions you will make that take you from where you are to where you want to be*. Hoboken, NJ: Wiley.

Thomas, J. (2009). *Working paper: Current measures and the challenges of measuring children's well-being*. Newport, RI: Office for National Statistics.

Traux, C. B., & Mitchell, K. M. (1971). Research on certain therapist interpersonal skills in relation to process and outcome. In A. E. Bergin & S. L. Hartfield (Eds.), *Handbook of psychology and behavior change*. New York, NY: Wiley.

Verrico, S. (2016). The value of the full title. *ASHA Leader, 21*, 6.

Wainwright, S. F., Shepard, K. F., Harman, L. B., & Stephens, J. (2010). A comparison of how reflection is used to inform the clinical decision-making process. *Journal of the American Physical Therapy Association, 90*(1), 75–88.

Westfall, C. (2012). *The new elevator pitch*. Dallas, TX: Marie Street Press.

Wilson, J. (2007). *The performance of practice: Enhancing the repertoire of therapy with children and families*. London, UK: Karnac Books.

World Health Organization. (1997). *WHOQOL Measuring Quality of Life*. Geneva, Switzerland: Author.

Zimring, C. M. (1981). The stress in the designed environment. *Journal of Social Issues, 37*, 145–171.

CHAPTER 15

Creation of a Learning Organization

1. THE LEARNING ENVIRONMENT

A Continuous Learning Track

A learning organization is one in which its members are on a *continuous learning track* for the good of the organization as well as their own individual professional growth. According to Kerka, learning organizations function best when learning is continuous, valued, and shared (1995). Every experience is viewed as an opportunity to learn. Learning organizations do the following (Kerka, 1995; Senge, 2006):

1. Link individual performance with organizational performance
2. Make it safe for individuals to openly share
3. Embrace creative tension as a source of motivation, energy, and transformation
4. Provide continuous learning opportunities
5. Use learning to facilitate their mission and vision

In 1990, Peter Senge, founding chair of the Society for Organizational Learning (SoL), popularized the concept of *the learning organization* as an organization within which both individual and collective learning take place. A learning organization can be described as the sum of individual learning for the good of the organization, but there must be vehicles in place for individual learnings to be transferred to organizational learning (Papir-Bernstein & Legrand, 1993; Wang & Ahmed, 2003).

In his 2006 book, *The Fifth Discipline*, Senge identified five disciplines that learning organizations seem to have in common. Each discipline provides principles and practices that we study, integrate and master in our lives, and include, systems thinking, personal mastery, mental models, building shared vision, and team leaning. *Systems thinking* and *mental models* have been discussed in Chapter 9, when we reviewed frameworks and maps. *Systems theory* is the cornerstone to the integration of theory and practice for learning organizations as it allows us to examine the interrelationship between the individual parts and the whole. We all need to look beyond our individual context and consider the impact of our actions on each other. In that way, we all play a part in the creation of ongoing feedback mechanisms that create the internal dialogue necessary for transformational learning (Bolman & Deal, 1997).

Personal Mastery, Shared Vision, and Team Learning

Personal mastery is seen as a commitment to the process of learning through the discipline of clarifying and deepening personal vision. This goes beyond competence and skills, but certainly involves both (O'Keefe, 2002). Mastery is viewed as a lifelong process and a type of calling. It is not developed simply because it is logical and a good idea, but rather because it is part of the chosen vocation (Senge, 2006).

When personal mastery becomes a discipline, it involves the process of continually clarifying what is important to us. People with a high level of personal mastery share several basic characteristics (Senge, 2006). They have a special sense of purpose that lies behind their goals. For such a person, a vision is a calling rather than simply a good idea, and they live in a continual learning mode. They are acutely aware of what they do not know and areas of needed growth. At the same time, they are deeply self-confident (Papir-Bernstein, 1995). *Personal mastery* can be perceived as a threat to any organization if individuals do not engage with a shared vision. Individual learning must be encouraged and valued, and an environment created where individuals can share what they have learned. Both individual and shared learning are key, and learning processes within organizations can be identified, promoted, and evaluated (Smith, 2001).

The development of a shared vision provides motivation for all levels of staff, generates a focus and common energy for learning, and creates a common identity (Senge, 2006). *Team or shared learning* facilitates learning in individuals, just as individual learning contributes to team learning. As a result, the team has improved problem-solving capacity through better access to knowledge and expertise (Argyris, 1999). The presence of organizational structures, such as ease of boundary crossing and openness, can facilitate team learning in learning organizations.

Beliefs and Attitudes

According to Fullan, all learning is predicated on four cornerstones (1990; Papir-Bernstein & Legrand, 1993):

- We learn by *doing*: by trying, evaluating, and modifying
- We learn by *connecting*: by linking new information to prior information
- We learn by *reflecting*: by monitoring our interpretations, perceptions, decisions, and behaviors
- We learn by *being in a supportive environment*: by receiving and incorporating feedback that acknowledges our individual and divers attitudes, cognitive styles, and experiences

This is true for our students as well as for us. There is a strong connection between student learning and our own thought processes and attitudes as well as our professional actions. Attitudes are molded by beliefs, culture, emotions, motivation, and reflection. Staff development, therefore, should target not only professional content but thought processes and professional attitudes as well. New information is best when paired with opportunities for change in beliefs and attitudes.

As leaders, we need to facilitate the development of both personal mastery and commitment. Over the years, I have learned that professionals with personal mastery do tend to be more committed. They take more initiative, have a deeper sense of accountability and responsibility about their work, and experience greater fulfillment within their work lives (Papir-Bernstein, 2002). We need to be relentless in our efforts to foster climates that allow personal mastery to be practiced and truly valued.

A.R.T.: A Learning Organization

Looking back, it is not surprising that I was the organizational member called upon for research and writing projects. Although I did not realize it at the time, I was developing the knowledge management and information design skill set to facilitate change from within. I saw a need, developed a vision, rallied the troops, and proceeded to develop theories, implementation models, and practical applications for the development of assessment and intervention methodologies. This type of approach exemplifies one of the principles in *learning organizations*.

I would get an idea from research journals, textbooks, or a source external to our field. Remembering that I worked within the largest and most complex school system (for students with severe and profound disabilities) in the country, the process that ensued went something like this: sell it to my supervisor who had to sell it to the director, survey the supervisors and speech therapists working in my organization to see who might be interested in a new project, organize a "committee," procure meeting space and a schedule of meeting dates, and begin the arduous task of leading a small group of seemingly motivated professionals. Membership in the committee presumed that each individual would need to agree upon a unique perspective, become fluent in the language of the content, and be willing to partake in the emotional process of creation.

Mindsets

Our attitudes about learning are very much connected to and reflected within our beliefs about human qualities and potential. Do we believe that qualities can be cultivated through effort, or do we believe they are "carved in stone" and are therefore highly resistant to modification and change? Throughout the ages, research has supported both points of view, but it is your adopted perspective that will impact your professional values and clinical decisions.

In her book, Dweck differentiates between two basic types of mindsets, a *fixed mindset*

and a *growth mindset* (2006). People with a fixed mindset believe that their abilities, intelligence, and talents are fixed qualities. That belief will impact their effort and expectations by devaluing challenge. People with a growth mindset think their abilities, intelligence, and talents can be developed through effort and persistence, and that "failure" is simply an opportunity to learn. The type of mindset we operate with will impact our orientation about learning for ourselves as well as for the students with whom we work.

2. PROGRAM EFFECTIVENESS

We Work in Complex Host Environments

Schools have been described as *complex host environments* that can potentially impact our work with the students in a variety of way (Schmitt & Justice, 2011). According to the research, peer influence and teacher self-efficacy (feelings about effectiveness) seem to be two variables that impact our intervention. Strategies have been suggested to maximize the quality of the school environments. Schmitt and Justice (2011) suggest empowering teachers by supporting language learning in the classroom, becoming an integral part of school committees, and increasing awareness of our own self-efficacy related to student outcomes (Papir-Bernstein, 2012).

We need to pull back our scopes and look at the wider context of the school environment, in addition to the more specific student factors that influence achievement of outcomes. Appendix D refers to some of these essential components or competencies that need to exist in your program. These areas are not related to any specific content area, but rather to the overall effectiveness of your therapy programs (Papir-Bernstein, 2001).

Professional Outcome Data

Whatever our reasons for using outcome data, whether they are for us (internal) or our clients (external), they will be evidence-based for one person at a time and offer us systematic feedback. It will most likely have evolved from something known as a *pluralistic perspective*, meaning that different people benefit from different practices at different times (Cooper & McLeod, 2011). Pluralistic perspectives honor idiosyncratic preferences, client strengths, cultural worldviews, and theory of change. As discussed in Chapter 11, *outcome measurement* ensures that nothing we do is left to chance. It also facilitates transparency and true partnership with clients, keeping their perspective as "the centerpiece" of the *clinical alliance* (Duncan & Sparks, 2016). Our work demands that we continue to "show up," and in order to do that we must continue the passion that drove us to this field in the first place.

We want to learn and improve from our experiences, rather than simply repeating them and hoping for the best. Our *professional development* is an essential part of our identity, and harvesting growth experiences will help us replenish and ensure that our work continues to be fulfilling. Our own perceptions, self-assessments, and feedback from the professional community about our work habits and clinical strategies teach us how to work better and smarter. Self-evaluation takes courage. Clients who are not benefitting from our services offer us the most opportunity for learning by encouraging us to step outside our comfort zone to look for a better *strategy fit*.

Performance Review

Any type of *performance review* has the potential to provide a system of accountability, promote professional development and growth, provide opportunities for improvement, promote rejuvenation and renewal, promote quality assurance, and ultimately promote performance improvement. At its best, the process fosters empowerment because it includes values and practices that align personal interests with organizational goals for the purpose of promoting growth, learning, and fulfillment (Schraeder, Amaryl, Cave, Hubert, & Green, 2008).

Performance review and professional growth has become associated with the concept of *empowerment*, facilitated by autonomy, responsibility, and continuous learning. Empowerment partners with the difficult *dimensions* of acknowledging vulnerability, culpability, and accountability. Becoming part of the decision-making process leading to *program improvement* fuels empowerment for the following reasons (Schraeder et al., 2008): expectations are clearly identified; outcomes are personally meaningful; responsibilities are defined; the SLP assumes ownership of the process; collaborative problem-solving and communication are promoted; and intrinsic motivation to learn is present.

According to ASHA, a *professional performance review process* is a multistep procedure including self-reflection, self-rating, open dialogue (about challenges and needs), and feedback (ideas and plans for professional development activities) (ASHA, 2014). *Self-reflection* is a dynamic process that allows us to view our environment with different lenses, different perspectives, and different vantage points. It helps us understand ourselves, our motivations, our drivers, and our contributions within the larger educational framework.

We need to assess our impact on student performance and our contributions to the success of the overall school community. One assessment model, called *Value-Added Assessment* or VAA, ensures that the evaluation measures accurately reflect our unique role in contributing to each student's overall vocational, social, and academic performance that impacts educational outcomes (ASHA PACE, 2014). Any evaluation system should consider our specific and unique roles and responsibilities, as outlined in the ASHA document Roles and Responsibilities of Speech-Language Pathologists in the Schools (ASHA, 2010), and our unique work environments.

Clinical Growth Plans Help Us Move Above the Line

Clinical education procedures have been developed to help students acquire self-supervision skills (Geller & Foley, 2009; Moses & Shapiro, 1996; O'Sullivan, Reaper-Fillyaw, Plante, & Gottwald, 2014). One such procedure is the development of a clinical growth plan, stipulating *areas of strength,* and *areas of requested growth.* Blosser and Neidecker, among others, refer to a professional development plan or professional growth plan as serving to specify role delineations, staff development needs, and student outcome accountability (2002; Ehren, 1999; Papir-Bernstein, 1995).

As *accountability* deepens and people move above-the-line within the organization, a shift occurs from "tell me what to do" to "here is what I am going to do, what do you think?" How can we move above the line (Conners, Smith, & Hickman, 1994; Papir-Bernstein, 2001)?

- Invite candid feedback about our performance.
- Muster the courage to see the reality, acknowledge the problems, and welcome the challenges.
- Don't waste time or energy on things we cannot control or influence.
- Commit 100% to what we are doing, and if commitment begins to wane, rekindle it.
- "Own" our circumstances.

- Recognize when we are dropping below the line, and act quickly to avoid the traps of the victim cycle.
- Enjoy opportunities to make things happen.
- Constantly ask yourself, "What more can I do to get the results I want."

3. COMPLIANCE, ADHERENCE, AND CONCORDANCE

Commitment and Compliance

We know that vision statements and organizational missions are part of *a learning organization.* A learning organization encourages people to develop "personal mastery" through commitment to the development of a personal vision. It is through the development of an individualized vision that professionals excel and learn, not because they are told to, but because they want to. If individuals do not have their own vision, they simply sign up for someone else's. The result is compliance, never commitment. Real commitment is quite rare.

Senge tells us that 90% of the time, what passes for commitment is compliance (2006). *Commitment* describes the state of feeling fully responsible for making the vision happen, and the creation of structures to support it. In some organizations, there are relatively few people truly enrolled and even fewer committed. The great majority of individuals are in a state of compliance. Compliant followers go along with a vision and do what is expected of them. Often, compliance is confused with enrollment and commitment because *compliance* has prevailed for so long it is difficult to recognize anything else.

In addition, there are several levels of compliance and some of the behaviors look quite similar. The hierarchy of attitudes, from *apathy to commitment,* looks something like this (Belasco & Stayer, 1993; Boldt, 1993; Papir-Bernstein, 1995; Senge, 2006):

- *Apathy:* The individual is neither for nor against the vision. There is no expressed interest, enthusiasm, or energy and the person is basically waiting for the discussion to be over so that they can go home.
- *Noncompliance:* The individual does not see any benefits of the vision, and will not do what is expected of them.
- *Grudging compliance:* The individual does not see benefits, but does not want to lose a position or a job, and so does what is expected because he or she feels they have to. They do make it known, however, that they are not on board.
- *Genuine compliance:* The individual does see the benefit of the vision, and does exactly what is expected but not one inch more. They follow "the letter of the law and could be described as "good soldiers."
- *Enrollment:* The individual totally buys into it and will do whatever can be done to make it happen within "the spirit of the law."
- *Commitment:* The individual will create new laws and structures to insure that it happens. They will do whatever it takes.

Student Adherence and Concordance

In medical conditions, *adherence* may be an issue of critical importance as it relates to health and safety instructions for the patient. *Nonadherence* may create risk for poor health outcomes, or even death. In the educational setting, adherence becomes less critical but just as necessary to achieve positive educational and clinical outcomes.

Client adherence refers to the person's ability to follow recommendations provided by the healthcare or educational provider (Rogus-Pulia & Hind, 2015). In previous decades, the term *compliance* was used to indicate the frequency and accuracy of followed recommendations. Of late, the terminology has shifted from *compliance to adherence* because it is felt that adherence more respectfully represents principals of person-centered care (PCC) that we talked about in Chapter 13 (Aronson, 2007).

Another term that is related to both compliance and adherence is *concordance,* which can be traced back to its Latin roots meaning "being of one mind" (Vocabulary, 2016). The term implies that practitioner and student should come to an agreement about goals of therapy and the course of treatment, thereby having the student take greater responsibility for his or her management. The student needs to be in the *driver's seat,* while the practitioner provides the *road map* and acts as *navigator* (Rogus-Pulia & Hind, 2015).

One of the client factors that has been shown to influence adherence is *perceived self-efficacy* (PSE). As discussed in Chapter 7, PSE refers to an ability to attain goals, expectations and outcomes by implementing situation-specific behaviors and strategies (Hoffman, 2013). It is influenced by three variables: having *knowledge* about one's condition; possessing the *skills* necessary to complete the specified task; and having *confidence and motivation* to perform the tasks (Rogus-Pulia & Hind, 2015).

A.R.T.: Self-Efficacy?

When I was a novice practitioner, one of my students had a severe lateral-emission (LE) lisp. He was highly motivated, and had both the knowledge and skills necessary to self-correct at this point in his therapy program; however, he reverted back to his LE every Monday morning. We were making no headway. I assumed the problem had to do with his lack of homework practice routines, although he promised me that he was doing his exercises at home every night.

> Parent-teacher conferences were approaching, and I was happy to discover that his mother was coming to speak with me. On the evening of our meeting, we shook hands, and as soon as she began to speak, I understood what the problem was. His mom was, in fact, practicing with him every evening —but she had the same LE lisp.

Collaborative Practices and Compliance

In Chapter 13, we discussed collaborative practices as dependent upon interactions and relationships with other professionals. Merritt and Culatta remind us that collaborative relationships are similar to personal relationships as they both involve differing stages and developing levels of comfort, trust, acceptance, and expectations (1998). Just as it is not possible to expect all friends to become "best" friends, it is not reasonable to expect that all professionals will become true collaborators. Here are some common sense starting points for establishing collaborative-shared visions for learning organizations (Kaufman, Braswell, Cohen, & Papir-Bernstein, 1995; Merritt & Culatta, 1998; Papir-Bernstein, Bernstein, Braswell, Kaufman, & Magnante, 1995):

- Recognize that *initial successes* will reinforce your expertise and reputation as a willing collaborator.
- Begin with professionals you *get along with*, and build from there.
- *Don't expect* to collaborate with everyone you meet, or even to sell the idea's value.
- Accept that lower levels of the collaborative ladder will *provide foundations* for higher levels of interaction.

Collaboration progresses through several levels or stages, and the developmental progression looks much like steps of a ladder. It begins with compliance, progresses to cooperation, and finally becomes true collaboration (Friend & Cook, 1992; Merritt & Cullatta, 1998; Kaufman et al., 1995). At the *compliance level*, interaction is minimal if at all out of a sense of "responsibility." There is verbal or digital communication only when absolutely necessary. At the *cooperation level*, professionals seek out each other for a variety of reasons. All have started developing knowledge about each other's roles and responsibilities, and have begun to exchange information. Meetings are usually formalized and planned. At the highest level of professional interaction, *collaboration*, professional expertise is valued and supported. Trust and mutual respect is evidenced through open, and sometimes informal, exchanges of needs, plans, and proposed actions.

Facilitating Student Adherence

Client adherence has been defined as an individual's motivation and ability to comply with clinical advice (Behrman, 2012). Research in our field about adherence is limited, but suggests that degree of client adherence is a strong predictor of successful therapy outcomes.

In Chapter 8, we discussed the importance of increasing student's ability to self-regulate through our use of prompts and cues. We spoke about our *responsibility to figure out* what is needed by our clients for achievement of *positive therapeutic outcomes*. The same is true for helping facilitate client adherence to therapy practices, which is equally as important as knowing about a particular therapeutic approach. One component of positive therapeutic outcomes is the client's ability and motivation to adhere to therapy instructions and directives. It has been suggested that through clinical expertise, our ability to integrate research with experiential knowledge facilitates positive therapeutic outcomes for our clients.

It is our responsibility to do things differently and thus facilitate client adherence (Behrman, 2012). Behrman offers the following practical suggestions (2012). Consider that clinical intervention is a *creative enterprise* between client and practitioner, and thus all you can do to foster your own creativity will assist your efforts. Fostering *self-reflection and mindfulness* will heighten our insights into the client's problems with adherence, and influence our decision-making process. Become introspective about *frames and perspectives* as they impact your client's thinking about speech and language therapy and impede adherence.

4. CLINICAL EXPERTISE

From the Inside Out

In the mid 1990s, Kamhi presented a case for focusing on the "internal' decision-making skills, interpersonal skills and attitudes (that help define clinical expertise) rather than the "external" technical and procedural aspects of treatment (1994, 1995). Practitioners and clients may define *clinical expertise* and *quality of services* differently. Frattali suggests that practitioners have defined quality by technical skill level, while clients define it in terms of humanistic traits (1991; Kamhi, 1994).

This same internal-external process applies to professional development. In typical school districts, research, development and diffusion (RD&D) models look fairly similar. Experts are hired or recruited from within, and present the topic often in standard lecture format. In the traditional model, practice sometimes assumes a subordinate relationship to theoretical knowledge. Knowledge comes from the outside in, whereas in reflective practice, knowledge is gained from the "inside" first (Osterman & Kottkamp, 1993). In the

traditional model, the practitioner becomes a passive consumer of knowledge. In the reflective practice model, the practitioner becomes a researcher and engages in a continuing process of self-education (Schön, 1983). Discussions sometimes begin with acknowledgment that something does not feel "right" in the program. Behavioral change must address the emotional dimension, and discussion includes ideas generated from tacit personal experience and intuitive knowledge as well as from explicit research.

Differentiating Emerging From Expert Professional

What is clinical expertise, and how do we differentiate expert from notice? Kamhi was one of the first researchers in our field to present a model of clinical expertise (1994). As described, clinical expertise is the acquisition of comfort level in each of four areas: self-monitoring skills, knowledge base, problem-solving skills, and interpersonal skills and attitudes.

Research from the fields of psychology and education has isolated distinctions between the cognitive styles of emerging and established professionals. Whereas *novices* tend to pay attention to irrelevant information and use disorganized schemas, experts solve problems with greater speed (Lewandowsky, Ecker, Seifert, Schwarz, & Cook, 2012). *Experts* tend to evaluate their own biases and assumptions through a self-reflection process that allows them to self-examine their own effectiveness.

Interest has peaked in additional areas of practitioner performance, called *skillfulness*. Milne and colleagues have devised competence scales for psychotherapists, and distinguish between 6 levels of competence (1999). Expert, the highest level of competence, defines a practitioner who no longer simply uses rules or guidelines, but has deep *tacit understanding* of the issues and is able to use novel problem-solving techniques. In addition, the expert employs a wide variety of self-monitoring and inward-attending tools (Bennett & Parry, 1998).

Professional Knowledge and Experience

Edgar Schein (1972) described three components to professional knowledge:

- The *basic science* behind the underlying discipline from which our practice developed and upon which it rests,
- The engineering component or *applied science* from which diagnostic and assessment procedures are derived,
- The *skills and attitudinal* component that concerns the professional performance and provision of services to clients through the application of basic and applied knowledge

Experience is certainly one factor that has an impact on clinical expertise. However, as was discussed in the Introduction to this book, Cornett and Chabon identified *three attitudes* they consider important to the provision of high-quality services: a scientific attitude, a therapeutic attitude, and a professional attitude (1988). In addition to knowledge and attitudes, much has been written concerning the importance of *technical skills and interpersonal skills*, sometimes referred to as *process or process-oriented skills* (Goldberg, 1997). Goldberg describes *technical skills* as defined by precise conditions and delineated steps for implementation. A *process-oriented skill* is less precise and therefore not as easily measured. They often involve the use of structured statements and elicited responses that indicate the client's desired perception about the practitioner, the therapy process, or their own clinical/educational outcomes. Please see Appendix E

for a detailed listing of Goldberg's technical and process skill breakdowns.

Kamhi presents a model of *clinical expertise* as including four factors: self-monitoring skills, knowledge base, procedural, and problem solving skills and interpersonal skills and attitudes (1994). Expertise is defined as an attained level of comfort in each of the four factors, hopefully acquired over time, and examined through ongoing self-reflection. In an article one year later reflecting interviews with practitioners working in a variety of settings, Kahmi indicated that clinical expertise categories clustered in one additional area he calls *clinical philosophies* (1995). He thus reframed *clinical expertise* as being comprised of *knowledge, technical/procedural skills, interpersonal skills/attitudes, and clinical philosophies*

Growth and Change

The aggressive pursuit of *lifelong learning* must be an ethical priority as it is key to the survival of our profession. It is one obvious indication to our membership and the public that our professions are dynamic, our scope of practice is expanding, and our services are consumer-oriented.

In Chapter 7, we discussed *growth and change* as one of the *philosophical pillars of practice*. The maintenance of clinical expertise is an ongoing commitment to learning and change. It is not an end product of our studies, but rather an ongoing process of striving to improve the effectiveness of the services we provide. Different factors influence the development of motivation for clinician change and growth: client needs, administrative demands, professional requirements, specific changes in work settings, and practitioner motivation. Practitioner motivation can be viewed in terms of a *cost/benefits ratio*. The amount of practitioner effort needed for the change to occur is viewed as the cost. The benefit can be linked to any of the above impacting job satisfaction and administrative relationships through improved client outcomes (Kamhi, 1995; Papir-Bernstein, 2001).

A.R.T.: Cost/Benefits Ratio

As speech supervisor and coordinator for the staff development unit of our speech therapy division in the New York City Department of Education, I led meetings to suggest topics for our staff development unit. Ideas would evolve around latest research, cost factors, district initiatives, and student needs. We never thought about "practitioner effort," because all they had to do was attend.

As I conducted follow-up visits to the field after what I considered to be a fabulous training day, it never ceased to amaze me how few practitioners implemented what they had been exposed to during the training. One day, during some reflective dialogue with a small group under my supervision, I discovered a new perspective. Because there was no "cost," for many there was no perceived value. Many of the practitioners felt that if they had to pay for a training it would be worth more than if they were receiving it for free. That bit of new knowledge motivated me to reframe our post workshop evaluation, suggesting that specific questions about implementation with students on their caseload be added to the questions. Something related to their effort and investment had to be reflected as part of the cost/benefits ratio.

Building Master Practitioners

While discussing the process for building master clinicians, Culatta parallels successful intervention with successful supervision with reference to conducting observations, facilitating learning, modeling, and providing feedback (1992; Papir-Bernstein, 1995).

- Both the practitioner and supervisor are *observing*: the first observes the students communication behaviors, and the second observes the service being provided.
- Both the practitioner and supervisor are *facilitating learning*: the first provides information about changing behaviors, and the second about improving service.
- Both the practitioner and supervisor are *modeling*: the first models the appropriate communication target for the student, and the second demonstrates clinical strategies.
- Both the practitioner and supervisor are *providing feedback*: the first evaluates change, and the second evaluates knowledge and skills.

Characteristics of Exemplary Practitioners

In a pilot study conducted by Goldberg in preparation of his textbook, he found that six critical characteristics of exemplary practitioners had been identified (1997): being a compassionate scientist, being a facilitator, having exquisite timing, using contingency thinking, using consistency, putting concentration on acquisition tasks, and having intense focus. A *compassionate scientist* is one with an overriding orientation that synthesizes two essential perspectives: one of intense care for the wellbeing of the client, and the other of commitment to using methodologies that are both scientific and practice-based (O'Donohue, Fisher, Plaud, & Link, 1989).

Another exemplary quality is to be a *facilitator of change*—someone who provides necessary conditions for an individual to develop a new attitude, change a behavior, or learn new information (Goldberg, 1997). A facilitator is a type of teacher, one who engineers the environment so that learning becomes possible.

A.R.T.: Teacher or SLP?

In choosing my career, I was clearly opposed to becoming "a teacher." I knew I wanted to work with children, and I loved my initial speech pathology classes, so my course of study was set. In the years that followed, I would correct people when they referred to me (quite proudly) as "a teacher." This distinction, and upset about why my family could not seem to get my title right, continued for most of the decades and role delineations of my career.

Just as things had begun to quiet down on that front, one day a close friend said to me "how's teaching?" I turned to her and replied, "after all of these years, I can't believe you still think I teach." To which she said, "I meant your university teaching." In that moment, and about 30 years too late, I knew I had to abandon the inappropriate "elitist" response when someone referred to me as a teacher rather than a *speech-language pathologist*.

Our *exquisite sense of timing* allows us to maximize the impact that a statement or a response has upon the behavior of our client. It helps us know when to present information, when to withhold information, and how long to wait before providing additional cues and supports (Goldberg, 1997). *Contingency thinking* is the ability to anticipate a response before it occurs. That ability develops only after years of knowledge and experience have been accumulated. It sometimes begins with intuition, but always involves critical thinking and seasoned decision-making. When we view a contingency thinker in action, we see a

person who is able to think on their feet and not get thrown off course (Patterson, Rak, Chermonte, & Roper, 1992).

One of the main differences between master practitioners and those with less experience involves *consistency* with regard to how skills are used. Another difference is the degree to which *acquisition skills* rather than retrieval skills are targeted. An acquisition skill involves facilitating the learning of a concept or rule through a strategy that can be internalized and used in other situations. One additional characteristic of exemplary practitioners that has been identified is *intense focus* on the clients and their needs. Focus is a combination of practitioner attentiveness, concentration and connectiveness (Goldberg, 1997).

A.R.T.: Consistency

The best example I can think of that illustrates the importance of consistency comes from the selection of wines. Years ago, one of my oenophile friends took me to a wine shop for a small educational seminar. They spoke about consistency, as one of the criteria that distinguishes a fine wine from the others. The next week when purchasing wine for a dinner party, I bought six bottles of a $10.00 wine. The shop owner tried to persuade me to upgrade to a $20.00 wine, but I didn't listen. On the night of the party, it was only when we opened the third and fourth bottles that I understood. We can all get lucky *sometimes* . . .

Developing Super-Vision

We discussed in Chapter 7 that growth was strongly connected to perception of self-efficacy. We also know that professional competence is directly related to and influenced by professional confidence. Confidence in part develops from exposure to exceptional staff development resources. However, the other part of what is needed to grow confidence is a bit more elusive: self-assessment, self-diagnosis, and self-remediation. How do we do that? We need to know what to look for. That is what I like to call super-vision (Papir-Bernstein, 2002). Super-vision is what we strive for, whether working with students, staff, or families. It is using what we know to further develop or skills so that new challenges can be met. It involves accurate self-assessment, implementation of best clinical and educational practices, and use of resources.

There have been numerous attempts to identify the super-vision that facilitates qualities of master clinicians who work in the helping professions, and include the following suggestions. Be in touch with your own feelings and reveal yourself to others. Regard each person as unique and understand them for who they are. Be realistic about your own knowledge and capabilities, and admit uncertainty. Lastly, be flexible and open to new information (Goldberg, 1997; Murphy, 1982; Satir, 1967).

5. COMMUNITIES OF PRACTICE

Dealing With Clinical Uncertainties

In Chapter 7, we talked about critical thinking, clinical reasoning, and rational thought as they relate to the clinical decision-making process. Inherent to that process is the balance of certainty with uncertainty, as our uncertainties drive us to seek new ideas and approaches to solve clinical problems (Clark & Flynn, 2011). Although certainty may be our preferred approach, that attitude can sometimes prevent us from considering all of the options.

An attitude of uncertainty centers the task on us rather than the student.

If we were to use the metaphor of Sherlock Holmes and Watson, the Watson system is the natural tendency of the mind to believe what we see and hear. The Holmes system is to question everything. We need to incorporate a health dose of skepticism, to observe not merely to see. The Holmes system helps us preserve a place of uncertainly and fight against the biases of intuition. That requires mindfulness, and the constant presence of mind to attend to the here and now (Konnikova, 2013; Lewis, 2016).

How can we incorporate uncertainty within our clinical approach? The answer ties in with the commitment for ongoing professional growth within *professional learning communities* (Kamhi, 1995). It may be difficult to admit uncertainly when working with other professionals because of the tendency to feel "at fault" for not being certain, but the opportunity rarely presents itself when working alone. In fact, it is virtually impossible to balance certainty with uncertainty when working alone, which is why we need to work within teams. On the other hand, although questioning our own actions is difficult, when we cast doubt on the actions of others it may be perceived as disrespectful or taken personally (Clark & Flynn, 2011).

The term *professional learning communities (PLCs)* are somewhat self-defined, as a group of professionals who come together as a self-created and supportive community for the purpose of learning. Effective PLCs in school-based programs can be characterized as containing four components: *shared beliefs* and a commitment to focus on student learning; *shared and supportive leadership*, including a shared authority for decision-making; *collective thinking and learning* that leads to creative solutions; and *shared personal practice*, including comfort with giving and receiving feedback (Clark & Flynn, 2011; Hord & Sommers, 2008).

As speech-language pathologists, we are invaluable members of school communities during each phase of the clinical and educational process with students: assessment, planning, implementation, and progress monitoring. Each phase of the process provides opportunities to question decisions and explore options from a multitude of lenses and perspectives. Rational thinking requires the use of a *metacognitive approach* through team interactions and shared approaches to practice. Below are some advantages of using this type of approach to draw out and confront uncertainties (Clark & Flynn, 2011):

- During the *assessment process*, discrepancies about educational and functional performance can be discussed that may result from testing methodologies (standardized, criterion-referenced, curriculum-based) used by different professionals.
- During the *planning process*, IEP goals and objectives can be integrated so that overall academic and functional needs for each student may be better addressed.
- During the *implementation process*, service delivery options will be considered that can best foster a team-based model (classroom-based and co-teaching or pullout, integrated or separated within the classroom). It is also the time to discuss shared methods and materials.
- During the *progress monitoring process*, team members will discuss student progress by questioning their beliefs and assumptions and any uncertainties related to the IEP.

Why We Sometimes Prefer Working Alone

It is not surprising that the concept for *professional learning communities* as collaborative work environments evolved from the world of business. In fact, PLCs reflect the evolv-ing collaborative culture that is happening in business, health care, and education. This is a change from long ago and more recent past history of most fields of practice, including education, which were characterized by *dominant paradigms of autonomy and isolation* (Banks & Knuth, 2013). Understanding our history will help us appreciate why it feels sometimes more difficult for us to work with each other than it does to work by ourselves.

In her book *The Field*, Lynne McTaggart explains that our stories define our lives, and help us make sense of all that goes on around us (2008). It is our scientific stories, and specifically those about our universe, that most define us. We have grown up thinking that science presents the ultimate truth. Isaac Newton and Charles Darwin were both major authors in the story of our world. Through the Newtonian vision, the universe was described as containing the movement of all mater within a three-dimensional space and time according to certain fixed laws. This worldview bolstered Charles Darwin's theory of evolution and the suggestion that survival is only available to the genetically fittest of us. Life is about winning and getting there first. Both of these stories idealized separateness, competition, winning, and losing—and that is how our world was fashioned. These theories formed the backbone of modern science, creating our worldview and overall frame of education and professional success: *all elements of the universe are wholly self-contained and isolated from each other.* From a spiritual and metaphysical perspective, these paradigms led to a desperate sense of isolation (McTaggart, 2008).

Quantum physics and the quantum energy field, identified in the 1970s, tell us a very different story. The quantum field binds us all together in a type of invisible web. At our universal essence, we exist in unity, in relationship, utterly interdependent with and affecting each part of the whole. There is a central organizing force, one underlying energy field, which governs our bodies as well as the entire cosmos (McTaggart, 2008). This newer vision empowers us with a larger sense of purpose and unity in our world, and a greater sense of importance. Everything we do and think matters, because we are a part of something much larger. If we are not really separate there can be no winning and losing, and we would therefore have to redesign the choices we make governing our communities, our interactions and our work practices. Although much of this research was conducted more than a third of a century ago, it seems that when it comes to our communities of practice, we are still catching up.

Professional Learning Communities (PLCs)

The PLCs are based upon the premise that reflections about daily experiences are enhanced when shared during interactions with other educational professionals. As a result, and as the adults increase their collective professional knowledge and skills, the student's capacity to learn and specific learning outcomes will improve as well (Banks & Knuth, 2013; Dufour, 2004).

The PLCs target student learning outcomes as well as the professional development of each person on the educational team. They facilitate greater use of research-based practices through connection and alignment of commonalities rather than highlighting differences. As PLC members engage with reflective dialogues and extend conversations about students, conceptions about *accountability* extend beyond individual students (Banks & Knuth, 2013). PLCs infer that professionals have a responsibility to be accountable to other team members as well. They provide us with opportunities to balance our personal styles, philosophies, and preferences with collaborative standards of practice.

Professional learning communities are infrastructures that model and implement methodologies for successful collaborations. The PLC process results in the development of a group of school-based professionals who collaborate for the purpose of *professional development* and overall *school improvement* in areas of teaching and learning. Some would say that unless a PLC involves a professional development model that incorporates action research and data collection, it is a simply a work committee or social network (Feger & Arruda, 2008; Rudebusch & Wiechmann, 2013). Professional learning is characterized by ongoing collaborations and shared experiences with other educators to achieve a common vision for school and student improvement.

When professional learning communities are discussed in the educational and speech-language pathology literature, five key attributes are often cited: shared values and vision, supportive conditions, shared leadership, collective creativity, and shared practice (Rudebusch & Wiechmann, 2013).

A.R.T.: Shared Leadership

As a speech supervisor for many years, I saw professional themes come and go as they yielded their influence on supervisory practices. One year, the conversation of "joint observations" came up at a staff meeting. In prior years, the speech supervisor observed the speech practitioners for reasons of professional support as well as administrative responsibility. It seems that some building principals had expressed the desire to observe and rate the speech practitioners in their schools, much the same way they observed and rated their classroom teachers.

Needless to say, this created a state of panic in the minds of some practitioners as well as speech supervisors. Although some chose to view this as a *power play*, I saw it as an opportunity to rally and show team support as well as share professional expertise. It allowed both of us to view the speech practitioners with different eyes and support them with different voices. It became a win-win for all.

Research about learning communities have identified the following positive outcomes for students, teachers, administrators, and support staff such as speech-language pathologists (Rudebusch & Wiechmann, 2013):

- Greater commitment to the school's mission and vision
- Shared responsibility for student educational outcomes
- Reduced isolation
- Increased understand of content provided by all professionals
- Higher morale and lower stress
- Increased appreciation of role differentiation and professional expertise
- Lower student dropout rate and absenteeism
- Greater student academic success

Our involvement with PLC's takes place at the local, state, and national levels. At the local level, our participation with our school learning communities helps establish successful learning pathways for the students. On a larger local district level, we can team with other SLPs for sharing research and experiences about therapy our programs. At the state and national levels, our involvement broadens to learning communities with our various associations and at conventions and conferences.

A.R.T.: PLCs at the Local Level

In the late 1990s and as a result of a two-year study about innovative practices, the Department of Education implemented changes in annual performance review procedures for all teachers (SLPs included). In my organization, one of the *annual performance options* was for the speech practitioners to design a research and practice based project, targeting communication needs through academic standards. Each project had to be motivating, functional, collaborative, and contain a delineation of assessment methodology for collecting outcome data.

This was one of the most creative implementation of PLCs at local school and district levels, although the phrase was not yet commonly used in our field. It provided opportunities for all members of the teaching and learning community, from students through administrators, to excel within collaborative projects.

Knowledge Sharing

The knowledge sharing process is complemented within organizational structures through the creation of "communities of practice." Although the term may be relatively new, the concept originated in ancient Greece through the middle ages as societies of craftsmen, masons, and guilds of workers that protected its members and maintained standards (Smith, 2001). *Communities of practice* are groups of workers dedicated to a mission, informally bound together by shared expertise and a passion for a joint enterprise. Members of these communities guide, drive, motivate and inspire ongoing work in the organization. Over time, communities of practice develop the knowledge assets of the organization, build knowledge for themselves and the organization, transfer their tacit and explicit knowledge, and stimulate innovation (Pascarella, 1997; Smith, 2001). The value and worth of intellectual assets grow exponentially when shared. On the other hand, human inertia is the biggest obstacle to knowledge-management efforts (Wah, 1999).

Knowledge Translation Using Mindlines

We learned, from Chapter 1, that evidence-based practice principles sometimes have the result of creating dilemmas in the world of health care. One of them is the fear that tacit knowledge-in-practice will be undervalued through the overprescription of "cookbook" therapy. Successful implementation of research evidence requires a process of "sense-making" so that knowledge from both explicit and tacit sources is collected and internalized into routine practice (Gabbay & Le May, 2010; Weick, 1995). In one study with primary care general practitioners and nurses, "mindlines" were defined as tacit guidelines that were internalized and reinforced by readings, observations, and interactions with other colleagues. These networking interactions were considered fluid and part of "communities of practice," and resulted in socially constructed "knowledge in practice" (Gabbay & Le May, 2010). Practitioner tacit knowledge is often referred to as knowledge in practice.

When health care professions are questioned about ways that evidence is obtained for the decision making process, they do not necessarily go through the steps that are traditionally associated with the linear-rational model of evidence-based practice (Gabbay & Le May, 2010; Trinder & Reynolds, 2000). Although they may have easy paper and digital access to guidelines, protocols, and manuals, discussions with colleagues was their primary method for gathering information about issues, new situations, or discrepancies. The following additional techniques were evidenced as well: *anecdotes* with a purpose, or

narratives about a clinical case; *Post-It stickers* on a white board in a shared space; and *informal networking* coffee meetings about some new research (Gabbay & Le May, 2010).

Clinicians rarely accessed and used the explicit evidence directly from research or other formal sources. In other words, rather than accessing information from the literature or other written sources, practitioners acquired their best evidence from the people they trusted. They seemed to work best in fluid *communities of practice* and combined with information from a wide range of sources into *mindlines*, or internalized and collectively reinforced tacit guidelines resulting largely from day to day practice patterns (Gabbay & Le May, 2010).

The following is a summary of mindlines and implications for their use (Choo, 1998; Gabbay & Le May, 2010):

- The development of mindlines seems reliant on professional interactions.
- They are learned and internalized sequences of thought and behavior (guidelines) that professionals find difficult to articulate.
- Mindlines seem to begin with research evidence, expand through *communities of practice*, and transform into *knowledge in practice*.
- The *opinion leaders* (those key leaders to whom other turn to for opinions) have a collective professional responsibility to ensure that their knowledge is based on research and experiential evidence.

Practice-Based Networks

Practice research networks (PRNs) involve another type of infrastructure that demonstrates possible applications of research in improving routine clinical practice in school-based settings. (Margison et al., 2000). They involve large numbers of practitioners who agree to collaborate for the purpose of collecting and reporting data. Sometimes PRNs are linked with academic centers, professional study groups, or university programs. The PRN structure provides an excellent match for the agendas of both evidence-based practice (EBP) and practice-based evidence (PBE) (Margison et al., 2000).

Although practice-based research networks (PBRNs) have been part of the National Institutes of Health (NIH) roadmap vision, they have served largely as a recruitment vehicle for clinical trials, because they provide access to large groups of patients. However, the practice-based context provides another laboratory for data collection via observational studies, surveys, and qualitative analyses. School-based intervention studies can contribute crucial knowledge that takes us beyond evidence of efficacy (Papir-Bernstein, 2012).

6. SELF-DIRECTED APPRAISAL PROCESS

A Reflective Approach to Professional Development

Reflective practice is often viewed as the *bedrock of professional identity* (Finley, 2003). Reflective practice has been included in official benchmark standards, explicitly and/or implicitly, in nursing, occupational therapy, physical therapy, medicine, speech-language pathology, and other health professional education. In essence, this process becomes a vital part of our trajectory for lifelong learning and professional development (ASHA, 2006; Health Professions Council, 2006).

Self-awareness is the first step of any change process that leads to self-direction. As part of a professional development program, any type of reflective practice strategy is highly effective in achieving behavioral change (Osterman & Kottkamp, 1993). As we

discussed in Chapter 2, the primary purpose of traditional staff development is knowledge acquisition, but with reflective staff development, the ultimate purpose is behavioral change leading to improved performance. The knowledge transmitted is useful, and allows the practitioner to make better sense of their experiences. It is viewed more as process knowledge than content or product knowledge. When we learn what is truly useful, we are acquiring knowledge of the artistry of our craft, and what Schön calls, knowing-in-action (Schön, 1983).

Adult Self-Directed Learning

Theories of adult learning are led by *constructivist and social theories of learning*, and suggest that active learning is best achieved by self-directed learners who have multiple opportunities to practice and gain experience, collaborate with others, participate with communities of practice, reflect upon their experiences, and formulate principles for practice based upon such reflections (Bandura, 1986; Gagne, 1985; Schön, 1991).

Self-directed learning is one of the most powerful principles in adult learning for several reasons. First, it relates to a larger concept called *self-actualization*, or sense of accomplishment. Second, it relates to a professional demand to keep up to date through lifelong learning and continuing education. And third, it allows learners to take responsibility for regulating and monitoring their own learning content and pace (Harris, 2011).

Whenever you are encouraging *self-directed learning* for children or adults, these recommendations will ease the process. Students *need to feel safe*, so use a supportive environment where they can admit gaps in their knowledge and ask questions. Students need *opportunity to collaborate* with master practitioner to formulate goals, select strategies, learn about resources, and assess progress. Students *need direction* with and opportunity for critical reflective practice. Students *need guidance* in the process of self-assessment, and will require knowledge of performance criteria and feedback from others (Knowles, 1990).

The central tenet of adult learning relates to active, self-directed learning in relation to authentic experiences (Knowles, 1975, 1990). In fact, this is one of the central tenets of all learning, and the idea can be traced as far back as in the work of Rousseau in his book about the education of children (Harris, 2011). Knowles, however, formulated five premises about adult learning, based on the assumption that adults have different life situations than children (1975).

1. *Self-directed learning:* As individuals mature and become more dependent on themselves and less on others, they have an increased desire to identify their own learning needs and ways to address them.
2. *Experience:* As adults develop a rich and diverse repertoire of experiences, these experiences provide an obvious resource for developing knowledge and competence.
3. *Motivation:* Adults are motivated to learn by envisioning immediate application of situation-specific skills.
4. *Authenticity:* The problems they solve must feel real to them, and applicable to their lives.
5. *Internal Factors:* Factors such as goal accomplishment and learning satisfaction can heighten motivation.

Self-Directed Appraisal Process

Self-directed programs for professional growth are advocated for and supported from different directions and diverse lenses: traditional models of supervision, changing standards

in criteria for evaluations, role juggling, and expansions of responsibilities, and research about adult learning (Papir-Bernstein, 1995). Self-reflection and self-assessment is a component of the formative assessment process in the ASHA Standards for Certification (ASHA, 2013; Daly, 2010). ASHA has developed a self-reflection tool to assist the practitioner in determining areas of strength and areas where additional professional development may be needed. The practitioner is asked to reflect on his or her own performance in each of the areas (PACE, 2014).

Self-directed development is a process by which the practitioner systematically plans for his or her own professional growth and carries out the plan over the course of the year. The program is carried out using available resources and creating expansive options. Self-directed staff development has three primary features: the practitioner *takes primary responsibility* for a program of professional growth; the practitioner develops and follows *professional improvement goals;* and the practitioner has access to a wide variety of *resources* (Glatthorn, 1984; Papir-Bernstein et al., 1995).

Self-directed study or self-managed professional development is all part of the self-appraisal process (O'Connell, 1997). It allows professionals to enter into a "contract" with oneself, and is similar in concept to a student's Individualized Educational Plan (IEP). It facilitates acquisition of new knowledge and skills and documenting professional growth objectives. The self-directed process consists of four steps (O'Connell, 1997; Papir-Bernstein, 1995):

1. Formulation of an open-ended list of *potential professional growth objectives*
2. Completion of a *professional growth plan* that includes self-analysis of the intervention program including strengths and areas of concern, targeted areas for

improvement, and professional improvement goals (Appendix F)

3. Completion of an *action plan* that breaks down areas into performance objectives, methods, resources, and time lines needed for achievement of objectives

4. Completion of a *summative conference* or self-evaluation

This type of approach is most useful with practitioners who are self-driven, feel competent, skilled in self-analysis, and enjoy independent work projects (Papir-Bernstein & Legrand, 1993). Research has shown us that professionals who are empowered with the belief that they have the capability and opportunity to effect what happen to themselves are more likely to be high achievers, assuming greater initiative and responsibility at work (Sparks-Langer & Colton, 1991). That sounds like you, doesn't it?

REFLECTIVE SUMMATIVE QUESTIONS

1. How would you insure that you have created a *learning environment* for your students and co-workers?

2. Do you see any place for ASHA's VAA in a speech therapy program? How would you implement this type of *evaluation system*?

3. Describe why compliance, adherence, and concordance are important concepts for our work. What strategies might you implement to insure *student adherence and concordance*?

4. What place does *clinical expertise* play in our overall continuum of professional happiness? What experiences have you had that reinforce your beliefs about expertise?

5. How might you expand your comfort with *communities of practice*?

6. When and why would you be motivated to pursue self-directed professional development?

REFERENCES

American Speech-Language-Hearing Association (ASHA). (2006). *Professional performance review process for the school-based speech-language pathologist* [Guidelines]. Retrieved from http://www.asha.org/policy

American Speech-Language-Hearing Association (ASHA). (2010). *Roles and responsibilities of speech language pathologists in schools* [Professional issues statement]. Retrieved from http://www.asha.org/policy

American Speech-Language-Hearing Association (ASHA). (2014). *Performance assessment of contributions and effectiveness of speech-language pathologists (PACE)*. Retrieved from http://www.asha.org/Advocacy/state/PACE

Argyris, C. (1999). *On organizational learning*. Oxford, UK: Blackwell.

Aronson, J. K. (2007). Compliance, concordance, adherence. *British Journal of Clinical Pharmacology, 63*(4), 383–384.

ASHA Council for Clinical Certification in Audiology and Speech-Language Pathology. (2013). *2014 Standards for the Certificate of Clinical Competence in Speech-Language Pathology*. Retrieved November 29, 2016, from http://www.asha.org/Certification/2014-Speech-Language-Pathology-Certification-Standards/

Bandura, A. (1986). *Social foundations of thought and action: A social cognitive theory*. Englewood Cliffs, NJ: Prentice Hall.

Banks, P., & Knuth, R. (2013). Working as a team: The new conception of professionalism. *ASHA SIG 16 Perspectives on School-Based Issues, 14,* 18–21.

Behrman, A. (2012). Fostering patient compliance by nurturing clinical expertise in graduate school. In R. Goldfarb (Ed.), *Translational speech-language pathology and audiology.* San Diego, CA: Plural.

Belasco, J. A., & Stayer, R. C. (1993). *Flight of the buffalo: Soaring to excellence and learning to let employees lead.* New York, NY: Warner Books.

Bennett, D., & Parry, G. (1998). The accuracy of reformulation in cognitive analytic therapy: A validation study. *Psychotherapy Research, 8,* 84–103.

Blosser, J., & Neidecker, E. (2002). *School programs in speech-language pathology: Organization and service delivery.* Boston, MA: Allyn & Bacon.

Boldt, S. G. (1993). *Zen and the art of making a living.* New York, NY: Penguin Group.

Bolman, L. G., & Deal, T. E. (1997). *Reframing organizations: Artistry, choice and leadership.* San Francisco, CA: Jossey-Bass.

Choo, C. W. (1998). *The knowing organization: How organizations use information to construct meaning, and create knowledge.* New York, NY; Oxford, UK: Oxford University Press.

Clark, M. K., & Flynn, P. (2011). Rational thinking in school-based practice. *Language, Speech and Hearing Services in Schools, 42,* 73–76

Conners, R., Smith, T., & Hickman, C. (1994). *The OZ principle: Getting results through individual and organizational accountability.* Upper Saddle River, NJ: Prentice Hall.

Cooper, M., & McLeod, J. (2011). *Pluralistic counseling and psychotherapy.* London, UK: Sage.

Cornett, B. S., & Chabon, S. (1988). *The clinical practice of speech-language pathology.* Columbus, OH: Merrill.

Culatta, R. (1992). Where has the master clinician gone? *ASHA, 40,* 49–52.

Daly, G. (2010). Formative assessment as a clinical supervision tool. *ASHA Perspectives on Administration and Supervision, 20*(3), 113–116.

Dufour, R. (2004). What is learning community? *Educational Leadership, 61*(8), 6.

Duncan, B. L., & Sparks, J. A. (2016). Systematic feedback through the Partners for Change Outcome Management System (PCOMS). In M. Cooper & W. Dryden (Eds.), *Handbook of pluralistic counseling and psychotherapy.* London, UK: Sage.

Dweck, C. S. (2006). *Mindset: The new psychology of success.* New York, NY: Ballantine Books.

Ehren, T. (1999). *Developing a professional growth plan for speech-language pathologists.* In-service meeting for Broward County School District, Ft. Lauderdale, FL.

Feger, S., & Arruda, E. (2008). *Professional learning communities: Key themes from the literature.* Providence, RI: The Education Alliance, Brown University.

Finlay, L. (2003). Mapping multiple routes. In L. Finlay & B. Gough (Eds.), *Reflexivity: A practical guide for researchers' social sciences.* Oxford, UK: Blackwell.

Frattali, C. (1991). In pursuit of quality: Evaluating clinical outcomes. *National Student Speech Language Hearing Association, 18,* 4–17.

Friend, M., & Cook, L. (1992). *Interactions: Collaboration skills for school professionals.* White Plains, NY: Longman.

Fullan, M. G. (1990). *Changing school culture through staff development.* Association for Supervision and Curriculum Development (ASCD). Alexandria, VA: ASCD.

Gabbay J., & Le May, A. (2010). *Practice-based evidence for health care: Clinical mindlines.* Oxon, UK: Routledge.

Gagne, E. D. (1985). *The cognitive psychology of school learning.* Boston, MA: Little, Brown.

Geller, E., & Foley, G. M. (2009). Broadening the ports of entry for speech-language pathologists: A relational and reflective model for clinical supervision. *American Journal of Speech-Language Pathology, 18,* 22–41.

Glatthorn, A. A. (1984). *Differentiated supervision.* Association for Supervision and Curriculum Development. Alexandria, VA: ASCD

Goldberg, S. (1997). *Clinical skills for speech-language pathologists.* San Diego, CA: Singular.

Harris, I. B. (2011). Conceptions and theories of learning for workplace education. In J. P. Hafler (Ed.), *Extraordinary learning in the workplace.* New York, NY: Springer.

Health Professions Council (HPC). (2006). *Your guide to our standards for continuing professional development.* London, UK: Author.

Hoffman, A. J. (2013). Enhancing self-efficacy for optimized patient outcomes through the theory of symptom self-management. *Cancer Nursing, 36*(1), E16–26.

Hord, S. M., & Sommers, W. A. (2008). *Leading professional learning communities: Voices from research and practice.* Thousand Oaks, CA: Corwin Press.

Kamhi, A. (1994). Toward a theory of clinical expertise in speech-language pathology. *Language, Speech, and Hearing Services in Schools, 25,* 115–119.

Kamhi, A. (1995). Research to practice: Defining, developing and maintaining clinical expertise. *Language, Speech, and Hearing Services in Schools, 26,* 353–356.

Kaufman, H., Braswell, Y., Cohen, M., & Papir-Bernstein, W. (1995). Citywide speech services collaborative consultation pilot project. *Journal of the New York State Association of Supervision and Curriculum Development (NYSASCD), 10,* 30–34.

Kerka, S. (1995). *The learning organization: Myths and realities.* Eric Clearinghouse. Retrieved September 9, 2016, from http://files.eric.ed.gov/fulltext/ED388802.pdf

Knowles, M. S. (1975). *Self-directed learning: A guide for learners and teachers.* New York, NY: Association Press.

Knowles, M. S. (1990). *The adult learner: A neglected species* (4th ed.). Houston, TX: Gulf.

Konnikova, M. (2013). *Mastermind: How to think like Sherlock Holmes.* New York, NY: Penguin Random House.

Lewandowsky, S., Ecker, U. K. H., Seifert, C. M., Schwarz, N., & Cook, J. (2012). Misinformation and correction: Continued influence and successful de-biasing. *Psychological Science Public Interest, 13,* 106–131.

Lewis, M. (2016). *The undoing project: A friendship that changed our minds.* New York, NY: W.W. Norton.

Margison, F. R., Barkham, M., Evans, C., McGrath, G., Clark, J. M., Audin, K., & Connell, J. (2000). Measurement psychotherapy. Evidence-based practice/practice-based evidence. *British Journal of Psychiatry, 177,* 123–130.

McTaggart, L. (2008). *The field.* New York, NY: HarperCollins.

Merritt, D. D., & Culatta, B. (1998). *Language intervention in the classroom.* San Diego, CA: Singular.

Milne, D. L., Baker, C., Blackburn, I. M., James, I., & Reichelt, F. (1999). Effectiveness of cognitive therapy training. *Journal of Behavior Therapy and Experimental Psychiatry, 30,* 81–92.

Moses, D., & Shapiro, D. (1996). A developmental conceptualization of clinical problem solving. *Journal of Communication Disorders, 29*(3), 199–221.

Murphy, A. T. (1982). The clinical process and the speech-language pathologist. In G. H. Shames & E. H. Wiig (Eds.), *Human communication disorders.* Columbus, OH: Merrill.

O'Connell, P. F. (1997). *Speech, language and hearing programs in schools: A guide for students and practitioners.* Gaithersburg, MD: Aspen.

O'Donohue, W., Fisher, J. E., & Plaudd, J. J., & Link, W. (1989). What is a good treatment decision? The client's perspective. *Professional Psychology Research and Practice, 20*(6), 404–407.

O'Keefe, T. (2002). Organizational learning: A new perspective. *Journal of European Industrial Training, 26*(2), 130–141.

O'Sullivan, J., Reaper-Fillyaw, R., Plante, A. & Gottwald, S. (2014). On the road to self-supervision. *SIG 11 Perspectives on Administration and Supervision, 24,* 44–50.

Osterman, K. F., & Kottkamp, R. B. (1993). *Reflective practice for educators.* Newbury Park, CA: Corwin Press.

Papir-Bernstein, W. (1995). *Supervision for the 21st Century: Facilitating self-directed professional growth.* NYSSLHA Mini-Seminar, New York, NY.

Papir-Bernstein, W. (2001, November). *Creating the perfect fit: Merging personal competence with program effectiveness.* Presented at ASHA Convention, New Orleans, LA.

Papir-Bernstein, W. (2002). *Developing AAC supervision: Essential components of speech/language therapy programs.* Presented at LIU/UCP AAC Conference, Brooklyn, NY.

Papir-Bernstein, W. (2012). The artistry of practice-based evidence (PBE): One practitioner's path—Part I. In R. Goldfarb (Ed.), *Translational speech-language pathology and audiology* (pp. 51–57). San Diego, CA: Plural.

Papir-Bernstein, W., Bernstein, S. W., Braswell, Y., Kaufman, H., & Magnante, P. (1995). *Col-*

laborative consultation: An adventure with alternative service delivery models. New York State Speech-Language-Hearing Association (NYS-SLHA), New York, NY.

Papir-Bernstein, W., & Legrand, R. (1993). *Differentiated systems for staff development: Self-direction and reflection*. Presented at ASHA Convention, Anaheim, CA.

Pascarella, P. (1997, October). Harnessing knowledge. *Management Review*, pp. 37–40.

Patterson, L. E., Rak, C. F., Chermonte, J., & Roper, W. (1992). Automaticity as a factor in counselor skills acquisition. *Canadian Journal of Counseling, 26*(3), 189–200.

Rogus-Pulia, N., & Hind, J. (2015). Patient-centered dysphagia therapy: The critical impact of self-efficacy. *SIG 13: Perspectives on Swallowing Disorders, 24*, 146–154.

Rudebusch, J., & Wiechmann, J. (2013). The SLP's guide to PLCs. *ASHA SIG 16 Perspectives on School-Based Issues, 14*, 22–27.

Satir, V. (1967). *Conjoint family therapy*. Palo Alto, CA: Science and Behavior Books.

Schein, E. (1972). *Professional education: Some new directions*. New York, NY: McGraw-Hill.

Schmitt, M. B., & Justice, L. (2011, June). Schools as complex host environments: Understanding aspects of schools that influence clinical practice and research. *ASHA Leader*, pp. 8–11.

Schön, D. (1983). *The reflective practitioner: Professionals think in action*. Hoboken, NJ: Jossey-Bass.

Schön, D. A. (Ed.) (1991). *The reflective turn: Case studies in and on educational practice*. New York, NY: Teachers College Press.

Schraeder, T., Amaryl, S., Cave, C., Hubert, F., & Green, T. (2008, November). *Making professional performance review work for you*. Presented at ASHA Convention, Chicago, IL.

Senge, P. (2006). *The fifth discipline: The art and practice of the learning organization*. New York, NY: Doubleday.

Smith, M. K. (2001). Infed. *The learning organization: Principles, theory and practice*. Retrieved October 13, 2016, from http://www.infed.org/biblio/learning-organization.htm

Sparks-Langer, G. M., & Colton, A. B. (1991). Synthesis of research on teachers' reflective thinking. *Educational Leadership*, 37–44.

Trinder, L., & Reynolds, S. (Eds.). (2000). *Evidence-based practice: A critical appraisal*. Oxford, UK: Blackwell Science.

Vocabulary. (2015). *Concordance*. Retrieved from https://www.vocabulary.com/dictionary/concordance

Wah, L. (1999). Making knowledge stick. *Management Review*, pp. 24–29.

Wang, C. L., & Ahmed, P. K. (2003). Organization learning: A critical review. *The Learning Organization, 10*(1), 8–17.

Weick, K. (1995). *Sensemaking in organizations*. Thousand Oaks, CA: Sage.

CHAPTER 16

Leadership Within Teaching and Learning

1. PROFESSIONAL DEVELOPMENT CONTENT

What Is Professional Development?

Professional development is conceived broadly to include any activity or process intended to improve skills, attitudes, comprehension, and performance related to professional roles and responsibilities. Traditional staff development vehicles include courses, workshops, committee projects, peer intervisitations, and one-on-one support. While large training sessions are appropriate vehicles for presenting new information and stimulating ideas, implementation often gets overlooked. Our charge is to create environments in which *professional growth is valued* and facilitated.

Although staff development programs may differ in content and format, they all share the common purpose of bringing about *change in three areas*: the beliefs and attitudes of the professional, the use of specific instructional and clinical practices, and individual student learning outcomes. Research indicates that experienced and highly competent professionals seldom feel committed to an innovation until they have seen that it works (Guskey, 1985). The most significant changes in attitudes and beliefs happen only after new practices are successfully implemented and changes in student learning are seen. Neither training alone nor training followed by implementation are sufficient conditions for change. Beliefs, attitudes, and motivational factors change only when training and implementation are combined with evidence of improved student learning outcomes.

Trends that are more recent include staff development approaches that sustain ongoing dialogue, reflection, and self-exploration. One of our challenges is to incorporate training approaches that validate and investigate our own attitudinal factors as well as reflect upon changes in student communicative behaviors. When we use *differentiated approaches*, we are better able to consider the needs of the practitioner at different stages of professional development. This ultimately leads to increased self-efficacy and a greater sense of autonomy. One of the major marketing strategies for using differentiated approaches to staff development and supervision is that all practitioners do not need the same approach by virtue of differing experiences and competencies. Just as we offer students choices of activities and materials for building their independent functions and providing the dignity of choice, so too can practitioners be offered choices (Papir-Bernstein & Legrand, 1993).

One of the responsibilities of leadership is to help professionals understand the importance of promoting the experience of reflective practices as a technique to facilitate our own clinical knowledge as well as a productive learning strategy for our students (Vera-Barachowitz, 2003).

A.R.T.: Intervisitations Encourage Learning Teams

Throughout the school year, we, as supervisors, encouraged our practitioners to arrange for visits with other nearby practitioners. The reasons were varied—it might have been for a boost of adrenalin, to exchange areas of expertise, to learn a new skill, or to observe someone work who was more seasoned. The outcomes of some of the visits provided learning experiences not just for the practitioners, but for me as well. For example, I learned that most people are uncomfortable being "observed," so better to call it "collaborative therapy." I learned that two practitioners working in the same program did not necessary take advantage of each other's presence. Therefore, I suggested they set up a "communication bulletin board" for exchange of ideas.

Feedback forms were completed after each visit by both the sending and receiving practitioners. They were asked to narrate their learnings, and reflect on further steps they would like to take for their own professional development.

Designing Professional Development Activities

Those of us involved with designing professional development materials have the responsibility of keeping it self-directed, rigorous, engaging, functional, sustainable, and quantifiable. We do that by targeting three dimensions: context, process, and content (Papir-Bernstein, 2004). *Context* refers to the environment in which the professional development takes place. At best, it supports and encourages research and learning through experimentation. *Process* refers to the delivery methodology of professional development, and includes the planning process, implementation, follow-up, and evaluation. At best, the participants are active designers as well as learners. *Content* refers to the skills and knowledge base. At best, it integrates theory with practice and focuses on product as well as process.

Quality professional development has been described as containing the following attributes (Csikszentmihalyi, 1997; Mundry, 2005; Papir-Bernstein, 2004):

1. *Results-driven:* The ultimate goal relates to improved student outcomes, but may also reflect positive changes in the environment, development of leadership skills, and changes in habits, attitudes, instructional, and clinical practices.

2. *Standards-based:* This relates to all the standards that drive our work, including student performance standards, curriculum standards, educational standards, and clinical standards.

3. *Differentiated:* It must be matched to individual needs, levels of expertise, learning styles, experiential development, and professional preference.

4. *Job-embedded:* Both the content and delivery are to be related to the real work challenges and day-to-day experiences of the participants.

5. *Collaborative:* Attention must be paid to the importance of learning communities, social context, and peer support.

6. *Reflective:* Time should be provided for participants to consider and apply new learning.

7. *Evaluative:* There should be evidence about how the activity will have positive impact.

Staff Development as Innovation

In Chapter 2, we discussed thinking about research as a type of innovation. The same can be said of professional development. Barriers to innovation effectiveness have been identified across a variety of professions and disciplines. They include too little time for professionals to learn new skills; lack of central administrative and supervisory support; trying to do too much with too little; lack of technical and financial assistance; staff turnover rate; failure to clarify roles and relationships of participants; and failure to fit innovation into existing structure (Fullan, 1990; Papir-Bernstein, 1995; Pink, 2012).

2. THE HIDDEN CURRICULUM

What Is the Hidden Curriculum?

A hidden curriculum is thought to be a secondary or side effect of intentions during the educational process. The *hidden curriculum* often impacts and imparts values and beliefs about cultural and social norms. It refers to the unwritten, unofficial, and unintended lessons, and perspectives that we learn in school. The hidden curriculum may not come across with words, and yet the students are picking up an attitude about learning as well as a global approach to living through the unspoken and implicit academic, social, and cultural messages (Abbot, 2014; Rosenbaum, 1976). The hidden curriculum refers to cultural mores that are transmitted through formal and informal practices, but not openly acknowledged (Hafferty & Hafler, 2011). One must consider the dynamics between different sources in instruction and explore how intensions interact with actual practices in the academic environments and workplaces. It involves socialization and relationships between learner and educator. For more information about how the hidden curriculum infiltrates your therapy program, please see Appendix G.

The hidden curriculum can reinforce or contradict the formal curriculum in a variety of different areas, such as cultural expectations, values and perspectives, curricular topics, teaching strategies, school structure, and administrative roles and responsibilities (Abbot, 2014). In recent decades, reform has focused on numerous fixes, including the multicultural and diversity educational shift. It is important to note that to some degree the hidden curriculum will always have a presence. Identity formation has been studied in medical education programs, and it was discovered that less distance between formal and hidden curriculums of professional preparation programs lead to greater internalization of a consistent professional identity and occupational autonomy (Hafferty & Hafler, 2011; Hirsh, Ogur, Thibault, & Cox, 2007).

The Implicit Curriculum

Staff development content defines an organization and shapes its members, and can be analyzed in much the same way that different curricula are evaluated. Eisner differentiates between the two types of information contained within a curriculum: an explicit information and implicit information (1985). The *explicit curriculum* contains the courses and most of the technical information. It contains information about the content and requirements. The *implicit curriculum*, however, includes values, beliefs, attitudes, and expectations. The implicit curriculum sometimes becomes the null curriculum, and reflects what is missing from our training. It might include courses not offered, skills related to professional responsibilities that are not taught, or neglected clinical settings (Shepard & Jensen, 1990).

Implicit variables influence professional actions, behaviors, and ways of thinking that ultimately enhance or inhibit professional growth (Papir-Bernstein, 2012b). The implicit curriculum is projected through the following (Eisner, 1985; Shepard & Jensen, 1990):

- relative importance of specific types of information
- discussions about the challenges that clients present
- what personal and professional behaviors are acceptable and unacceptable
- effective stress management
- effective caring skills
- balance of personal and professional
- critical thinking,
- expectations for lifelong learning and lifelong service to the profession
- respect for and trust in one's colleagues
- openness to innovation

The implicit curriculum includes modeling ways of thinking that ultimately lead to continued professional growth or a lack thereof (Shepard & Jensen, 1990). Implicit messages can profoundly influence our fate as practitioners. We all model personal and professional behaviors about how professionals are supposed to behave. One of the professional behaviors that is often modeled in training programs is *patient primacy*, the belief that the patient always comes first (Scully & Shepard, 1983). This applies to all aspects of our work, so patient primacy becomes student primacy for us, and practitioner primacy for field-based supervisors.

Knowledge Distinctions

There are two types of knowledge that we impart. One is *technical knowledge*, the know-what and the know-why, and that includes principles, examples, and rules. This basic and applied knowledge is an absolute necessity for clinical training and practice, and is abundant in the explicit curriculum (Shepard & Jensen, 1990).

The second type is called *reflective, tacit or intuitive knowledge*, focusing on the actual performance of everyday clinical practice or the know-how. This type of knowledge comes out during our spontaneous actions, but may not follow conscious rules. Schön calls this *the indeterminate zone of practice* (Schön, 1987). He states that these zones of practice escape the guidelines of *technical rationality*. He tells us that when practitioners recognize a situation as unique, they cannot handle it solely by applying theories or techniques derived from their store of professional knowledge. As situations arise with conflicts of beliefs and values, there are no clear and consistent theories to guide the technical selection of solutions. We as professors, students, and practitioners, and leaders must be prepared for the unknown. This is not a field where cookbooks suffice.

In earlier chapters, also, we talked about *technical rationality* and its influence on traditional thinking about academic knowledge. Technical rationality viewed professional practice as problem solving through application of theory and research. It included an assumption that once you *knew something*, knowing it would help you know how to *do something*. In other words, we hoped that knowledge about theory and research should and would inform practice. However, what we now know is that *knowing about something* is not the same type of knowing as *knowing how to do something*.

Extraordinary Workplace Learning

The hidden curriculum is central to learning, and that is true for us as well as for our students. It consists of what is implicitly taught by example on a day-by- day basis, and many of us are blind to it, and to its impact. This sometimes results in troubling educational scenarios. In health care, as well as education, *professional standards* have been known to function more as *suggestions* than as normative mandates, largely due to the influence of union delegations and their accompanying strategies to protect the practitioners from the demands of the bureaucracy (Ginsberg, Regehn, Stern, & Lingard, 2002). Practitioners sometimes view inconsistencies and disconnects between what was said in the classroom (the formal curriculum) and what is done in the school-based practice setting (the hidden curriculum).

Although any training format may look and feel good, sometimes both the giver and receiver of this approach suffer, as it may create feeling of burden, overresponsibility, entitlement, and dependence. Self-care involves a commitment to professional growth that includes the joy of acquisition of professional knowledge, the excitement of research, and the sense of community that comes from service to one's profession.

Why does this happen? Most educational and health care settings view their own workplace activities as *hallmarks of effectiveness*, and people working within would never consider themselves unprofessional because of the culture within which they work. There are *cultures of silence and social control*, as professionals would rather avoid messy confrontations with others whose practices need remediation. There are still cultures of *overhelping and overdoing*, which prevent students from achieving necessary outcomes and lead to institutional rather than educational attitudes. There are existing cultures of *defensiveness and denial* when practitioners are approached by an administrator (Groopman, 2007; Hafferty & Hafler, 2011). What makes

this even more difficult, we are often unaware of how frustrated we are becoming until it is too late. Acknowledging and appreciating *the overly demanding implicit and hidden curriculum* is the first step for creating an extraordinary workplace.

3. SHARING THE IMPLICIT AND TACIT

Describing Tacit Knowledge

The sharing of *tacit knowledge* in an educational setting is a difficult task largely because its very nature prevents it from being easily articulated. Studies about expert teachers have shown consistent findings and isolated the following variables: clarity of presentation, enthusiasm, command of subject matter, preparation, organization of materials, stimulating student interest for engagement in learning, creating a positive learning environment, and approachability (Havita, Barak, & Simhi, 2001; Kane, Sandretto, & Heath, 2004; Shim & Roth, 2008). However, lacking from these studies are indications of how expert teachers do what they do. One of the key differences between expert teachers and novice teachers lies not with "what" they do, but with "how" they do it. Although teachers may possess the tacit knowledge of how they do their job, they often struggle with the attempt to bring this knowledge to the surface and explain it to others (Polanyi, 1967; Shim & Roth, 2008).

Although scholars have investigated the importance and benefits of sharing tacit knowledge, the relationship between tacit and explicit knowledge is not always clear (Nonaka & Takeuchi, 1995; Shim & Roth, 2008). Tacit knowledge has been described in the literature as sometimes codified and sharing a continuum with explicit knowledge (Nonaka &

Takeuchi, 1995; Kane et al., 2004). However, the question remains—*how* is this deep procedural knowledge codified and shared with less seasoned professionals or mentees?

In one study by Shim and Roth (2008), the learning theory known as *constructivism* provides insight. Within this theory of learning, cognitive apprenticeship is described as a method that helps novices acquire expertise (Charon, 1979). When learners interact with each other, they actively construct knowledge that may be used functionally in other contexts. Tasks by apprentices are completed as experts model, scaffold, coach, and thus *mold their tacit knowledge in context* (Shim & Roth, 2008).

In this same study, descriptions by seasoned professionals were elicited about the tacit nature of their expertise (Shim & Roth, 2008). They used phrases such as "a mixture of art and science, a lack of awareness about performance, and the innate perspective of teaching expertise" (p. 11). They did not recognize their teaching expertise as formal knowledge. They expressed their skill development as more art than science, taking place largely through intuition and instantaneous situational adjustments. The art of practice is individual and highly personalized. One of the main characteristics of expert performance is *fluidity*. Fluid performance happens when experts perform their work without consciously thinking about what they are doing. It appears natural and seamless (Dreyfus & Dreyfus, 1986).

Articulating Tacit Expertise

Tacit expertise is articulated through modeling, observing, using probing questions, describing intentions, and reflecting on actions (Shim & Roth, 2008). Two categories for sharing tacit knowledge have been identi-fied. One is to involve learners in *real practices* without actively transforming tacit expertise into explicit knowledge. This happened largely via observations of the raw practices that allow the observers to see where tacit knowledge lives. Observation was a passive way to communicate tacit knowledge.

A second way allowed tacit knowledge to come to the surface by applying metacognitive skills, *storytelling, or metaphors*. This method forces tacit knowledge to the surface by actively questioning and probing the content of the observations. One effective meta-cognitive skill is "talking out loud" or narrating everything that you are watching (during or after the observation) (Smith, 2001). Metaphors are helpful because you are transforming the context of what you are seeing into an everyday experience that contains greater comfort and familiarity. An example would be describing the sequence of activities that you observed as if in the context of a dance, or a cooking activity.

Whether through passive observation or active "bringing it to the surface" (BIS), reflection on the practices and that type of *process experience* needs to follow. The sharing of tacit knowledge facilitates a process of *personal creation*. There is no recipe, and no detailed instructions. The first step is building background and knowledge, but the rest has to be worked out by itself. Theories, supervision, guidance, and suggestions all can help. Ultimately, you have to choose a path—simply because tacit knowledge interacts with personality and resides differently with each person's mind (Shim & Roth, 2008).

The sharing of tacit knowledge requires more intention and focused reflection than the sharing of explicit knowledge. Expertise can be viewed from the perspective of art and practice implicit in the artistic and intuitive processes that some practitioners naturally bring to their teaching contexts (Schön,

1983). It should also be noted that expertise is deeply influenced by culture and work settings, therefore *knowledge sharing* needs to be valued within the organization (Smith, 2001).

Knowledge Sharing Techniques

As Kamhi investigated the question of *clinical expertise* in our field, he describes research about *teaching and learning* from the fields of psychology, education, and medicine (1994). It was surprising to discover that more than any other variable related to content or methodology, student involvement and engagement depended on environmental aspects such as pace, momentum, and expectations. Most educational and clinical methodologies had a higher rate of success if they were presented through an enthusiastic delivery with demonstrated strength of belief and support both from school personnel and home caregivers.

The real question is how do we gather data about clinical expertise as reflected by how practitioners think about clinical problems? Some suggested methodologies would be to obtain verbal protocols, rating scales, or descriptive analyses from practitioners as they observe clinical activities or perform those same activities. Formats might include thinking aloud narratives, questions, and answers, or running commentaries (Kamhi, 1994). The following strategies for organizational and personal knowledge sharing come from a variety of business and social science disciplines. They include (Pascarella, 1997; Smith, 2001; Thomas, 2000; Wah, 1999):

- Instill a corporate-wide culture that integrates knowledge resources into every organizational process.

- Encourage and support training, interactive learning experiences, and give and take communications
- Encourage knowledge sharing by connecting people by expertise in content topic or geography
- Create idea bulletin boards.
- Create communities of practice.
- Organize a human-talent exchange.
- Use extraordinary recruitment methods to attract, hire, and retain the most motivated and knowledgeable people.
- Create peer to peer networks.

4. ENGAGED SCHOLARSHIP

The Scholarship of Teaching and Learning (SoTL)

Many of the same tools identified and utilized in clinical and educational training programs may be applied throughout our work with students and our lifelong learning journeys. For example, much of the same current SoTL investigations relate to the spheres of higher education, professional development, and enhancement of student learning (Bowen, 2010; Boyer, 1990). We now know that science of teaching and learning extends far beyond academic settings. The SoTL research seeks to minimize the divide between research and practice by enhancing functional applications and learning practices through process analysis and self-reflection (McKinney, 2007).

The SoTL has been described as containing a deep knowledge base, critical reflectivity, going public with insights and innovations, conducted within a framework of continuous evaluation and improvement, and an inquiry process linked to creativity and change (Kreber, 2007; Robinson et al., 2011). Its purpose is to shine a light on the strategies, tools, and techniques of clinical and academic instruction because the integrity of our discipline begins in the classroom as we investigate effective teaching and learning. From the SoTL perspective, research into teaching and learning is as important as disciplinary research (Robinson et al., 2011).

Pedagogical Scholarship

In the light of recent evidence about the scholarship of teaching and learning (SoTL), the value and credibility of what is sometimes called "pedagogical scholarship" is now on our professional radar screens. It is defined as scholarly work about teaching and learning, published within fields *other than* education (Weimer, 2011). The SoTL is based upon both scholarly research, as well as reports of practice-based experience generated by and relevant to cross-discipline communities of professionals, and by definition occupies a seat in the translational arena (Papir-Bernstein, 2012b).

Weimer identifies one category of pedagogical scholarship as "wisdom of practice" or experience-based scholarship, which is published work based upon professional experience. Such experience may include: personal accounts of change resulting from the implementation of new instructional practices or policies; recommended practices reports; and personal narratives reflecting opinions and concerns (2011; Papir-Bernstein, 2012b).

These all become the building blocks of practice-based evidence, as long as we remember to share our evidence. The practitioner's task is to interpret external evidence from research in relation to a client's preferences, culture, environment and values regarding health and well-being. *Evidence-based practice* is the dynamic integration of clinical expertise (internal, experiential, or *practice-based evidence*) with external evidence in everyday

practice (Dollaghan, 2007; Kamhi, Vanleer, Lundgren, Verdolini, & Bernstein-Ratner, 2009). Although EBP focuses on methodology and measurement, we know that there is usually more than one recommended course of clinical action, and we sometimes get little direction about targeting goals and objectives from external research.

The Scholarship of Application and Integration

Commitment to service as part of education and learning is a natural baseline for the scholarship of application (Shulman, 1999). The term "scholarship" has an expanded definition of intellectual and academic life that pertains to the processes of *discovery, integration, application, service, and teaching* in addition to its original reference to *research* (Boyer, 1990; Glassick, 2000). Excellence in scholarship, or published or professional rewarded work, has been defined by the Carnegie Foundation in the following way and as meeting the following standards: it must have clearly defined goals, use appropriate methods of research, meet standards of significant results, be presented within professional circles, and be reflectively critiqued for future improvement (1989).

As we reflect on learning, we are carried into new areas relating to our understanding about the nature of knowledge. Perhaps today it is best described as the pursuit of and the process of knowing, which implies an active creative process. The educational bottom line is that old academic categories about fields of study no longer make sense. Malloch and Massey tell us that because knowledge is growing exponentially, theories are continuously reshaped, and disciplines are intersecting in new and unpredictable ways (2006). *Hyphenated disciplines* are appearing as overlapping academic neighborhoods, and knowledge is being reshaping so that all teachers and students (of all ages) would be using the same categories of knowing across disciplines (Boyer, 1987; Polanyi, 1967).

The scholarship of integration implies the process of making connections within and across disciplines. The process is closely related to the scholarship of discovery, when research is conducted in areas where disciplines converge. We fit our thinking about our work into larger intellectual patterns, which brings new interpretations and insights to our own patterns of practice.

Participatory Action Research (PAR)

There have been many changes in traditional views about academic knowledge and its relationship to practice. We are considering ways that scholarship can be more clearly grounded and translating into everyday practice by drawing on the participatory, experiential and procedural experiences of practitioners (Kielhofner, 2005).

Engaged scholarship requires a new way of thinking about how knowledge is generated, and include innovative approaches such as *participatory action research* (PAR). It seeks to discover new ways of addressing issues related to everyday practical problems grounded in real life contexts. At best, it uses a collaborative model in which researcher and practitioner share responsibility in shaping the research process, thus bridging the academic world with the world of practice (Suarez-Balcazar & Harper, 2003). Practitioners are viewed as research stakeholders who help shape the research into areas such as what questions are addressed, what data is to be collected, and how finding should be best interpreted and disseminated.

Action research is defined as a tool of curriculum development and consists of continuous feedback that targets program improvement. The educator becomes researcher and role model and encourages students to put theories into practice as they report their field experiences and analyze teaching strategies with mentors, peers, and colleagues (Moon, 2004).

A.R.T.: Participatory Action Research

Looking back, it is not surprising that I was the organizational member called upon for many of our research and writing projects. In addition to having "assignments," I would develop ideas from journal articles, textbooks, or sources external to our field and form a curriculum committee.

One such committee project was called *Assessment Strategy Sourcebook for Evaluating Special Students* (with each word carefully chosen for the acronym ASSESS) (Papir-Bernstein, 1993). We worked with university training programs, journals, and textbooks, and surveyed published assessments and intervention programs compiled for students with

severe and profound disabilities. The purpose was to develop an assessment resource for our students, because in the early 1990s there was very little already published. The committee was comprised of practitioners, staff developers, and one supervisor (that was me).

My involvement with university teaching, research, and writing placed me in the practitioner-researcher role. I thought all was going well, until one day I found a change of title sitting on my desk—with the final S omitted. That became the first day of integrating feedback and re-evaluating power differentials. We eventually came out with a wonderfully useful product.

Scholarship Behind Integrity and Authenticity

The challenges of this century require institutions of higher education to prepare discipline specialists to be independent thinkers and productive leaders (Kreber, 2007). For some, SoTL is viewed relevant only to concerns of higher education. For others, it must include broader agendas and relates to the learning experiences of students in all learning settings. We are all working as students and teachers, and sometimes simultaneously. Palmer reminds us that the role of teachers is to generate *a sense of connection and community* between themselves and their students, themselves and their subject, and eventually between their student and the subject (1998). In doing this, we communicate not only enthusiasm for the subject, but we also communicate how and why the subject matters (Kreber, 2007).

Palmer, Zajonc, and Scribner use the word "integrity" to describe the quality that we discover through our efforts with building those vital connections, as we courageously express aspects of our *selfhood* when we share what matters to us, what we truly care about, and how that fits with our lives (2010). Our enthusiasm about this field—whether communicated through our therapy, our teaching, our professional development, or our work within communities—expresses the fact that our work matters beyond the walls of the setting. Kreber uses the term *authenticity* to express a similar sentiment (2007).

When is an idea or action deemed authentic? It has been proposed that an identity becomes authentic when up against a background of substantial issues that crucially matter. Such issues, as the needs of our fellow human beings, then qualify as being part of a *horizon of significance* (Kreber, 2007; Taylor, 1991). Our work creates a huge horizon of significance, as we balance our love of the field with care about the interests of the people it serves and the people we teach.

---

5. FORGING TRANSLATIONAL PATHWAYS

Dealing With the Gap

The Centers for Disease Control and Prevention (CDC) have defined *translational research* in public health as it relates to accepted and evidence-based public health interventions. The principle that research is important and needs to be translated is not in dispute, but the remaining questions relate to everyday applications in clinical practice (Papir-Bernstein, 2012a). Cases have been made for the synthesis of evidence from practitioners working in other sectors (such as architects and teachers), input from a wider range of disciplines, and expansion of practice-based applications (Ogilvie, Craig, Griffin, Macintyre, & Wareham, 2009; Westfall, Mold, & Fagnan, 2007).

However, those of us who have studied the dynamics of change (or simply work within large bureaucracies) know that there are many reasons personal and professional growth attempts are thwarted in organizations—some having to do with the organizational culture and others with individual attitudes and preferences (Papir-Bernstein & Legrand, 1994). One of the hallmarks of a successful *translational process* is the establishment of cultures that enable collaboration and cooperation across the continuum of professional diversity (Feldman, 2008). Another hallmark is facilitation of professional development (for those who are providing and/or supervising the service) in the areas of accountability, self-direction, leadership, personal mastery, and commitment (Papir-Bernstein, 2012a).

In the world of medicine, there is a growing consensus that the transfer of knowledge from discovery to development to dissemination and through implementation should be accelerated (Thornicroft, Lempp, & Tansella, 2011). *Translational research* requires different skill sets applied to a unified goal, and sets up a demand for stakeholders to bridge the gap and join forces so that biomedical achievements are translated into practical benefits. There have been many changes in traditional views about academic knowledge and its relationship to practice. We are considering ways that scholarship can be more clearly grounded and translating into everyday practice by drawing on the participatory, experiential, and procedural experiences of practitioners (Kielhofner, 2005).

Surveys of rehabilitation practitioners across a variety of medically related fields revealed that they felt that research lacked real-life relevance to clinical situations, that it addressed topics not necessarily relevant to practice, and that results were not easily applied to practice (Keilhofner, 2005). They often felt torn between being *client-centered* and *science-centered*, as the evidence does not always match their perception of client needs (DiLollo, 2010; Dubouloz, 1999).

The Science Behind Research Dissemination, Implementation, and Diffusion

What do we actually mean by *dissemination, implementation, and diffusion of research*? Each one has a scientific underpinning supported by theories and models (Rosenbek, 2012). We must do whatever we can to insure that clinical discoveries--whether made in the university clinics, hospital labs, or educational arenas—are disseminated, implemented, and diffused through staff development programs and enhanced clinical practices of the pro-

fessionals who are both supervising the programs and directly working with the students (Papir-Bernstein, 2012a). As we discussed in Chapter 1, a *practice-based educational arena* provides opportunity for the essential link to be established between research discoveries and research dissemination, diffusion, and clinical implementation. This is known as the *translational process*.

According to The Centers for Disease Control and Prevention (CDC), *dissemination* refers to the spread of knowledge and distribution of the information, resulting in behavioral change. *Implementation* refers to the integration of activities and strategies for adoption within specific settings (such as a community center or school), and *diffusion* refers to the study of factors necessary for successful adoption and use of new practices (NIH, 2009; Papir-Bernstein, 2012a). Each one is essential in practice-based leadership and will be greatly impacted by individual and organizational variables, such as readiness for change, packaging of information, organizational leadership attitudes, and staff resources (Flay et al., 2005).

Dissemination, implementation, and diffusion will be greatly impacted by individual and organizational variables, such as readiness for change, packaging of information, organizational leadership attitudes, and staff resources (Flay et al., 2005). Staff development is the most effective application platform for enhancing "organizational learning" and individual behaviors and attitudes. It will impact the clinical and educational practices of the professionals who are both supervising the programs and directly working with the students (Papir-Bernstein, 2012a).

Both *knowledge management and information design* need to be carefully considered before this translational process can even begin (see Chapter 1). Most importantly, and before all else, we need to get the ball rolling from within our clinical and educational programs. It has been well acknowledged that although school-based practitioners place a high value on principles related to evidence and evidence-based practice (EBP), they are not frequent sources for original research, publications, assessment protocols or practice guidelines. Collecting and sharing evidence is at least equally as important as knowing where to find it in the world of scientific research.

A.R.T.: In the Early Days

Through most of the 1970s, I was the speech-language therapist in a New York City Department of Education school program called School for Language and Hearing-Impaired Children (SLHIC). Many of these students were referred to as "rubella babies," born of mothers who had contracted German measles in their first trimester of pregnancy. Needless to say, this population was largely underrepresented in research. The same was true for the second population of students I worked with beginning in the early 1980s, now as a speech therapy supervisor—children with Autism Spectrum Disorder (ASD) and/or Pervasive Developmental Disability (PDD). Although in both of these instances, I had access to fascinating populations of low-incidence students, research in these and other areas of our field was sorely lacking and what we now call evidence-based practice (EBP) had not yet been born (Papir-Bernstein, 2012a). If only I could turn back the clock . . .

Why Is Translation So Difficult?

As we learned in Chapter 1, the *translation of research into practice* is a complex process that involves many steps including dissemination and implementation of the information to and for practitioners. *Implementation science* is the study of methods that impact the integration of evidence-based interventions into practice settings. Effective implementation ensures that practices validated in the laboratory produce similar "real-world" outcomes.

A.R.T.: From Training to Real World

Professional development was one of my main passions, and I was involved with formulating training seminars as a practitioner, staff development specialist, and speech therapy supervisor. It became clear to me pretty early on, that many people sitting in the room saw this simply as an opportunity to *not* be in their school buildings and working with the students. Some even pretended to take notes. Before the age of technology had arrived, I spent days photo copying and collating materials, and each practitioner left the workshop with a thick looseleaf filled with what I considered to be essentials for a therapy program (the "curse of knowledge"). I was painfully aware that we had to build a bridge—strategies to ease the transition from workshop to therapy program.

I decided to work the process the other way—I began with my visits out to the field, and chose training topics based upon where I either saw the need, or the opportunity to ask the practitioners to share what was really working. The agenda for our next meeting was set from those topics, and I began the discussion with the research. It continued with the examples from the "real world," presented by the practitioners. This format was so successful, that we applied for and were granted Continuing Education Provider status by The American-Speech-Language-Hearing Association. At the time, we were one of the few school districts in the country awarded such an honor.

Knowledge translation complements implementation science, as the process through which new evidence is synthesized and adopted into current practice procedures. As professionals, if we knew what to do and were doing it, there would be no need for knowledge translation or implementation science (Redle, 2016). Redle cites the example of hand-washing practices, which one might assume is a combination of common sense leading to consistent best practice in health care and educational settings. However, we learned over the years that implementation strategies (even for something seemingly as simple as hand-washing) are context dependent and vary across participants and settings.

Although educators and practitioners may more easily define and identify evidence-based practices, we still question methodologies for disseminating and utilizing such practices to communicate findings in meaningful and useful ways and thus reduce the research-to-practice gap (Cook, Cook, & Landrum, 2013). We can learn much from the fields of social marketing and management about how to think differently about research dissemination.

Tonelli describes that the gap between clinical research and clinical practice can be understood in two ways (1998, 2006). First, the knowledge we look for in each endeavor is different. In the first, we are looking for "average," because all background noise created by individual variations is eliminated. In the second, the application must be individualized and unique. The second way they differ is ethical, and relates to values and preferences. In order to make the leap from research to practice, we must consider the *goals and values of the client*, the setting and society in general. Therefore, research alone cannot provide us with the type of knowledge we need to make decisions about client care. Clinical decision-making must also include clinician experience and knowledge about the educational system.

One common shortcoming of the conception of the translational pathways is that they are mainly professionally driven, within which the scientists deliver inventions to clinicians, and the clinicians in turn deliver treatments to patients (Rabin, Brownson, Haire-Joshu, Kreuter, & Weaver, 2008). This unidimensional movement has not yet integrated the concept of patient and public participation in health care. In addition, there are few investigations about patient-related factors that accelerate or impede knowledge transfer (T3). For example, well-informed patients can become active *stakeholders* as well as demanders of treatment expectations (Thornicroft et al., 2011). Scientists, on the other hand, are motivated by professional incentives, such as the desire to publish research findings in peer-reviewed journals, which are most often read by their scientific peers. They struggle, as we all do, with clarity about who takes the responsibility to get this information into clinical routines, and to the clients (Rabin et al., 2008).

Another challenge is the lack of a theoretical paradigm for implementation studies. However, increasing attention to this theoretical deficit has been given through the formulation of an integrative framework with clinical guidelines, called the "knowledge to action" model (Thornicroft et al, 2011). This model considers three states of knowledge: discovery, invention, and innovation. It is based on the notion that stakeholders adopt and use knowledge that has a perceived utility (Lane & Flagg, 2010).

Memetic Theory

What we are really talking about here are ideas, and how we nurture them, grow them, and share them so that they will succeed by living on in the world. How do we get messages to make a difference through their lasting impact on opinions and behaviors? In Chapter 14, we began this discussion with *memetic theory*, and examples of successful *memes*. Now, through the work of the Heaths, we investigate why some ideas stick and others do not (2007). Some ideas are born more interesting than others (nature), while some are designed to be more interesting and useful (nurture). Those seem to be the ones that stick. Why are some ideas stickier than others, or put another way, what causes some information to "catch on" and make the leap from small groups to big groups (Cook et al., 2013; Gladwell, 2000)? The right audiences and contexts certainly do make a difference, but the *stickiness factor* seems to be the most important attribute.

Perhaps we might think about *dissemination of information* by maximizing its stickiness. Six principles for implementation have been identified that can be summed up with one acronym SUCCESs: *a simple, unexpected, concrete, credentialed, emotional story* (Cook et al., 2013; Heath & Heath, 2007).

1. *Simplicity*—Strip an idea down to its core, and make it resonate with the audience. Simply crafted powerful messages can be profound, and used to guide behaviors in a variety of situations. Professional development should translate and control amount of information disseminated.

2. *Unexpectedness*—Use the elements of surprise, to increase alertness and focus and generate interest. Few things grab our attention like surprise. Information that conforms to expectations can be predictable, lack stimulation, and generate boredom. Create curiosity by opening gaps and identifying "cognitive holes" in the knowledge base, and then filling the gaps.

3. *Concreteness*—Explain ideas in terms of meaningful human actions, rather than ambiguous strategies and visions. Vivid content can enhance the persuasiveness of the message. As it holds attention and

excites imagination, new information is more readily connected to existing knowledge.

4. *Credibility*—Sticky ideas have to be able to carry their own credentials, and should allow people to test the idea for themselves rather than relying on data. Academic degrees do not always translate into trust or convey credibility. Credibility often flows best from personal and experiential relationships in real-life situates and contexts, rather than from research and data.

5. *Emotions*—We are wired to feel for people rather than concepts, to harness and convey those emotions with an affective lens.

6. *Stories*—We act on ideas more easily when stories provide the models. As we discussed in Chapter 2, storytelling is a part of science, and its power should be harnessed for disseminating research findings.

These strategies can be illustrated with the following explanation. Research findings can be presented in the form of a narrative (story) by a real practitioner (credible) who crafts a core message (simple) that contains vivid details about implementing a specific practice (concrete) with a surprising twist that impacts outcomes (unexpectedness) and culminates with a heartfelt response by a parent (emotional) (Cook et al., 2013; Dearing, 2008)

The use of these principles combats a cognitive bias known as *the curse of knowledge*, the difficulty we have sharing what we know because we cannot imagine what it is like not knowing it. The *curse of knowledge* sometimes acts as our villain, interfering with our ability to create ideas using these commonsensible principles. This natural psychological tendency can be illustrated by the simple game of "tappers and listeners." The listeners find it very difficult to piece together the song that is being tapped, which the tappers predict that the song will be easily guessed. The tappers think that the song is obvious because they are hearing it in their heads, and it is impossible for them to imagine what it's like for the listeners to hear just the isolated taps. That is the curse of knowledge (Birch & Bloom, 2007; C. Heath & D. Heath, 2007).

6. SIGNATURE PEDAGOGY

What Is Signature Pedagogy?

The term "signature pedagogy" was coined by Lee Shulman, who noted that distinctive *teaching and learning practices* in specialized professions defined learning experiences within that profession (Youatt & Wilcoxx, 2008). Today, and in view of our demanding cognitive age, the new signature pedagogies need to be characterized as "discovery-centered, interdisciplinary, integrative, translational, and contextual" (Youatt & Wilcox, 2008, p. 25). It is the responsibility of both teachers and learners to integrate these characteristics into the most meaningful learning experience.

- *Discovery-centered learning* targets original work that contributes to the knowledge in a discipline. It involves generating *practice-based evidence* as well as remaining lifelong learners.
- *Interdisciplinary learning* involves the investigation of a topic of interest from a broad and diverse range of disciplines that naturally cut across restrictive boundaries.
- *Integrative learning* requires us to connect knowledge and skills evolving from a wide variety of sources and types of experiences. In essence, it bridges knowledge to experience and theory to practice by promoting *ways of knowing*.
- *Translational learning* encourages the utilization of information and research in

new ways, beyond the specific applications designed in the clinic or lab. It involves adapting the research for real-world *practice based educational arenas* or the "blue highways" as described in Chapter 1.
- *Contextual learning* considers the natural, social and human factors of an environment as they relate to *ethical, moral, and responsible practices*.

Why Is It Important For Us to Know About?

Every profession has its favored approaches for professional training programs where we teach disciplinary habits of mind, ways of knowing, and values respected by experts in the field (Chick, Haynie, & Gurung, 2012; Gurung, Chick, & Haynie, 2009). Students have been prepared by educators for professional practices for centuries, but only recently have we taken a hard look at our *signature pedagogies*. Lee Shulman defines signature pedagogies as the forms and styles of teaching and learning experiences that organize the fundamental ways our future practitioners are being educated (2005).

The *purpose of professional education* is preparation for the "good work" of *acting both accomplished and responsible in service to others*. Signature pedagogies form not only habits of the mind, but habits of the heart and of the hand (Shulman, 1999; 2005). Signature pedagogies include pedagogic approaches and distinctive practices. Distinctive practices are not just about knowledge, they are about *habits of mind*: the ways of thinking about a subject, doing it, and being a professional in the area (Thomson, Hall, Jones, & Sefton-Green, 2012). Overall, the signature pedagogy of a particular field teaches us about its personality and culture (Shulman, 2005).

Signature pedagogies ultimate determine the *architectural design of a field*. A signature or distinctive pedagogy has three dimensions of structure referred to as *surface, deep, and implicit.* Surface structure refers to concrete acts of teaching and learning, whereas deep structures reflect assumptions about how to communicate knowledge and know-how. The implicit structure includes beliefs about attitudes and values, and translates to the moral dimension (Gurung et al., 2009; Shulman, 2005).

How It Ties In With Professional Development

Shulman conceptualized professional development in terms of the intertwined processes of the development of clinical skills and specialized knowledge referred to as *signature pedagogies* (2005). Our signature pedagogies are pedagogies that are special and unique to our field. In addition, effective professional practice requires the development of *practical knowledge* allowing one to respond to situations characterized by conditions of "complexity, uniqueness, uncertainty, ambiguity, and conflicting value and ethics orientations" (Hafler, 2011, p. 5). Furthermore, the *reflective competencies* learned in practice situations within *communities of practice* facilitate the application and generalization of formal knowledge in a specific situation to other related situations. All of these contribute to *extraordinary learning experiences.*

Learning has been deemed *extraordinary* when there is congruence and synergy between the preparation of professionals through the formal curriculum and the informal and tacit learning that takes place within the hidden curriculum that is embedded in professional training and workplace settings (Hafler, 2011). Self-directed and practice-based methodologies facilitate extraordinary learning.

7. USING REFLECTIVE PRACTICE FOR TEACHING AND LEARNING

A Tool for Self-Direction

Reflection is a tool for *self-direction,* and provides a process of viewing one's successes and targeting future critical issues. It is a professional development strategy that equips practitioners with opportunities to explore, articulate and represent their own ideas and knowledge in unique ways (Moon, 2004; Osterman & Kittkamp, 1993). Reflection helps us understand what we do and why we do it. It is an attitude of mind that is cultivated through relational exchanges, thus allowing us to view interchanges from a variety of perspectives (Geller, 2013).

As Caty and colleagues posit, *reflective practice* draws attention to how knowledge is generated from practice and experience (2016). Our reflection about clinical relationships, clinical situations, or organizational issues are sources of professional learning that get embedded into our practice-based evidence knowledge base. This becomes part of our *epistemology of practice,* Schön's term for knowledge derived from reflection about experiences in the workplace that help us make sense of our professional decisions and actions and those of others (1983, 1987). Reflective tasks include (Geller, 2013):

- Relating and experiencing emotionally significant events,
- Examining feelings, thoughts, intentions, and actions evoked by these events,
- Considering how to best use this understanding for continued professional growth.

As with any new concept, there was a period of pendulum swings as researchers cautioned against sacrificing content when incorporating reflective practices in the curriculum and professional development programs of schools, colleges and departments of education (SCDEs). This "baby with the bathwater" tendency in educational institutions is not unusual—it reminds us that new information must go through a careful integration process to insure that previous information is simply not discarded for the new.

A.R.T.: The Baby and the Bathwater Syndrome

I have worked with a variety of practitioners, staff developers, and supervisors who were tempted to fall into this pattern. Something new came along, such as the Content-Form-Use paradigm, and everything that was previous known about language frameworks went down the drain. Gathering the new and discarding the old is much easier than culling and integrating. Do your best to work with professionals who understand this.

As times and paradigms shift, new generations emerge who will be both providing and consuming our services. Professional zeitgeist watchers and celebrated trend masters report a disconnect between theory they hear and behaviors they see (Walker, 2009). In Chapter 3, we discussed the concept of *zeitgeist* as one of the guiding principles for all that we do, and reflect much about the spirit and sensibility of an era. Students today are brighter than ever, and want to understand the importance of the content they are taught. We are writing a *new mythology*, affecting both our sense of individuality and the way we define community and balance collective needs. We *want* to know what needs to change, but *need* to know the essential principles that must be maintained and grown.

Beginning a Reflective Process About Our Practices

Here are some guiding questions for *reflection-on-action* (ROA):

- Did the session meet the expected outcomes?
- How did I feel about the session?
- How did the students react?
- Was there anything I could have done more effectively?
- Were there any unresolved problems?
- Would I feel comfortable with other professionals watching this session?
- Did the students have fun?
- Did I have fun?

Here are some additional guiding questions for *reflection-for-action*:

- How can I improve outcomes?
- Should I track talk-time ratio (me to student)?
- How can I make the session more motivating?
- What new materials and activities can I use?
- What is my next step?
- How can I improve the learning environment?
- How can I improve my clinical methodologies?
- How can I develop this into a research study or presentation?

REFLECTIVE SUMMATIVE QUESTIONS

1. Think about a recently attended professional development event and evaluate it based upon some of the criterion in this chapter.

2. How has the implicit curriculum within some professional context impacted your thinking about school or work-related activities and people?

3. What are your preferred modalities for expressing your tacit and experiential knowledge?

4. As you reflect on information dissemination in your classes or work setting, how have the SUCCESs principles been implemented?

5. In what ways might the signature pedagogy of our discipline be expanded and improved?

REFERENCES

Abbot, S. (Ed.). (2014, August). *The glossary of education reform: Hidden curriculum*. Retrieved November 16, 2016, from http://edglossary.org/hidden-curriculum

Birch, S. A., & Bloom, P. (2007). The curse of knowledge in reasoning about false beliefs. *Psychological Science, 18*(5), 382–386.

Bowen, G. (2010). Service learning in the scholarship of teaching and learning: Effective practices. *International Journal for the Scholarship of Teaching and Learning, 4*(2), 1–15.

Boyer, E. L. (1987). *College: The undergraduate experience in America.* New York, NY: Harper & Row.

Boyer, E. L. (1990). *Scholarship reconsidered: Priorities of the professoriate.* Princeton, NJ: Carnegie Foundation for the Advancement of Teaching.

Caty, M., Kinsella, E. A., & Doyle, P. C. (2016). Reflective practice in speech-language pathology: Relevance for practice and education. *Canadian Journal of Speech-Language Pathology and Audiology, 40*(1), 81–91.

Charon, J. M. (1979). *Symbolic interactionism: An introduction.* Upper Saddle River, NJ: Prentice-Hall.

Chick, N. L., Haynie, A., & Gurung, R. A. R. (Eds.). (2012). *Exploring more signature pedagogies: Approaches to teaching disciplinary habits of mind.* Sterling, VA: Stylus.

Cook, B. G., Cook, L., & Landrum, T. J. (2013). Moving research into practice: Can we make dissemination stick? *Council for Exceptional Children, 79*(2), 163–180

Csikszentmihalyi, M. (1997). Flow and education. *NAMTA Journal, 22*(2), 2–35.

Dearing, J. W. (2008). Evolution of diffusion and dissemination theory. *Journal of Public Health Management and Practice, 14*(2), 99–108.

DiLollo, A. (2010). Business: The crisis of confidence in professional knowledge. *SIG 11-Perspectives on Administration and Supervision, 20,* 85–91.

Dollaghan, C. (2007). *The handbook for evidence-based practice in communication disorders.* Baltimore, MD: Brookes.

Dreyfus, L., & Dreyfus, S. E. (1986). *Mind over machine.* Oxford, UK: Basil Blackwell

Dubouloz, C., Egan, M., Vallerand, J., & von Zweck, C. (1999). Occupational therapists' perceptions of evidence-based practice. *American Journal of Occupational Therapy, 53,* 445–453.

Eisner, E. (1985). *The educational imagination: On design and evaluation of school programs.* New York, NY: Macmillan.

Feldman, A. (2008). Does academic culture support translational research? *CTS: Clinical and Translational Science, 1*(2), 87–88.

Flay, B. R., Biglan, A., Boruch, R. F., Castro, F. G., Gottfredson, D., Kellam, S., . . . Ji, P. (2005). Standards of evidence: Criteria for efficacy, effectiveness and dissemination. *Prevention Science, 6*(3), 151–175.

Fullan, M. G. (1990). Changing school culture through staff development. *Yearbook of the Association for Supervision and Curriculum Development.* Alexandria VA: ASCD.

Geller, E. (2013, November). *Broadening ports of entry for speech-language pathologists: A reflective model of supervision.* Presented at ASHA Convention, Chicago, IL.

Ginsburg, S., Regehr, G., Stern, D., & Lingard, L. (2002). The anatomy of the professional lapse: Bridging the gap. *Academic Medicine, 77,* 516–522.

Gladwell, M. (2000). *The tipping point: How little things can make a big difference.* Boston, MA: Little, Brown.

Glassick, C. E. (2000). Boyer's definitions of scholarship, standards for assessing scholarship, and elusiveness of the scholarship of teaching. *Academic Medicine, 75*(9), 877–880.

Groopman, J. (2007). *How doctors think.* New York, NY: Houghton Mifflin.

Gurung, R. A. R, Chick, N.L., & Haynie, A. (Eds.). (2009). *Exploring signature pedagogies: Approaches to teaching disciplinary habits of mind.* Sterling, VA: Stylus.

Guskey, T. R. (1985). Staff development and teacher change. *Educational Leadership, 42*(7), 57–60.

Hafferty, F. W., & Hafler, J. P. (2011). The hidden curriculum, structural disconnects and the socialization of new professionals. In J. R. Hafler (Ed.), *Extraordinary learning in the workplace.* New York, NY: Springer.

Hafler, J. P. (Ed.). (2011). *Extraordinary learning in the workplace.* New York, NY: Springer

Havita, N., Barak, R., & Simhi, E. (2001). Exemplary university teachers: Knowledge and beliefs regarding effective teaching dimensions and strategies. *Journal of Higher Education, 72*(6), 699–729.

Heath, C., & Heath, D. (2007). *Made to stick.* New York, NY: Random House.

Hirsh, D. A., Ogur, B., Thibault, G. E., & Cox, M. (2007). Continuity as an organizing principle for clinical education reform. *New England Journal of Medicine, 356*(8), 858–866.

Kamhi, A. G. (1994). Research to practice: Toward a theory of clinical expertise in speech-language pathology. *Language, Speech, and Hearing Services in Schools, 25,* 115–118.

Kamhi, A., Vanleer, E. Lundgren, K. Verdolini, K., & Bernstein-Ratner, B. (2009, November). *EBP: The promise and the reality.* Presented at ASHA Convention, New Orleans, LA.

Kane, R., Sandretto, S., & Heath, C. (2004). An investigation into excellent tertiary teaching: Emphasizing reflective practice. *Higher Education, 47,* 283–310.

Kielhofner, G. (2005). Scholarship and practice: Bridging the divide. *American Journal of Occupational Therapy, 59*(2), 231–239.

Kreber, C. (2007). What it's really all about? The scholarship of teaching and learning as an authentic practice. *International Journal for the Scholarship of Teaching and Learning, 1*(1). https://doi.org/10.20429/ijsotl.2007.010103

Lane J. P., & Flagg, J. L. (2010). Translating three states of knowledge—discovery, invention, and innovation. *Implementation Science, 5*(9), 1–14.

Malloch, T. R., & Massey, S. T. (2006). *Renewing American culture: The pursuit of happiness.* Boston, MA: M & M Scrivener Press.

McKinney, K. (2007). *Enhancing learning through the scholarship of teaching and learning: The challenges and joys of juggling.* San Francisco, CA: Jossey-Bass/Anker.

Moon, J. A. (2004). *A handbook of reflective and experiential learning.* New York, NY: Routledge.

Mundry, S. (2005). Changing perspectives in professional development. *Science Educator, 14*(1), 9–15.

National Institutes of Health. (2009). *Translational research.* Retrieved July 11, 2011, from http://nihroadmap.nih.gov/clinicalresearch/overview-translational.asp

Nonako, I., & Hirotaka, T. (1995). *The knowledge creating company: How Japanese companies create the dynamics of innovation.* Oxford, UK: Oxford University Press.

Ogilvie, D., Craig, P., Griffin, S., Macintyre, S., & Wareham, N.J. (2009). A translational frame for public health research. *BMC Public Health, 9*(116), 1–10.

Osterman, K. F., & Kottkamp, R. B. (1993). *Reflective practice for educators.* Newbury Park, CA: Corwin Press.

Palmer, P. (1998). *The courage to teach: Exploring the inner landscape of a teacher's life.* San Francisco, CA: Jossey-Bass.

Palmer, P. J., Zajonc, A., & Scribner, M. (2010). *The heart of higher education: A call to renewal.* San Francisco, CA: Jossey-Bass.

Papir-Bernstein, W. (Ed.). (1993). *Assessment strategy sourcebook for evaluating special students (ASSESS).* New York City Department of Education (NYCDOE).

Papir-Bernstein, W. (1995, April). *Supervision for the 21st century: Facilitating self-directed professional growth.* Presented at NYSSLHA Convention, New York, NY.

Papir-Bernstein, W. (2004). *Standards for professional development.* NYC District 75: Citywide

Speech Services Staff Development, New York, NY.

Papir-Bernstein, W. (2012a). The artistry of practice-based evidence (PBE): One practitioner's path —Part I. In R. Goldfarb (Ed.), *Translational Speech-Language Pathology and Audiology* (pp. 51–58). San Diego, CA: Plural.

Papir-Bernstein, W. (2012b). The artistry of practice-based evidence (PBE): One practitioner's path —Part II. In R. Goldfarb (Ed.), *Translational Speech-Language Pathology and Audiology* (pp. 83–90). San Diego, CA: Plural.

Papir-Bernstein, W., & Legrand, R. (1993, November) *Differentiated systems for staff development: Self-direction and reflection.* Presented at ASHA Convention, Anaheim, CA.

Papir-Bernstein, W., & Legrand, R. (1994) *Removing barriers: Creating diversity consciousness through self-regulatory process training.* Presented at ASHA Convention, New Orleans, LA.

Papir-Bernstein, W., & Rosaly-Santos, M. (2004). *Diversity training for providers of speech therapy.* NYCDOE District 75: Citywide Speech Services Staff Development.

Pascarella, P. (1997, October). Harnessing knowledge. *Management Review*, pp. 37–40.

Pink, D. H. (2012). *To sell is human: The surprising truth about moving others.* New York, NY: Riverhead Books.

Polanyi, M. (1967). *The tacit dimension.* New York, NY: Doubleday.

Rabin, B. A., Brownson, R. C., Haire-Joshu, D., Kreuter, M. W., & Weaver, N. L. (2008). A glossary for implementation research in health. *Journal of Public Health Management Practice, 14,* 117–123.

Redle, E. E. (2013, November). *Improving practice through implementation science and knowledge translation.* Retrieved November 27, 2016, from http://www.asha.org/Academic/questions/Improving-Practice-Through-Implementation-Science-and-Knowledge-Translation/

Robinson, T. L., McCrea, E., Flahive, M., Johnson, A., Schulman, B. B., Kimbarow, M. L., & Ginsberg, S. M. (2011, November). *Why the scholarship of teaching and learning and ASHA.* Presented at ASHA Convention, San Diego, CA.

Rosenbaum, J. E. (1976). *The hidden curriculum of high school.* New York, NY: John Wiley & Sons.

Rosenbek, J. C. (2012). The science of dissemination. In R. Goldfarb (Ed.), *Translational speech-language pathology and audiology.* San Diego, CA: Plural.

Schön, D. (1983). *The reflective practitioner: How professionals think in action.* New York, NY: Basic Books.

Schön D. (1987). *Educating the reflective practitioner.* Hoboken, NJ: Jossey-Bass.

Scully, R., & Shepard, K. (1983). Clinical teaching in physical therapy education: An ethnographic study. *Physical Therapy, 63,* 349–358.

Shepard, K. F., & Jensen, G. M. (1990). Educating the reflective practitioner. *Journal of the American Physical Therapy Association, 70*(9), 566–573.

Shim, H. S., & Roth, G. L. (2008). Sharing tacit knowledge among expert teaching professors and mentees. *Journal of Industrial Teacher Education, 44*(4), 5–24.

Shulman, L. S. (1999). The scholarship of teaching. *Change, 31*(5), 11.

Shulman, L. S. (2005). Signature pedagogies in the professions. *Daedalus, 134,* 52–59.

Smith, E. A. (2001). The role of tacit and explicit knowledge in the workplace. *Journal of Knowledge Management, 5*(4), 311–321

Suarez-Balcazar, Y., & Harper, G. (Eds.). (2003). *Participatory and empowerment evaluation: Multiple benefits.* New York, NY: Haworth.

Taylor, C. (1991). *The ethics of authenticity.* Cambridge, MA: Harvard University Press.

The Carnegie Foundation for the Advancement of Teaching. (1989). *The condition of the professoriate: Attitudes and trends.* Princeton, NJ: The Carnegie Foundation.

Thomas, K. W. (2000). *Intrinsic motivation at work.* San Francisco, CA: Berrett-Koehler.

Thomson, P., Hall, C., Jones, K., & Sefton-Green, J. (2012). *The signature pedagogies project: Final report.* Newcastle, UK : CCE.

Thornicroft, G., Lempp, H., & Tansella, M. (2011). The place of implementation in the translational continuum. *Psychological Medicine, 41*(10), 2015-2021. https://doi.org/10.1017/S0033291711000109

Tonelli, M. R. (1998). Philosophical limits of evidence-based medicine. *Academic Medicine, 73,* 1234–1240.

Tonelli M. R. (2006). Integrating evidence into clinical practice: An alternative to evidence-based approaches. *Journal of Evaluation in Clinical Practice, 12,* 248–256.

Vera-Barachowitz, C. (2003). Book nook: Review of the reflective practitioner. *ASHA SIG Administration and Supervision. 13,* 14–15.

Wah, L. (1999). Making knowledge stick. *Management Review,* 24–29.

Walker, R. (2009). *Buying in: What we buy and who we are.* New York, NY: Random House.

Weimer, M. (2011). A primer on pedagogical scholarship. *Perspectives on Issues in Higher Education, 14*(1), 5–10.

Westfall, J., Mold, J., & Fagnan, L. (2007). Practice-based research: Blue highways on the NIH road map. *Journal of the American Medical Association, 297*(4), 403–406.

Youatt, J., & Wilcox, K. (Fall, 2008). Intentional and integrated learning in a new cognitive age. *Association of American Colleges and Universities Peer Review, 10*(4), 24–26.

CHAPTER 17

Practice-Based Leadership

1. TRANSFORMATIONAL LEADERSHIP

Why Lead?

One of the most important questions to consider is what motivates people to become a leader. Some say it is expected as part of professional development, or that it enhances their personal effectiveness. Other reasons might include external motivators such as pay raise or career progression, or internal rationales such as desire to give back or sense of obligation to serve their organization (Kolditz, 2007).

> **A.R.T.: Bulldogs**
>
> The question can be answered in several ways. One of my most beloved dogs happened to have been an English bulldog. One day in a shopping mall, I saw a poster about leadership that really caught my eye. It stated, "lead, or suffer the consequences" and below the sentence were two English bulldogs, one following the other . . .
>
> Sheryl Sanberg, CEO of Facebook, said it a bit differently (2013). She defined leadership as *making others better as a result of your presence, and making sure that impact lasts in your absence.* Ted Turner, on the other hand, gives some choices. He says, *"lead, follow, or get out*

of the way" (2009). Effective leadership sometimes involves all three. One of the best ways of leading is to let others do it.

Management Is Different From Leadership

Miller and Thoresen describe two Latin verbs that differentiate well between the two different attitudinal styles in any type of relationship: *docere* and *ducere* (2003). *Docere* relates to a deficit model, and implies that "I have what you need and I will impart it to you." *Ducere* means, "to call forth from or pull out of" such as drawing water from a well. It is a verb used to describe another person's wisdom, and the process of taking advantage of the vast store of knowledge and experience that each person has. This relates to how we think about leadership.

Administration, management, and leadership are sometimes used interchangeable, but can have very different interpretations. According to Ackoff, *administration* consists of directing others to carry out the will of a third party. *Management* is the means by which to do so, and *leadership* is the guidance, encouragement, and facilitation to accomplish it all. Leadership requires an ability to bring the will of followers into agreement with that of the leader. The end result will be voluntarism, enthusiasm, and dedication—none of which are necessarily present in management or administration (2010).

Leadership studies conducted by John Kotter at Harvard (2012) distinguish between management and leadership. *Management* refers to the ways complex organizations are kept orderly, nonchaotic, and productive. *Leadership*, by contrast, refers to effectively handling the changes that the competitiveness and volatility of the times have wrought. Kotter describes leadership as an emotional craft, by using *motivation and inspiration* to energize people. Rather than push people in the right direction, as leaders we satisfy the basic human need for achievement, a sense of belonging, a feeling of control over one's life, and the ability to live up to one's ideals (Kotter & Rathgeber, 2016; Papir-Bernstein, 2001).

A Newer Type of Leadership

Leadership has been around for thousands of years, has many definitions, and is constantly evolving. One of the most widely written about theories of leadership is *transformational leadership* because it focuses on motivating the followers to higher levels of performance (Ackoff, 2010; DePree, 1989). This type of leadership can be found in most professions and types of organizations around the globe. It is one of the most inspiring and empowering types of leadership, driven largely by the belief that we can all improve our performance with the right type of motivation (Ackoff, Addison, & Bibb, 2007).

The concept behind this type of leadership was first introduced by James MacGregor Burns. He described it as a process rather than a set of behaviors, whereby both the leaders and followers elevated each other to higher levels of motivation and morality by appealing to higher ideals, values, purpose, and meaning (1978). He was the first theorist to integrate an ethical and moral dimension into a model of leadership. When the book *Emotional Intel-*

ligence appeared in 1995, the acknowledgment of "transformational leadership" techniques was well underway. For organizations riding the waves of change, and we are certainly members of those, traditional leadership is not enough. Transformational leaders are able to rouse people through the sheer power of their own enthusiasm. Such leaders do not order or direct, they inspire, and are committed to nurturing relationships with those they lead. Such leaders mobilize people for organizational change by arousing their emotions about the work they do. Leadership of this kind is an *emotional craft* (Goleman, 1998; Papir-Bernstein, 2001).

Leadership Goals and Components

The goal of transformational leadership is to align people with organizations by transforming them in mind and heart, enlarging the vision, clarifying purposes, and building momentum (Covey, 2004). Transformational leadership appeals to social values and encourages people to collaborate, rather than to work as individuals competing with one another. Authentic transformational leaders recognize that leadership needs to be demonstrated by everyone in the organization. Leadership and "followership" in transformational organizations are predicated less on political authority and more on work relationships centered on common purpose.

Factor analytic studies have identified the following four components of this type of leadership to include (Bass & Riggio, 2006):

1. *Charismatic or idealized influence:* leaders behave in ways that allow them to serve as role models because they take stands and display convictions. They are admired, respected, and trusted so that followers want to emulate their behavior. At the same time, they demonstrate high

standards of ethical conduct. Charisma, however, is not to be confused with "skill" (Ripich & Whitelaw, 2014).

2. *Inspirational motivation:* leaders are able to communicate vision and encourage team spirit. They motivate and inspire by facilitating meaning and value within the work setting.

3. *Intellectual stimulation:* leaders encourage innovation and creativity as part of the problem-solving process. The leader's vision provides the followers with a framework for connecting to the larger organizational picture and to each other.

4. *Individualized consideration:* leaders pay special attention to the individual needs of each person through coaching, as they relate to individual needs for achievement and growth. Interactions address self-actualization, self-fulfillment, and self-worth.

Lenses of Responsibility

In her book about ethical leadership, Thornton describes our seven lenses of responsibility as profit, law, character, people, communities, the planet, and the greater good (2013). She explains the following guiding principals that honor all seven lenses, and should be implemented in our daily leadership activities: be morally aware; stay competent and generate effective performance; model expected performance and leadership; respect others and boundaries; trust others and be trustworthy; communicate openly and authentically; work for mutually beneficial solutions; and improve our global society for the future.

Ethical Leadership

Ethical leadership as a *learning journey* that begins and ends with what Aristotle called "moral excellence," and develops as a result of *habit*. The doing of just acts facilitates *the habit of justice*, just as the doing of brave acts facilitates the *habit of bravery* (Thornton, 2013). As we sift through the mountains of never-ending information, we need to synthesize and discover the hidden meanings that will help us consider the ethical implications of every decision we make. There is no one reference book to use because we are lighting the way across many professional communities at once: government, business, academia, and medicine (Knapp, 2007; Northouse, 2016).

Ethical leadership reminds us that certain mindsets prepare us better than others, and impact how we think, behave, and perform our work. The four principles that foster ethics in leadership are (Thornton, 2013):

- Lead with a moral compass
- Lead in ways that bring out the best in others
- Lead with positive intent and impact
- Lead for the greater good

Servant and Invitational Leaders

Servant leaders are people of character, filled with principles, ethics, and insights. Their egos are in check, and they are in it for more than themselves. They put other people first and are skilled persuasive communicators. They are compassionate and authentic collaborators who use foresight and systems thinking (Sipe & Frick, 2015).

Servant leadership is transformational and transformative because it is the leader's commitment to serve others that always comes first and matters the most. It is a shift away from traditional autocratic and hierarchical modes of leadership toward a model based on community and teamwork. The natural feeling of wanting to serve happens first (Robinson et al., 2013). The aspiration to lead is a conscious choice we make in order to help others grow as people, and become healthier, wiser, and more autonomous. Leadership must be about service, as both an attitude and a behavior (Greenleaf, 1998). Leadership, as a service, is more about process than content. It is more about activity, than position.

Invitational leadership is similar to servant leadership, as they both shift away from emphasizing "leadership as control" to leadership that focuses on *connectedness, cooperation, community, caring, and communication.* It is an internal holistic process based upon principles such as intentionality and trust, and is reflected in how we lead our lives rather than in activities we do at work. As we "invite" others to this concept of leadership, we are enrolling them in our vision with purpose and generosity (Purkey & Siegel, 2003).

Reawakening the Spirit of Leadership

Hawley suggests that the *new currency of leadership* demands integration of four agendas: that of head, heart, body, and spirit (1993). A visual map might look something like a four-ring pretzel, with the upper left as the *head agenda* (intellectual), the upper right as the *heart agenda* (feelings), the lower left as the *body agenda* (wellness), and the lower right as the *spirit agenda.*

The components of what Hawley calls "*organizational dharma*" are the *core commandments* that provide support for leadership responsibilities (1993). They evolved from the teachings of Panasonic's founder, Konosuke Matsushita, and were embedded in the culture of his organization. Values such as these can establish one set of drivers within our own work culture as well.

1. *Contribution to society* (national service): actions and commitment that impact more than yourself
2. *Fairness and honesty:* human justice and equity when dealing with people

3. *Cooperation and team spirit:* seeking unity and peaceful amity
4. *Relentless efforts for improvement* (struggle and betterment): for growth of the individual and team
5. *Courtesy and humility:* including the need for respect and dignity
6. *Adaptability and assimilation:* selflessness, teamwork, and being one of the family
7. *Gratitude:* appreciation and expression of such

2. QUALITIES OF EFFECTIVE LEADERS

Leaders Are Gift-Givers

Personal qualities of effective professionals have been identified in the literature, with similarities across a variety of medical, social science, and educational professions (Flasher & Fogle, 2012; Fogle, 2013). They provide foundational skills for effective leadership in our field. Leaders are encouraging. *Encouragement* helps professionals believe in their potential for improvement. Leaders are *self-aware*, which helps maintain emotional stability. Leaders are *patient,* and are able to adjust feedback systems accordingly. Finally, leaders are *sensitive* to the needs of others and empathic to diverse perspectives.

Leaders are often perceived as people who are supposed to provide direction. A more spiritual interpretation would say that leaders are *gift-givers* who facilitate feelings of love, power, authorship, and significance. According to Bolman and Deal, *the gift of love* includes caring and compassion. *The gift of power* includes autonomy and influence. *The gift of authorship* includes accomplishment and craftsmanship. *The gift of significance* includes working with others at something to make the world better (1995).

Kouzes and Posner identify the five practices of exemplary leadership as (2007):

1. *Model the way* by clarifying values and setting the example.
2. *Inspire a shared vision* by envisioning the future and enlisting others.
3. *Challenge the process* by searching for opportunities and taking risks.
4. *Enable others to act* by fostering collaboration and strengthening others.
5. *Encourage the heart* by recognizing contributions and celebrating values and victories.

The Charisma Behind Leadership

In a 2011 article from the *New York Times*, Zachary Woolfe begins his discussion about the phenomena of *charisma* from the perspective of musical performances. He quickly generalizes to all areas of life and accomplishments. He describes it as something that you cannot look away from, as a physical presence with a spark that empowers. When you watch, you feel elevated, focused, and enlarged. You actually lean forward into it, as a type of surrender. If you have it, at any age, you have no choice but to exude it.

Charisma has quite a fascinating history. In Christian theology, it is seen as a gift from God, such as knowledge, hearing, or prophecy. In the field of social sciences, Max Weber used it to describe leadership of divine origin (Eisenstadt, 1968; Woolfe, 2011). Unlike Woolfe who concludes that this sort of compelling charisma is a gift, I believe that charisma can be developed through the expression of a deep and learned passion. However, we must find those things that we connect with so vehemently. That is our challenge.

We recognize a charismatic performance when we see it, whether on stage, at a meeting, or behind a podium. We instantaneously appreciate the heart's deep connection to something that matters, and compels continued inquiry, emotional investment, and spiritual reverence (Glassman & Swatos, 1986). We are watching and sharing a moment with someone who has the alignment of their intellect, their heart, and their soul—to participation in a subject area, issue, or concern. We are experiencing full engagement in which someone loses themselves and their ego to share the results of their hard work and preparation—a transformative moment when we connect to their passion.

Charisma can be cultivated by pursuing interests and passions, as we lose ourselves to a deeper understanding, mystery, and mastery. Charisma in this sense is a higher order expression of transformative knowledge and understanding which, when coupled with a personal connection and shared with others, becomes compelling and authentic. Finding something we care to invest ourselves in is the first step in cultivating the possibility of charisma.

Charismatic Communicators

Aspects of nonverbal behaviors such as gesture use and speech rate have been shown to influence how charismatic an individual is perceived to be, and how likely someone is to want to engage in conversation with that person (Jones & Turkistra, 2011). Charisma is derived from an ancient Greek work meaning "gift of grace" (Oxford English Dictionary, 1989).

A charismatic communication style is perceived as "strong" as opposed to "weak," and contains animation, openness, friendliness, and attentiveness. Charisma is sometimes paired with the concept of *sparkle*, communication features that emote enthusiasm and foster motivation among communication partners to stay engaged (Jones & Turkistra, 2011; Peterson & McCabe, 1983). Charismatic leaders use intimate and personalized styles of interaction (Antonakis et al., 2011). According to the *Charismatic Leadership Communication Scale (CLCS)*, the following qualities have been linked to conversational partners perceived as having charisma (Antonakis, Fenley, & Liechti, 2011; Levine, 2008):

- Can empathize with others
- Knows when to talk and when to listen
- Maintains eye contact during communication
- Puts others at ease
- Understands what people need
- Asks others to share ideas and opinions
- Communicates confidence

Intuitive Leadership

The "new normal" is a leader who is both responsive and intuitive. An intuitive leader has the ability to respond with greater speed than their peers, the ability to challenge existing fundamentals, and to establish bold drivers for change (Wagstaff, 2011).

An intuitive leader makes decisions informed by *informational feeds* within research and practice, from practitioners and clients, related to past practices and future trends. Knowledge is gleamed from within and across the disciplines. Intuitive leaders understand the power of engaging younger generations, encouraging new ideas, and allowing space at the front of lines.

A.R.T.: Intuitive Leadership

When I was providing speech therapy services to students who had been placed in a special school for children with language disabilities, I began to realize that classroom teachers were looking for a standardized language curriculum. (This was right before all of those special education laws were enacted, beginning with P.L. 94-142, which virtually transformed our professional lives.) I had become very friendly (that is code for you know what) with one of the teachers, and the two of us decided to form a "language curriculum committee," or the LCC. The principal was thrilled, the teachers were looking forward to the meetings, and I, of course, was chairing the committee. My speech supervisor came shortly thereafter to visit, and she had no idea of this latest venture. I described my thinking, and the process that had just barely begun . . . to which she said, "Yes, but why do *you* have to chair it? Why can't you just be on it?" To which I replied, "Why does a sculptor sculpt?" I had little choice but to lead the venture, if it was in fact ever going to happen . . .

Natural Leadership

Leadership qualities and skills are useful not only for administrative leadership positions in the school setting, but for practitioner positions as well. You can use them as a vantage point for guiding your own thinking, aligning team members, developing others, and building unity in a time of change.

It is not difficult to find lists of leadership skills from books or websites. Here is one such list with questions that follow will help you think about the importance of that quality in your professional life (Christensen, Hall, Dillon, & Duncan, 2016):

- *Integrity:* How deep are your beliefs? To what extent do your guiding values and principles align with your behaviors and the choices you have made?
- *Vision:* Do you understand your place in your community, team, or organization? Are you inspired by your organization?

- *Persuasion:* Do you consider yourself to be charismatic, persuasive, and influential? To what extent do people value your opinion and follow your lead?
- *Coaching and development:* How do you nurture and empower those around you? Do you feel threatened by others, or jealous of their success?
- *Decision-making:* Are you comfortable making bottom line decisions after gathering opinions and data?

3. EMOTIONAL INTELLIGENCE

A New Romanticism

In this age fueled by technological advances, we sometimes find ourselves wondering how we, as humans, can remain valuable. This question has prompted the emergence of what Brooks calls *a new romanticism*, an attitude of inspiration, subjectivity, intuition, and belief in the importance of the individual (2015). It has been suggested that the best strategy for retaining value is to ask yourself what activities we humans will insist be performed by other humans, even if computers were able to do them (Colvin, 2015).

The answers are relational, and boil down to the following predictions. *Humans will remain in charge* because individuals will be held accountable for important decisions. *Individuals must work together* to set collective goals, because our concept of what the problem is and what our goals are keeps changing. Problem solving becomes a necessity, and groups solve problems faster and better than any individual can.

Only humans can satisfy deep interpersonal needs. Our essential human nature demands that there are tasks that we must do with or for other humans. We are hardwired as social beings and equate personal relationships with survival. We love to solve problems with others, tell our stories, and create new ideas with others. These are all deeply human abilities: building community, storytelling, building relationships, collaborating, and brainstorming. We need to interact (Colvin, 2015; Pinker, 2007).

Our Relational Society Needs Soft Skills

To look into someone's eyes is the key to high-value work in the new economy (Colvin, 2015). Employers' top priorities are the right-brain skills of social interaction (Basford, Schaninger, & Viruleg., 2015). Big picture data on how Americans work today versus how they worked in the 1970s tell us that biggest changes have been seen in education and health services. Empathy is one of the most critical 21st-century skills. Relational jobs are expanding, and the ability to sense what another human being is sensing or feeling becomes an important workplace skill (Brooks, 2011). The cluster of social graces, interpersonal skills, the leadership awareness in conjunction with specific personality characteristics, are sometimes referred to as *soft skills*. Soft skill attributes are strongly connected with people skills and can be reflected as our *emotional intelligence* (EI) or *emotional intelligence quotient* (EQ as opposed to IQ).

In a 1989 survey by the Department of Labor Employment and Training Administration, American employers reveal that more than half the people who work for them lack the motivation to keep learning and improving in their job (Carnevale, Gainer, & Meltzer, 1990). Four in ten are not able to work cooperatively with their fellow employees. When employers were asked what they were looking for in entry-level workers, specific technical skills are now less important than the underlying ability to learn on the job. In addition, employers listed:

- Listening and oral communication
- Adaptability and creative responses to setbacks and obstacles
- Personal management, confidence, motivation to work toward goals, a sense of wanting to develop one's careers and takes pride in accomplishments
- Group and interpersonal effectiveness, cooperation and teamwork, skills at negotiating disagreement
- Effectiveness in the organization, wanting to make a contribution, leadership potential

The Newer Competence

It is clear that the rules for our work are changing, and that we are going to be judged by a new yardstick. The new measures were related to people or "human competencies." They accounted for what "human abilities" make up the greater part of the ingredients for excellence at work, especially for the leadership roles we were assuming (O'Boyle, Humphrey, Pollack, Hawver, & Story, 2011).

In McClelland's 1973 paper, "Testing for Competence Rather than Intelligence." the argument was presented that traditional academic aptitude, school grades, and advanced credentials simply did not predict how well people would perform on the job. Instead, he proposed that a set of specific competencies include empathy, self discipline, and initiative. A competence, in this tradition, is defined as a personal trait, or set of habits that leads to more effective or superior job performance. This provided the basis for much of later research about what we now call *emotional intelligence.* Howard Gardner was another pioneer who helped us think differently about the emotional link to intelligence (1983). His book became a manifesto about the multiplicity of intelligence, and set the stage for later works with his description of Personal Intelligence as interpersonal (turning outward and relating to other people) and intrapersonal (turning inward and relating to self-knowledge).

These qualities had been talked about loosely for decades under a variety of names such as character, personality, and soft skills. There is, at last, a more precise understanding of these human talents, a new name for them coined by Daniel Goleman: emotional intelligence (1995). These ideas are not new to the workplace and are central to much classic management theory. They refer to managing feelings so that they are expressed appropriately and effectively, enabling people to work together smoothly toward their common goals. Emotional intelligence impacts leadership, as it helps us understand the biological and neurological underpinnings of "people interactions" (Ripich & Whitelaw, 2014).

Our Emotional Life

Our emotional life is a domain that can be handled with greater or lesser skill dependant upon a unique set of competencies. Our emotional aptitude is a type of meta-ability, determining how well we can use whatever other skills we have. People who are emotionally adept, that is, who know and manage their own feelings, and who read and deal effectively with other people's feelings, are at an advantage in any domain of life.

The good news about emotional intelligence is that it can improve throughout life. In the normal course of a lifetime, emotional intelligence (EI) tends to increase as we learn to be more aware of our moods, to handle distressing emotions better, to listen, and empathize, in short, as we become more mature. To a large extent, maturity itself describes this process of becoming more intelligent about our emotions and our relationships. Emotional

Intelligence develops with age and experience from childhood to adulthood. This potential for improvement puts emotional intelligence in sharp contrast to IQ, which remains largely unchanged throughout life (Goleman, 1995, 1998). For ideas about *student behaviors as they reflect emotional intelligence*, please see Appendix H.

Our emotional competence shows how much of that potential we have translated into on-the-job capabilities. It should be noted that the emotional intelligence capacities are independent, meaning that each makes a unique contribution to job performance. They are also considered interdependent, meaning each draws to some extent on certain others with many strong interactions. They are considered hierarchical, because that they build upon one another. Each is considered necessary but not sufficient. Having an underlying EI ability does not guarantee people will display the associated competencies such as collaboration or leadership. Factors such as the climate of an organization for a person's motivation will also determine how the competence manifests itself. Lastly, they are considered generic, which means that to some extent applicable to all fields of work (Goleman, 1998; Papir-Bernstein, 2001).

Five Elements of EI

Our emotional intelligence is based on five elements: self-awareness, self-regulation, motivation, empathy, and adeptness at relationships. Being skilled in these emotional competencies can certainly affect our work. Please see Appendix I for one example of an emotional competency questionnaire. Our emotional intelligence determines our potential for learning the practical skills in areas of *personal competence* and *social competence* (CREIO, 2015; Goleman, 1995, 1998; Papir-Bernstein, 2001). *Personal competence* determines how we

manage ourselves, and is based on three areas: self-awareness, self-regulation, and motivation. *Self-awareness* consists of *emotional awareness* (recognizing our own emotions and their effects), *self-assessment* (knowing one's strengths and limitations), and *self-confidence*. *Self-regulation* consists of *self-control* (keeping impulses in check), *trustworthiness* (maintaining standards), *conscientiousness* (taking responsibility for performance), *adaptability* (flexibility in handling change) and *innovation* (comfort with novel ideas). *Motivation* consists of *achievement drive* (striving to improve in order to meet a standard of excellence), *commitment* (aligning with organizational goals), *initiative* (readiness to act on opportunities), and *optimism* (persistence in pursuing goals despite obstacles and setbacks).

Social competence determines how we handle relationships, and is based on two areas: empathy and social skills. *Empathy* consists of *understanding others* (sensing feelings and perspectives), *developing others* (sensing developmental needs), *service orientation* (anticipating and meeting needs), *leveraging diversity* (cultivating opportunities involving differences), and *political awareness* (reading power relationships). *Social skills* consists of *influence* (using persuasive tactics), *communication* (speaking and listening openly), *conflict management* (resolving disagreements), *leadership* (inspiring and guiding others), *change catalyst* (managing change), *building bonds* (nurturing relationships), *collaboration and cooperation* (working with others), and *team capabilities* (pursuing collective goals).

Program Effectiveness Is Impacted By Our Emotional Intelligence

In the previous chapter, we described schools as *complex host environments* that impact our own self-efficacy, as well student outcomes.

Emotional intelligence, with all of its components, seems to provide both the bridge and the glue. The essential components of program effectiveness, as discussed in Chapter 15 and Appendix D, tend to improve in numerous areas when combined with an approach that strengthens emotional quotients. As practitioners under my supervision strengthened social and emotional variables, the clinical effectiveness of their therapy programs was impacted in the following ways (Papir-Bernstein, 2001, 2012b):

As *Personal Competence* improved (how we manage ourselves), a variety of Program Effectiveness variables improved as well: *Self-Awareness* impacted self-advocacy, awareness of student progress, and self-image; *Self-Regulation* impacted balance of service delivery, space organization, use of materials, student independence, and paperwork management; and *Motivation* impacted student outcomes, professional growth, and staff development implementation.

As *Social Competence* improved (our ability to handle relationships), so did the following Program Effectiveness variables: *Empathy* impacted communication with administrators, the school-home connection, diversity consciousness, and involvement with school community; and *Social skills* impacted classroom involvement, peer communication, relationship with evaluation and instructional support teams, integration of curriculum and standards, and student carryover (Papir-Bernstein, 2012a).

A.R.T.: Cognitive Frameworks

My formal study of what I liked to call "thinking" began years before I was introduced to the concepts of either Goleman's emotional intelligence or Gardner's multiple intelligences. I came across the works of J. P. Guilford and Mary Meeker. Guilford formulated his "Structure of Intellect" (SOI) model that organized cognitive abilities along three dimensions: content, products, and operations (Guilford, 1967, 1977). Meeker adapted Guilford's model for educational use (Meeker, 1968).

Most of my assessment and intervention creations have had a strong linear component—a visual roadmap, a taxonomy, a framework, a paradigm, or simply a strong visual perspective. It is not surprising that I connected to Structure of Intellect. According to SOI, intelligence is classified and organized according to the content of information dealt with, the operations performed on the information, and the resulting products. The four content areas (figural, symbolic, semantic, and behavior), five operations (cognition, memory, divergent production, convergent production, and evaluation), and six products (units, classes, relations, systems, transformations, and implications) interact to form a three-dimensional 120-cell model, with each cell representing one relatively discrete cognitive ability (Papir, Perez, Kessler, & Mavretich, 1979).

Guilford, Gardner, and Goleman all created paradigms for aspects of behavioral, personal and social/emotional intelligence. Coleman's voice was the loudest, as he shared the research regarding the relationship that personal and social competencies have on job performance across fields.

An Emotionally Intelligent Leader

Goleman tells us that the primary tasks of leadership involve directing the attention of others, understanding biases, and cultivating a *triad of awareness* (2013). This triad consists of three simultaneous areas of focus: *inward focus* on knowing self, *outward focus* on knowing the larger world, and *other people focus* on knowing the team (Ripich & Whitelaw, 2014).

One of the simplest definitions of leadership states it is a process of social influence, which maximizes the efforts of others toward an achievement of a goal (Kruse, 2016).

An emotionally intelligent leader (Lemke, Robinson, Prelock, & Meehan, 2016):

- Believes that leadership is about serving others
- Knows their own personality strengths and weaknesses
- Is aware of concerns of people they are leading
- Knows when to take a stand
- Uses values to guide daily interactions
- Pays attention to how others feel
- Builds trust by being reliable and authentic
- Takes time to reflect
- Uses criticism as feedback for self-improvement

Learning leaders seek to improve a variety of personal and professional attributes (Csik-szentmihali, 2003; George, 2003; Sawyer & Villaire, 2007):

- Listening, being present, and being truly engaged in the conversation
- Enhancing ability to navigate "white water" in which unplanned events occur
- Participating with experiential learning and reflection, without the need to always quantify
- Developing an ability to ask better questions
- Learning to say "yes, and" instead of "yes, but"
- Understanding our role as leaders, and the link between leadership skills and our personal lives
- Making connections between all we experience in every facet of our lives
- Tapping into our flow state to access experiences and knowledge in a more effortless way

4. LEARNING LEADERS

Living As Learning Leaders

In our school programs, we are often viewed as educational leaders. Leadership is one of our most valuable assets, and can be applied to every work environment and by every professional in our field (Robinson et al., 2013). Until recently, leadership has rarely been covered in graduate school and, consequently, few of us are aware of how important clinical leadership is with regard to our work. In a 2012, school-based surveys of 180 SLP leaders, the following traits were cited as *common qualities*: they listen, they insist on teamwork, they have school-based crossover knowledge and skills, they have an academic end-point for all their work with students, they understand change, and they are risk-takers (Secord, 2014).

Apprenticeship

In ancient times, apprenticeship was the vehicle for transmitting the knowledge that practitioners needed to know. It took place across fields, from farming to cabinet making, from sculpting to tailoring, and even to medicine and law. *Cognitive apprenticeship* allows learners to see the processes at work, because it is a model of instruction that *makes thinking visible* (Aziz, 2003).

Cognitive apprenticeship is different from *traditional apprenticeship*. Within the traditional apprenticeship process, we model, scaffold, fade, and coach (Anderson, 1983). We show the apprentice how to do a task, watch as they practice, and turn over more and more responsibility as we fade our assistance and slowly give the apprentice greater responsibility (Brown, Collins, & Duguid, 1989). Coaching is one of the most crucial components of the apprenticeship experience, as the master helps the apprentices by scaffolding hints for their success, offering encouragement, and giving feedback. It is the process of *overseeing learning* (Abbott, 2014; Fitts & Posner, 1967).

Cognitive apprenticeship adds a couple of pieces to the learning puzzle. The first is that the thinking of the teacher must become visible to the student, and vice versa. In other words, the *metacognitive processes and tacit experiences* that are often hidden must be brought to the surface. Second, learning must move from the artificial classroom experience to the *real-life authentic setting*. Third, learning is no longer specific to just one context, so *generalization and transfer* occur in novel situations.

Sounds familiar, doesn't it? It is the way we learn, and it is also the way our students learn within the clinical intervention process. Let's look at the similarities between apprenticeship and the clinical intervention process (Robbins, 2015):

1. We oversee learning experiences by observing, scaffolding supports, fading assistance, and facilitating independent practice.
2. We provide supports to help the learner develop self-monitoring and correction skills.
3. We structure activities, and offer encouragement, and feedback.
4. We consider social contexts so that learning takes place with a variety of people and in a variety of environments.
5. We view learning as an incrementally staged process and provide concrete benchmarks for measuring learning outcomes and progress.
6. We integrate our won tacit experiences and focus on facilitating metacognitive processes to encourage higher level cognition.
7. We generalize through attention to authentic and naturalistic best practices.

Peer Coaching

In addition to coaching our students, we coach each other. *Peer coaching* has been described as a process by which two or more colleagues work together to *reflect on current practices*. The process can include sharing ideas, building new skills, teaching one another, conducting research, and brainstorming (Abbott, 2014; Robbins, 2015). Coaching has little to do with status, titles, fixing problem behavior, or evaluation.

Peer coaching can take many forms, including inter-visitations that were discussed in Chapter 16. It can involve coplanning, conferencing, materials development, live or pre-recorded technique analysis, action research, study groups, and storytelling. In fact, it can be as individualized and unique as the people sharing the coaching experience.

A.R.T.: Watching Others Work

The process of "observation" is something that most practitioners associate with a speech supervisor or administrator of a school building. To ease their comfort, and encourage more peer coaching, I arranged to be present during an intervisitation when another practitioner was watching a therapy session. By doing that (of course with everyone's agreement), we destigmatized the word, and removed the title distinctions. My presence helped facilitate the dialogue that followed, and my knowledge about both practitioners and how they worked added much to the conversation.

Leader As Designer

In Chapter 15, we talked about the learning organization. Learning organizations demand a new view of leadership. Belasco and Stayer describe leadership seminars in which supervisors and managers had been asked to imagine and describe their role as leader as if their organization were *an ocean liner* (1993). The most common answer was the *captain*, as the person in charge, or the *navigator* who sets the direction. Others say the *helmsman* who controls the direction, or the *engineer* who stokes the fire and provides the energy. The neglected leadership role was the ship's *designer*.

The designer is the one person who has sweeping influence, yet it is often the neglected dimension of leadership. Why? Possibly, because little credit goes to the designer, and in fact, the design process often takes place behind the scenes. Those of us who aspire to lead out of a desire to control, gain fame, or simply be at the center of all the action, will find little attraction to the design work of leadership. However, those who practice leadership design find deep satisfaction with its ultimate outcome: empowering others (Papir-Bernstein, 1995).

Leader of the Journey

Another metaphor that Belasco and Stayer use pertains to the leadership paradigms described by a *herd of buffalo* and a *flock of geese* (1993). According to this paradigm, the job of the lead buffalo was to plan, organize, command, coordinate, and control. Buffaloes are loyal followers of one leader, and they wait for the leader to show them what to do. If the lead buffalo is slaughtered, the rest of the herd is easily killed as well. In this type of organization, people are waiting for their boss to issue the next instruction. Geese, on the other hand, fly in a V formation with leadership easily shifting. Each team member is comfortable with assuming ownership and responsibility.

According to this type of leadership model, the journey leader facilitates four types of learning for each situation: determine a focus and develop a vision, remove obstacles, develop ownership, and stimulate self-directed

actions. In turn, each situation has two owners of responsibility: the leader and the performers. The responsibility for performance lies with the performer, and it must be owned as such. The responsibility for empowerment lies with the leader (Belasco & Stayer, 1993; Papir-Bernstein, 1995). This can be summed up with an ancient quotation by Chinese philosopher, Lao Tze. Loosely translated, it means (Boldt, 1993):

The *bad leader* is he who the people despise.

The *good leader* is he who the people praise.

The *great leader* is he who the people say, "we did it ourselves."

5. THE CHALLENGES OF LEADERSHIP

Difficult Conversations

As leaders in our field, we are sometimes faced with the task of needing to confront difficult situations that call for dialogues containing emotionally-charged topics, and responses may become "reactive" (Whitelaw, 2012). The reasons that conversations may be perceived as "difficult" are varied, and can include power differentials, philosophical divides, or differing diversity perspectives.

One might think, as communication specialists, that the communication process would be easier for us than for others. Of course, most of us have discovered such generalizations are never true. It is not unheard of for marriage counselors to have marital issues, or for psychiatrists to have cognitive and emotional dysfunction. In fact, sometimes our knowledge and membership in a helping profession makes those kinds of conversations even more difficult. It brings to mind the expression, "the shoemaker's children have no shoes . . . "

There are numerous frameworks and tools that encompass leadership areas, such as consensus-building, negotiation, and conflict resolution (Whitelaw, 2012). *Triad Consulting Group* has gathered and made available a variety of Web-based leadership resources, including worksheets and suggested readings from the fields of psychology, organizational theory, economics, law, and neuroscience (2015). Most authors agree that a first step is the purposeful decision to either avoid or confront the situation by considering relationships and organizational consequences (Heath & Heath, 2010; Stone, Patton, & Heen, 2010). The use of tact and diplomacy, although helpful, may not ease the emotional impact of the conversation—which explains why feedback is so often underappreciated and thus ineffective for remediating "problematic" behaviors (Heen & Stone, 2014).

Another step in the conversational process is to become familiar with the structural aspects of all three categories of difficult conversations: *what happened* conversations, *feelings* conversations, and *identity* conversations (Stone et al., 2010; Whitelaw, 2012). When discussing *what happened*, conversational participants often debate the facts of "what happened to whom" because of differing perspectives and viewpoints. Common behaviors include scapegoating, assigning blame, and demonizing intention. An effective strategy would be to *jointly address* the causes of disagreement and remediation plans.

When participating in conversations about *feelings*, conversational participants often express emotions that may be irrational or unrelated to the facts of the situation. However, emotions must be valued as an integral part of the conversation before they become unraveled.

When participating in conversations about *identity*, self-esteem and competence may feel threatened. Any strategy that rebalances our sense of identity would be encouraged.

The Learning Conversation

The Harvard Negotiation Project has developed a research-based intervention framework for engaging with difficult conversations called "the learning conversation" (Stone et al., 2010). Whitelaw summarizes some of the programs most effective strategies. The learning conversation begins with motivation to understand what has taken place from the other person's point of view, rather than to assign blame. Multiple perspectives and viewpoints are encouraged with an "and" stance. The learning conversation acknowledges multiple sources of responsibility and joint contributions. The most effective framework for initiating difficult conversations should incorporate learning the story of each participant, expressing perspectives and feelings, and creating a partnership for problem-solving and joint decision-making (2012).

Pitfalls of Leadership

Some of the more common pitfalls of leadership include (Welsh & Welsh, 2015):

1. *Not placing value on self-confidence:* It is more difficult for people who lack confidence to develop innovative approaches and express creativity. Great leaders need to work relentlessly to develop self-confidence in others.

2. *Muffling the voices of others:* We all tend to over-talk and some of us tend to over-sell ourselves. We need to encourage all voices, and actively listen when they speak.

3. *Acting phony:* Nothing is more important than authenticity. People easily see through our facial expressions and our vocal tone, if not our words.

4. *Lacking the ability to differentiate:* When it comes to effort and accomplishments, all people are not created equal. Everyone

needs encouragement, but recognition should be given to those who deserve it.

5. *Skipping the fun part:* Everyone loves fun. Celebrate whatever and whenever you can.

6. LEADERSHIP DEVELOPMENT

Service Learning

Universities in this country are just beginning to understand the value of "service learning" as a means to embed a culture of partnership with professional and neighborhood associations. In addition to the obvious benefit of helping students develop *people skills*, it raises the place of volunteering in society as well as supporting organizations in need. It is an expression of active citizenship that enriches our democracy and contributes to social cohesion (EUCIS-LLL, 2011).

Civic engagement is working to make a difference in the quality of civic life of our communities (Ehrlich, 2000). Civic learning is framed by personal identity, diversity perspectives, values, motivation, and commitment. Civic engagement can take the form of volunteerism to organizational involvement and *community-based learning* (AAC&U, 2016).

Cultivating Leadership

Our state and national professional associations are excellent resources for leadership training programs and opportunities to flex your leadership muscles. For example, the ASHA Leadership Development Program (LDP) was designed in 2010 to help practitioners drive change, become leaders within and give back to professional associations, extend professional networks, and develop advocacy skills. A second leadership program, the Minority Student Leadership Program

(MSLP), was established for undergraduate, graduate, and doctoral students. It provides leadership activities and networking opportunities for participants who are chosen through an application process (Flynn, Robertson, & Smiley, 2013).

Since the mid-1950s, the National Association of Colleges and Employers (NACE) has been the leading source of information about employment of college graduates. Employers considering new college graduates for job openings are looking for leaders who can work as part of a team. When employers were asked which attributes they look for on a candidate's resume, the biggest group of respondents (77.8%) chose "leadership." Further evidence that having leadership skills can make or break a hiring decision is that when employers are forced to choose between two equally qualified candidates, they will choose the one with experience in a leadership position over the other (NACE, 2016).

In 2012, ASHA formed a Committee on Leadership Cultivation (CLC). One of its charges was to develop a survey to collect data in areas related to leadership qualities, activities, and strategies for developing a pool of volunteer leaders (Robinson et al., 2013). The survey was fielded to close to 900 volunteer leaders. When questioned about their own volunteer involvement, over half of the respondents were recruited to ASHA volunteer service by someone else, and about 30% evolved from volunteer positions in other professional associations.

Organizational research suggests that many talented people get overlooked in our search for new leadership. Leaders sometimes emerge in unexpected ways and places, and may not look as you might have expected. It is important first to understand how to create a context or "culture" whereby people are not only able to lead but willing to do so. Nelson Mandela called this "leading from behind" (Hemp, 2008).

Volunteer Leadership

Volunteer leadership is on our professional radar, and ASHA has some excellent resources. On the website, if you search for "volunteer," the *Become a Volunteer* page pops up. When you click "get involved," the following opportunities (most with their own links) present themselves:

- Join a committee, board, or council (currently more than 35 standing committees)
- Volunteer as a writer (for information handouts, journals, online resources, etc.)
- Become a mentor (in various ASHA leadership or research programs)
- Become an ASHA member representative (with subject expertise or speaking engagements)
- Get involved with grassroots advocacy (with neighborhood groups, visiting congress, etc.)
- Participating on a review panel (for grants, self-study programs, and awards)
- Assist with technology (assisting with the practice portal, offer feedback on the website)
- Participate in a focus group (share experiences and information)
- Help with the accreditation process (conduct site visits, establish policies)

Some of the best reasons to pursue volunteer leadership positions include driving change in our professions, giving back, contributing to best practices, impacting our professional associations, learning new skills, and advancing career opportunities (ASHA CLC, 2016). Opportunities present themselves on the student level and continue throughout your career.

The way we think about and practice leadership has changed. It is no longer about "you and them." It is now about "we." Being a great leader starts with being yourself. You need to see yourself as a leader, because in communities, each one of us leads and each one of us follows. Each one of us has important skills to offer, and each one of us crafts a vision and sets a direction (Moxley, 2015). Becoming a leader is the path to being you.

A.R.T.: Volunteer Leadership

My own volunteer experiences began with ASHA, and my nomination and election to Legislative Council in my state. To this day, I have no idea who nominated me. I will never forget my first council meeting. As I walked around the room and glanced at the names of people sitting at tables representing each state, it felt like the Academy Awards of our field. I was honored to be sitting in a room with so many of my professional heroes —admired researchers and authors.

From there, I moved on to Advisory Council, and an assortment of committees including Nominations and Elections, and Leadership Cultivation. Each experience was better than the last, as I learned from the best in our field and expanded my circles of personal friendships and professional colleagues. Thank you ASHA.

REFLECTIVE SUMMATIVE QUESTIONS

1. Which personal qualities needed for effective leadership do you feel are your strongest and your weakest? How could you use your strongest to strengthen your weakest?
2. What is your greatest fear when having difficult conversations?
3. When you think about moving into a leadership role, what about that is appealing to you?

4. How do you envision leadership in the field changing in the future?
5. Do you think of yourself as a leader? Why or why not?

REFERENCES

Abbott, J. (2014). *Battling for the soul of education: Moving beyond school reform to educational transformation.* Bath, UK: The 21st Century Learning Initiative.

Ackoff, R. L. (2010). *Differences that make a difference.* Dorset, UK: Triarchy Press.

Ackoff R. L., Addison H. J., & Bibb S. (2007). *Management f-Laws.* Dorset, UK: Triarchy Press.

American Association of Colleges and Universities (AAC&U). (2016). *Civic engagement.* Retrieved December 12, 2016, from https://www.aacu.org

Anderson, J.R. (1983). *The architecture of cognition.* Cambridge, MA: Harvard University Press.

Antonakis, J., Fenley, M., & Liechti, S. (2011). Can charisma be taught? Tests of two interventions. *Academy of Management Learning and Education, 10,* 374–396.

ASHA. (n.d.). *Become a volunteer.* Retrieved July 10, 2012, from http://www.asha.org/About/governance/Volunteering/

ASHA Committee on Leadership Cultivation (CLC). (2016). Why CSD programs encourage volunteer leadership. *The ASHA Leader, 28.*

ASHA Leadership Development Program (LDP). (n.d.). Retrieved July 14, 2015, from http://www.asha.org/About/governance/Leadership-Development-Program/

ASHA Minority Student Leadership Program (MSLP). (n.d.). Retrieved March 10, 2014, from http://www.asha.org/Students/MSLP-Award/

Aziz, G. (2003). Cognitive apprenticeship, technology, and the contextualization of environments. *Journal of Educational Computing, Design and Online Learning, 4.* Retrieved from https://wss.apan.org/jko/mls/LearningContent/Aziz-Cognitive Apprenticeship.pdf

Basford, T., Schaninger, B., & Viruleg, E. (2015). The science of organizational transformation. *McKinsey Quarterly.* Retrieved December 10, 2016, from http://www.mckinsey.com/business-functions/organization/our-insights/the-four-building-blocks--of-change

Bass, B. M., & Riggio, R. E. (2006). *Transformational leadership.* New York, NY: Psychology Press.

Belasco, J. A., & Stayer, R. C. (1993). *Flight of the Buffalo: Soaring to excellence-learning to let employees lead.* New York, NY: Warner Books.

Boldt, S. G. (1993). *Zen and the art of making a living.* New York, NY: Penguin Group.

Bolman, L. G., & Deal, T. E. (1995). *Leading with soul: An uncommon journey of spirit.* San Francisco, CA: Jossey-Bass.

Brooks, D. (2011). *The social animal.* New York, NY: Random House.

Brooks, D. (2015). *The road to character.* New York, NY: Random House.

Brown, J. S., Collins, A., & Duguid, P. (1989). Situated cognition and the culture of learning. *Educational Researcher, 18,* 32–42.

Burns, J. M. (1978). *Leadership.* New York, NY: Harper & Row.

Carnevale, A. P., Gainer, L. J., & Meltzer, A. S. (1990). *Workplace basics: The essential skills employers want.* San Francisco, CA: Jossey-Bass.

Christensen, C. M., Hall, T., Dillon, K., & Duncan, D. S. (2016). *Competing against luck: The story of innovation and customer choice.* New York, NY: HarperCollins.

Colvin, G. (2015). *Humans are underrated.* New York, NY: Random House.

Consortium for Research on Emotional Intelligence in Organizations (CREIO). (2015). http://www.eiconsortium.org

Covey, S. (2004). *The 7 habits of highly effective people.* New York, NY: Free Press.

Csikszentmihali, M. (2003). *Good business: Leadership, flow, and the making of meaning.* New York, NY: Penguin Books.

DePree, M. (1989). *Leadership is an art.* New York, NY: Doubleday.

Ehrlich, T. (Ed.). (2000). *Civic responsibility and higher education.* New York, NY: Oryx Press.

Eisenstadt, S. N. (1968). Introduction. In S. N. Eisenstadt (Ed.), *Max Weber on charisma and institution building* (p. ix). Chicago, IL: University of Chicago Press.

European Civil Society Platform on Lifelong Learning (EUCIS-LLL). (2011). Retrieved December 16, 2016, from http://www.eucis-lll.eu/

Fitts, P. M., & Posner, M. I. (1967). *Human performance.* Belmont, CA: Brooks Cole.

Flasher, L. V., & Fogle, P. T. (2012). *Counseling skills for speech-language pathologists and audiologists* (2nd ed.). Clifton Park, NY: Delmar Cengage Learning.

Flynn, P., Robertson, S., & Smiley, D. F. (2013, November). *Empowering members: A windjammer cruise.* Presented at ASHA Convention, Chicago, IL

Fogle, P. T. (2013). Essentials of communication sciences and disorders. New York, NY: Delmar.

Gardner, H. (1983). *Frames of mind: The theory of multiple intelligences.* New York, NY: Basic Books.

George, B. (2003). *Authentic leadership: Rediscovering the secrets to creating lasting meaning.* New York, NY: Penguin Books.

Glassman, R. M., & Swatos, W. H. Jr. (Eds.). (1986). *Charisma, history and social structure.* Westport, CT: Greenwood Press.

Goleman, D. (1995). *Emotional intelligence.* New York, NY: Bantam Books.

Goleman, D. (1998). *Working with emotional intelligence.* New York, NY: Bantam Books.

Goleman, D. (2013). *Focus: The hidden driver of excellence.* New York, NY: Harper.

Greenleaf, R. K. (1998). *The power of servant leadership.* San Francisco, CA: Berrett-Koehler.

Guilford, J. P. (1967). *The nature of human intelligence.* New York, NY: McGraw-Hill.

Guilford, J. P. (1977). *Way beyond the I.Q.* Buffalo, NY: Creative Education Foundation.

Hawley, J. (1993). *Reawakening the spirit in work.* New York, NY: Simon & Shuster.

Heath, C., & Heath, D. (2010). *Switch: How to change things when change is hard.* New York, NY: Broadway Books.

Heen, S., & Stone, D. (2014). *Thanks for the feedback: The science and art of receiving feedback well.* New York, NY: Viking/Penguin.

Hemp, P. (2008). Where will we find tomorrow's leaders? *Harvard Business Review, 86*(1), 123–129.

Jones, C. A., & Turkstra, L. S. (2011). Selling the story: Narratives and charisma in adults with TBI. *Brain Injury, 25*(9), 8–16.

Knapp, J. C. (2007). *For the common good: The ethics of leadership in the 21st century.* Westport, CT: Praeger.

Kolditz, T. A. (2007). *In extremis leadership: Leading as if your life depended on it.* New York, NY: Leader to Leader Institute.

Kotter, J. P (2012). *Leading change.* Harvard, MA: Harvard Business Review Press.

Kotter, J. P., & Rathgeber, H. (2016). *That's not how we do it here.* New York, NY: Penguin.

Kouzes, J. M., & Posner, B. Z. (2007). *The leadership challenge.* San Francisco, CA: Jossey-Bass.

Kruse, K. (2016). *Employee Engagement: How to motivate your team for high performance.* Richboro, PA: The Kruse Group.

Lemke, A., Robinson, T.,Prelock, P., & Meehan, A. (2016, November). *Dream more, learn more, do more, become more: Leadership lessons from the CLC.* Presented at ASHA Convention, Philadelphia, PA.

Levine, K. J. (2008, May) *Communicating charisma: Developing the charismatic leadership communication scale.* Paper presented at the annual meeting of the International Communication Association, Montreal, Quebec.

McClelland, D.C. (1973). Testing for competence rather than intelligence. *American Psychologist, 28*, 1–14.

Meeker, M. (1968). *The structure of intellect: It's interpretations and uses.* Columbus, OH: Charles E. Merrill.

Miller, W. R., & Thoresen, C. E. (2003). Spirituality, religion, and health: An emerging research field. *American Psychologist, 58*(1), 24–35.

Moxley, R. S. (2015). *Becoming a leader is becoming yourself.* Jefferson, NC: McFarland.

National Association of Colleges and Employers (NACE). (2016). Retrieved March 15, 2015, from http://www.naceweb.org

Northouse, P. G. (2016). *Leadership theory and practice.* Los Angeles, CA: Sage.

O'Boyle, E. H., Humphrey, R. H., Pollack, J. M., Hawver, T. H., & Story, P. A. (2011). The relation between emotional intelligence and job performance: A meta-analysis. *Journal of Organizational Behavior, 32*(5), 788–818.

Oxford English Dictionary Online: Charisma. (1989). Retrieved from http://oed.com

Papir-Bernstein, W. (1995). *Supervision for the 21st century: Facilitating self-directed professional growth*. NYSSLHA Mini-Seminar, New York, NY.

Papir-Bernstein, W. (2001, November). *Creating the perfect fit: Merging personal competence with program effectiveness*. Presented at ASHA Convention, New Orleans, LA.

Papir-Bernstein, W. (2012a). The artistry of practice-based evidence (PBE): One practitioner's path —Part I. In R. Goldfarb (Ed.), *Translational Speech-Language Pathology and Audiology* (pp. 51–58). San Diego, CA: Plural.

Papir-Bernstein, W. (2012b). The artistry of practice-based evidence (PBE): One practitioner's path —Part II. In R. Goldfarb (Ed.), *Translational Speech-Language Pathology and Audiology* (pp. 83–90). San Diego, CA: Plural.

Papir, W., Perez, E., Kessler, L., & Mavretich, M. (1979). *Instructional-management systems (IMS) for cognitive-semantic language development*. New York, NY: Board of Education for the City of New York-Division of Special Education.

Peterson, C., & McCabe, A. (1983). *Developmental psycholinguistics: Three ways of looking at a child's narrative*. New York, NY: Plenum Press.

Pinker, S. (2007). *The stuff of thought*. New York, NY: Penguin Group.

Purkey, W. W., & Siegel, B. L. (2003). *Becoming an invitational leader: A new approach to professional and personal success*. Atlanta, GA: Humanics Trade Group.

Ripich, D., & Whitelaw, G. (2014, April). *Intentional leadership: Harnessing potential in people and programs*. Presented at CAPSD Conference, Orlando, FL.

Robbins, P. (2015). *Peer coaching to enrich professional practice, school culture and student learning*. Alexandria, VA: ASCD.

Robinson, T. L., Papir-Bernstein, W., Chabon, S. S., Diefendorf, A. O., Franklin, T. C., Lubinsky, J. . . . Falzarano, A. (2013, November). *Leadership: It's more than a position*. Presented at ASHA Convention, Chicago, IL.

Sandberg, S. (2013). *Lean in: Women, work, and the will to lead*. New York, NY: Knopf.

Sawyer, C., & Villaire, M. (Fall, 2007). Recapturing relevance in a graduate leadership program: Self-directed learning. *Leadership Review: Kravis Leadership Institute, 7,* 111–121.

Secord, W. (2014). 10 skills you need to be a school leader. *ASHA Leader, 19*(5), 28–29.

Sipe, J. W., & Frick, D. M. (2015). *Seven pillars of servant leadership: Practicing the wisdom of leading by serving*. New York, NY: Paulist Press.

Stone, D., Patton, B., & Heen, S. (2010). *Difficult conversations: How to discuss what matters most*. New York, NY, NY: Penguin.

Thornton, L. F. (2013). *7 lenses: Learning the principles and practices of ethical leadership*. Richmond, VA: Leading in Context LLC.

Triad Consulting Group. (2015). *Help yourself: Resources for improving your conversations*. Retrieved from http://triadconsultinggroup.com/help-yourself

Turner, T. (2009). *Call me Ted*. New York, NY: Grand Central.

Wagstaff, C. (2011). *Informed intuition: Beyond convention wisdom*. Retrieved December 11, 2016, from http://www.criticaleye.com/insights-servfile.cfm?id=2774

Welsh, J., & Welsh, S. (2015). *The real-life MBA*. New York, NY: HarperCollins.

Whitelaw, G. M. (2012). Leadership challenges: Difficult conversations. *ASHA SIG 11 Perspectives on Administration and Supervision, 22*(1), 40–44.

Woolfe, Z. (2011, August). "A gift from the musical gods." *The New York Times*. Retrieved from http://www.nytimes.com

Conclusion

The same types of questions have puzzled mankind throughout the ages, and lie at the heart of fields of practice such as medicine, education, science, politics, art, philosophy, psychology, social work, as well as speech-language pathology (Ricard & Thuan, 2001). Why am I doing this work? How do I infuse my best work within the best aspects of society? How can I satisfy my sense of universal responsibility through my perspective as a professional and as an individual? While scientific research provides us with information, it does not provide us with *all we need to know.* We must enhance our understanding through personal experiences, and this transformation from theoretical knowledge to direct experience is the key to ethical solutions. "When our ethics reflect our inner qualities and guide our behavior, then they are naturally expressed in our thoughts, words, and deeds. They thus inspire others." (Ricard & Thuan, 2001, p. 20)

All researchers have *a sacred charge*, that of seeking and illuminating "truth" (Rendon, 2000). Academic cultures rely on empirically supported interventions as the roadmap for practice. This "Newtonian lens" is based upon a universal interpretation of strict causality and absolute space and time (Mansfield, 1995). Western epistemology has shaped our understanding of truth as a principle largely driven by reason and the intellect. This way of thinking has sometimes placed value on quantitative numbers over qualitative practices, research over scholarship, theory over practice, data over personal reflections, and outer views over inner ways of knowing (Greenspan, 1997; Tarnas, 1998).

Any type of therapeutic experience, however, is a creative collaboration that cannot always be quantified and measured. The therapeutic enterprise has been described as a process similar to a moment-to-moment dance, where the practitioner must be attuned to subtle changes and shifts in order to direct intervention (Smith, 2012). The dance involves not only the movement, but the relationship. While there is no question that the medical and educational models dominate our profession, we need to leave space for the *art of practice,* and that art form is anything but linear. Most of what occurs in the therapeutic relationship does so within "the spaces in between" practitioner and client (Smith, 2012).

My desire in writing this book has been driven largely by a belief that "understanding" must begin inside of us, with our heart and spirit as well as our mind. All that we learn, in every context of our lives, then connects through *the soul of our work.* There is no deadline for understanding. As we develop and grow our attitudes and practices, new meanings take shape from previously heard or learned ideas. We hear differently, when we *look in* as well as *look out.* The practitioner's path is a personal and inner experience. Sometimes when we try to explain it with words, the descriptions move to our heads rather than our hearts. In order to feel it, you must experience it. My use of metaphorical incidents presented as Autobiographical Reflective Tales (A. R. T.) conveys the spirit of those experiences. It is my hope that you get from the stories what you need at that moment, rather than what I may have intended. Let the book invite you to examine its stories and find the lessons within, as you forge associations and discover your own stories.

Consider the shape of this book like a spool, with each idea knitted together into one string, and that string is *the practitioner's path* (Solnit, 2013). The stories serve as scaffolds, and hold up the *principles of practice,* for they are the true storylines of this book. Through the process of creating *the practitioner's path*, I imagined how Einstein may have felt in his quest for a unified theory of the universe. The search never completes itself just as your path is never complete. Continue to build upon each of the four components, so that they extend and support your discoveries of uncharted *pillars of practice* and pathways to leadership.

REFERENCES

Greenspan, S. I. (1997). *The growth of the mind.* Reading, MA: Perseus Books.

Mansfield, V. (1995). *Synchronicity, science, and soul-making: Understanding Jungian synchronicity.* Chicago, IL: Open Court.

Rendon, L. I. (2000). Academics of the heart: Reconnecting the scientific mind with the spirit's artistry. *The Review of Higher Education, 24*(1), 1–13.

Ricard, M., & Thuan, T. X. (2001*). The quantum and the lotus: A journey to the frontiers where science and Buddhism meet.* New York, NY: Three Rivers Press.

Smith, H. (2012). *The spaces in-between: How the art of intuition informs the science of evidence-based practice in psychotherapy.* Master of Social Work Clinical Research Papers. Paper 93. Retrieved from http://sophia.stkate.edu/msw_papers/93

Solnit, R. (2013). *The faraway nearby.* New York, NY: Penguin Books.

Tarnas, R. (1998). The passion of the Western mind. In H. Palmer (Ed.), *Inner knowing* (pp. 14–20). New York, NY: Jeremy P. Tarcher/Putnam.

APPENDIX A

Activity-Based Language Experiences (ABLE)
(Papir-Bernstein, 1992)

Arts and crafts: making puppets out of paper, fabric, socks, or bags; making picture frames out of wrapping paper, foil, fabric, or shells; making season gifts for holidays, special occasions, for specific family members or friends based upon interests; origami (inexpensive books and digital resources available); collages; greeting cards; jewelry-making using clay, paper mache, beads, or ribbon; sewing small pillows, ornaments, or personalized gifts; string art

Shopping trips: supermarket, gift store, post office, department store, toy store, bookshop

Hobbies: building a model (boat, airplane, car, etc.), knitting and crocheting, quilting, hooking a rug or pillow, embroidering and sewing, collecting (baseball cards, stamps, coins, dolls, cars, comic books, etc.), photography, performing magic tricks, ceramics and pottery, drawing and painting, gardening, woodworking, reading or writing, leather work, camping, cooking or baking and technology

Music and movement: performing a song, writing a song, moving to the beat of music, playing a musical instrument, listening to music, karaoke, and learning dance steps

Sports: individual or team sports, participatory or spectator sports, sports equipment, planning a trip to a game, practicing a skill, and game rules

Work: job interviews, completing forms, attitude on the job, banking, using a computer, visiting work sites, and travel training

Grooming and personal hygiene: washing, shaving, manicuring, hair preparation, makeup, oral hygiene, and planning a diet

Fashion: selecting seasonal clothing, clothing for various occasions, buying clothing, coordinating accessories, and dressing routines

History and current events: reading the newspaper and magazines, reporting the news, listening to a news broadcast, writing a newsletter, understanding parts of a newspaper, answering an ad, determining fact from opinion, personal experiences as they relate to the news, consumer knowledge and awareness, our legal system, and cultural awareness

Generic activities: making a bulletin board, telling a joke, or teaching someone something new

REFERENCE

Papir-Bernstein, W. (Ed.). (1992) *Activity-Based Language Experiences (ABLE)*. NYCDOE City-wide Speech Services, D.75: New York, NY.

APPENDIX B

Multicultural Activities
(Papir-Bernstein, 1992)

All of these activities have been field tested by speech therapy practitioners in educational programs for children with disabilities across various grade levels.

- *I am somebody special* multicultural theme day
- Multicultural *bulletin boards*
- International *festivals* with dance, music, and food of other cultures
- Role-playing and *storytelling* events about other cultures
- *Family tree* art projects
- *Map*-making
- Formulating *rules* that facilitate respect for oneself and people from other cultures
- *Pen-pal letters* to peers from other countries
- Learning about people from various cultures who have made *significant contributions*
- Discussing *similarities and differences* across cultures
- Language and vocabulary exercises, examining multicultural word roots and *idiomatic expressions*

- *Community walks* to cultural and ethnic shops
- *Parent meetings* about cultural experiences from other countries
- *Field trips* to various ethnic history museums
- Observation and celebration of multicultural *holidays*
- Constructing *calendars* incorporating ethnic celebrations
- Starting a *recipe club* and multicultural cookbook
- Learning *dances* of different countries
- Planning multicultural *assembly* programs
- Beginning a *cultural awareness* club

REFERENCE

Papir-Bernstein, W. (Ed.) (1992) *Activity-Based Language Experiences (ABLE)*. NYCDOE Citywide Speech Services, D.75: New York, NY.

APPENDIX C

Diversity Perspective: Self-Assessment
(adapted from Cech, 1991)

(With *YES* as 5 and *NO* as 1, circle the appropriate number on each scale)

SETTING THE MOOD: **Start with the arrangement and use of space.**

1. Does the arrangement of space encourage cooperative group learning?

    5----------------4----------------3----------------2----------------1

2. Do the cultures presented visually reflect the multicultural reality of the world rather than just your classroom reality?

    5----------------4----------------3----------------2----------------1

3. Are members of minority groups shown as individuals with distinct features rather than stereotypes?

    5----------------4----------------3----------------2----------------1

4. Are all of the visual props equally aesthetically appealing?

    5----------------4----------------3----------------2----------------1

5. Do the props stretch imagination by suggesting alternative methods of living?

    5----------------4----------------3----------------2----------------1

6. Are some of the props contributed or made by the students or their families?

    5----------------4----------------3----------------2----------------1

MUSIC AND MOVEMENT: **Music and psychomotor games and exercises encourage cooperating and acceptance.**

7. Are the games drawn from many cultures rather than just one or two?

    5--------------4--------------3--------------2--------------1

8. Do the props and materials used reflect these cultures?

    5--------------4--------------3--------------2--------------1

9. Is cooperation rather than competition the basis for group games?

    5--------------4--------------3--------------2--------------1

10. Is music used with movement on a regular basis?

    5--------------4--------------3--------------2--------------1

11. Are musical instruments accessible and do they reflect the multicultural reality?

    5--------------4--------------3--------------2--------------1

ART: **Art can be a first step to appreciating other cultures, because it encourages the same qualities needed for living in a multicultural society: creative, experimentation, flexibility, and involvement.**

12. Are examples of art drawn from various cultures rather than just one?

    5--------------4--------------3--------------2--------------1

13. Are practical art projects a regular part of the program?

    5--------------4--------------3--------------2--------------1

14. Are projects, made by the students, exhibited in various parts of the room?

    5--------------4--------------3--------------2--------------1

15. Are papers and crayons/markers used that reflect color differences?

    5--------------4--------------3--------------2--------------1

16. Do art materials and projects reflect those from a variety of cultures?

    5--------------4--------------3--------------2--------------1

DISCOVERY GAMES: **These include puzzles, manipulatives, games, and toys, all of which can be quiet activities but elicit lots of language.**

17. Do individual puzzles depict people of all backgrounds?

    5---------------4---------------3---------------2---------------1

18. Are small toy figures multicultural in appearance in terms of facial features, skin color, and dress?

    5---------------4---------------3---------------2---------------1

19. Do counting materials and game cards represent objects from a wide variety of cultures?

    5---------------4---------------3---------------2---------------1

20. Do manipulatives encourage cooperative play?

    5---------------4---------------3---------------2---------------1

FOODS TO SHARE: **Food activities and snack time is the perfect time to broaden multicultural experiences.**

21. Is there a cultural variety of foods presented and discussed every day?

    5---------------4---------------3---------------2---------------1

22. Are various ways of eating or preparing foods modeled and practiced?

    5---------------4---------------3---------------2---------------1

23. Are negative comments about food handled sensitively?

    5---------------4---------------3---------------2---------------1

24. Are parents involved with food preparations for multicultural festivals?

    5---------------4---------------3---------------2---------------1

REFERENCE

Cech, M. (1991). *Globalchild: Multicultural resources for young children.* Boston, MA: Addison-Wesley.

APPENDIX D

Program Effectiveness
(Papir-Bernstein, 2001)

These essential components are not related to specific content, but rather to the overall effectiveness of your therapy program.

1. **Classroom Involvement:** planning and conducting successful collaborative sessions in the classroom
2. **Peer Communication:** having a working system for exchanging information among fellow speech providers regarding student information and staff development ideas
3. **Balance of Service Delivery Options:** meeting both individual student needs and overall programmatic needs through your use of service delivery options
4. **Space Organization:** optimizing space through organization and storage
5. **Self Advocacy:** expressing your professional needs to appropriate school personnel in productive ways
6. **Communication With Your Administrators:** establishing and maintaining open lines of communication with building and speech administrators
7. **Student Outcomes:** establishing an ongoing system for tracking student outcomes through assessment, observation, and use of informal protocols
8. **School-Home Connection:** being involved with successful parent workshops, IEP meetings, telephone conferences, and homework routines

9. **Use of Materials:** Being familiar with everything in your closet, rotating materials, and using/adapting what you have
10. **Professional Growth:** taking advantage of staff development offerings and pursue additional professional growth opportunities
11. **Awareness of Student Progress:** feeling that your work has impact upon the improvement of the student's ability to communicate
12. **Student Independence:** moving each student along the therapeutic continuum of service delivery
13. **Technology:** Being confident and competent using available technology
14. **Relationships with teams:** feeling comfortable with interdisciplinary conferences and meetings
15. **Curriculum and Standards:** Being able to infuse speech, language, and communication targets into themes and activities related to educational standards and curriculum areas
16. **Diversity Consciousness:** meeting the diverse needs of your students through curriculum modification, material adaptation, and use of support personnel
17. **Staff Development Implementation:** using the information from workshops to the benefit of your students and your instructional program

18. **Image:** feeling comfortable with the way staff members perceive your diverse roles and work with the students
19. **Paperwork Management:** fulfilling paper requirements on time and with little or no anxiety
20. **Involvement with the School Community:** participating with school committees, special projects, and staff meetings
21. **Carryover:** expanding your involvement with inclusionary programs and transition meetings

REFERENCE

Papir-Bernstein, W. (2001, November). *Creating the perfect fit: Merging personal competence with program effectiveness.* Presented at ASHA Convention, New Orleans, LA.

Technical and Process Intervention Skills

(adapted from Goldberg, 1997)

1. PLANNING INTERVENTION
   - 1.1 Contingencies (reinforcement, schedules, criteria)
   - 1.2 Materials (appropriateness, motivating, safety, organization)
   - 1.3 Goals (objectives, target behaviors)
   - 1.4 Stimulus Configuration (adaptations, rate, variation, redundancy, context)

2. APPLYING TECHNICAL INTERVENTION SKILLS
   - 2.1 Organizing Statements (purpose of activity, how activity was conducted, behavior consequences)
   - 2.2 Modeling (types, sequence)
   - 2.3 Controlling the Session (interactions, material and activity design, contingencies)
   - 2.4 Response Differentiation (successive approximations, multiple cueing)
   - 2.5 Parental Involvement (consultation, training)
   - 2.6 Process of Learning (stages, phases, levels)
   - 2.7 Changing Attitudes (discussions, demonstrations)
   - 2.8 Monitoring (clinician, students)

   - 2.9 Using Strategies (considerations, general strategies, applications, areas)
   - 2.10 Generalization (timing, stimulus, response, activities)
   - 2.11 Maintenance (things to maintain)
   - 2.12 Error Analysis (general conditions, types)
   - 2.13 Correct Response Analysis (confirmation of prior learning, self-analysis)
   - 2.14 Rephrasing (positive effects, methods)
   - 2.15 Confrontation (effectiveness, methods, problems)

3. APPLYING PROCESS INTERVENTION SKILLS
   - 3.1 Rapport (benefits, methods, limitations)
   - 3.2 Empathy and Compassion (types, uses)
   - 3.3 Speech Characteristics (intonational patterns, paralanguage)
   - 3.4 Communicating at the Students' Own Levels (style, comprehension)
   - 3.5 Showing Respect (cultural values, personal needs, interaction style)

3.6 Maximizing Response Opportunities (timing, cueing)

3.7 Being Attentive (conversational follow-through, asking relevant questions)

3.8 Being Flexible (areas of flexibility, components of flexibility)

3.9 Involving Clients in Decision Making (models for improvement, determining goals, selecting methods and materials, selecting reinforcers)

3.10 Nonverbal Behaviors (student behaviors, control, functions, clinician behaviors)

3.11 Acknowledgement (verbal, vocal, nonverbal)

3.12 Acceptance (withholding judgments)

3.13 Effective Use of Time (minimizing extraneous activities, maximizing responses)

3.14 Matching Activities to Learning Styles (cognitive styles, cultural styles)

3.15 Group Therapy (settings, leadership issues, interactions, functions)

3.16 Providing Feedback (student to clinician, clinician to student, types)

3.17 Professional Collaborations

3.18 Use of Professional Authority (charisma, competency)

REFERENCE

Goldberg, S. (1997). *Clinical skills for speech-language pathologists*. San Diego, CA: Singular.

APPENDIX F

Professional Growth Plan
(Papir-Bernstein, 1995)

NAME:

1. How would you describe the effectiveness of your speech and language therapy program this year?
   - Please describe specific *strengths and highlights*.

   - Please describe specific *areas of concern*.

2. Which area related to your professional abilities would you like to target for improvement and/or change? Please prioritize them by number.

   ___ adapting techniques/materials   ___ organization of professional resources

   ___ assessment   ___ parent/home contact

   ___ changing mandates   ___ planning for therapy

   ___ classroom collaboration   ___ problem solving

   ___ community integration   ___ scheduling

   ___ conflict management   ___ staff consultation/training

   ___ documenting student progress   ___ therapy techniques

   ___ implementing new information   ___ use of materials

   ___ interpersonal communication   ___ vocational integration

   ___ involvement with conferences   ___ other (please specify)

   ___ objective/goal setting

3. Based upon the above areas, formulate two goals you would like to accomplish by the end of the school year.

REFERENCE

Papir-Bernstein, W. (1995). *Supervision for the 21st century: Facilitating self-directed professional growth.* NYSSLHA Mini-Seminar, New York, NY.

APPENDIX G

Assessing Diversity Aspects of the Hidden Curriculum

(Papir-Bernstein & Rosaly-Santos, 2004)

VISUAL/WRITTEN COMMUNICATIONS

- How are the *decorations in your therapy space* reflective of members of the "Federal Five" (African Americans, Asian Americans, European Americans, Latin/Hispanic Americans, and Native Americans) and other diverse groups?
- How are the *handouts and worksheets* reflective of the diverse communities?
- How is the *content in your books* reflective of the diverse communities?
- How are the authors of the written material you provide representative of diverse communities?

VERBAL/NONVERBAL COMMUNICATIONS

- When reading or using people's names, are the names inclusive of diversity?
- How do you deal with put-downs or slurs within your therapy space?
- How do you and other students get comfortable and accurate with students' names that are difficult to pronounce?
- Are your assessment and evaluative procedures inclusive of diverse learning styles?
- Are your intervention strategies inclusive of diverse learning styles?

REFERENCE

Papir-Bernstein, W., & Rosaly-Santos, M. (2004). *Diversity training for providers of speech therapy.* NYC-DOE District 75: Citywide Speech Services Staff Development.

Observation of Student Behavior As It Reflects Emotional Intelligence

(adapted from Goleman, 1998)

(Using the carrier phrase, "Does the student . . . " please circle the appropriate number on each scale)

Practitioner's Name: _____

Student's Name: _____   **Date:** _____

1. Recognize his/her strengths and limitations (accept feedback and suggestions)

    (Yes) 1----------------2----------------3----------------4----------------5 (No)

2. Demonstrate self-confidence (act self-assured)

    (Yes) 1----------------2----------------3----------------4----------------5 (No)

3. Exhibit self-control (manage impulsive feelings and moods)

    (Yes) 1----------------2----------------3----------------4----------------5 (No)

4. Maintain honesty and trustworthiness (act ethically and admit mistakes)

    (Yes) 1----------------2----------------3----------------4----------------5 (No)

5. Show conscientiousness (work with care, organization, and punctuality)

    (Yes) 1----------------2----------------3----------------4----------------5 (No)

6. Respond well to change (demonstrate adaptability and flexibility)

    (Yes) 1----------------2----------------3----------------4----------------5 (No)

7. Exhibit innovativeness (show enthusiasm and openness to new ideas)

    (Yes) 1--------------2--------------3--------------4--------------5 (No)

8. Strive to improve (set goals and seek out information)

    (Yes) 1--------------2--------------3--------------4--------------5 (No)

9. Show commitment (support the goals of a larger group)

    (Yes) 1--------------2--------------3--------------4--------------5 (No)

10. Demonstrate initiative (go above and beyond what is expected)

    (Yes) 1--------------2--------------3--------------4--------------5 (No)

11. Remain optimistic (persevere despite obstacles and setbacks)

    (Yes) 1--------------2--------------3--------------4--------------5 (No)

12. Understand emotional cues (attentive and sensitive to tone of voice/facial expressions)

    (Yes) 1--------------2--------------3--------------4--------------5 (No)

13. Acknowledge the effort of others (offer feedback and praise)

    (Yes) 1--------------2--------------3--------------4--------------5 (No)

14. Anticipate the needs of others (offer assistance)

    (Yes) 1--------------2--------------3--------------4--------------5 (No)

15. Respect diversity (relate well to people from other backgrounds)

    (Yes) 1--------------2--------------3--------------4--------------5 (No)

16. Influence and persuade others (win consensus and support)

    (Yes) 1--------------2--------------3--------------4--------------5 (No)

17. Share information clearly and effectively (participate in give-and-take conversations)

    (Yes) 1--------------2--------------3--------------4--------------5 (No)

18. Resolve disagreements and conflicts (handle difficult people and tense situations)

    (Yes) 1--------------2--------------3--------------4--------------5 (No)

19. Exhibit leadership (inspire enthusiasm and lead by example)

    (Yes) 1--------------2--------------3--------------4--------------5 (No)

20. Recognize when change is needed (challenge the status quo and remove barriers)

    (Yes) 1----------------2----------------3----------------4----------------5 (No)

21. Cultivate and nurture relationships (establish friendships that are mutually beneficial)

    (Yes) 1----------------2----------------3----------------4----------------5 (No)

22. Collaborate and cooperate (work with others toward shared goals)

    (Yes) 1----------------2----------------3----------------4----------------5 (No)

23. Display team qualities (acknowledge the group and share credit)

    (Yes) 1----------------2----------------3----------------4----------------5 (No)

EI CODE:

Personal Competence (how we manage ourselves)

- Self-awareness: #1–2
- Self-regulation: #3–7
- Motivation: #8–11

Social Competence (how we handle relationships)

- Empathy: #12–15
- Social Skills: #16–23

REFERENCE

Goleman, D. (1998). *Working with emotional intelligence.* New York, NY: Bantam Books.

The Emotional Competency Questionnaire

(Papir-Bernstein, 2001; adapted from Goleman, 1988)

PERSONAL COMPETENCE (How we manage ourselves)

I. SELF-AWARENESS (Knowing your internal states, preferences, resources, and intuition)

A. Emotional Awareness (Recognizing your emotions and their effects)

1. Do you know what you are feeling and why?
2. Do you realize the connections between your feeling and what you think and say?
3. Do you recognize how your emotions affect your performance?

B. Accurate Self-Assessment (Knowing your strengths and weaknesses)

1. Are you aware of your strengths and weaknesses?
2. Are you reflective and do you learn from experience?
3. Are you open to feedback, new perspectives, and self-development?

C. Self-Confidence (Sureness about your self-worth and capabilities)

1. Do you present yourself with self-assurance?
2. Can you voice and defend views that are unpopular?
3. Are you able to make sound decisions despite uncertainties and pressures?

II. SELF-REGULATION (Managing your internal states, impulses, and resources)

A. Self-Control (Managing disruptive emotions and impulses)

1. Do you manage your impulsive feelings and distressing emotions well?
2. Do you stay composed and positive even in trying moments?
3. Do you think clearly and stay focused under pressure?

B. Trustworthiness *(Maintaining standards of honesty and integrity)*

1. Do you act ethically?
2. Do you build trust through your reliability and authenticity?
3. Do you admit your own mistakes?

C. Conscientiousness *(Taking responsibility for personal performance)*

1. Do you meet commitments and keep promises?
2. Do you hold yourself accountable for meeting your objectives?
3. Are you organized and careful in your work?

D. Adaptability *(Flexibility in handling change)*

1. Do you smoothly handle multiple demands and shifting priorities?
2. Do you adapt your responses and strategies to fit changing circumstances?
3. Are you flexible in how you view actions and events?

E. Innovativeness *(Being comfortable with and open to new ideas)*

1. Do you seek out fresh ideas from a wide variety of sources?
2. Do you entertain original solutions to problems?
3. Do you generate new ideas and take fresh perspectives?

III. MOTIVATION (Emotional tendencies that facilitate reaching goals)

A. Achievement Drive *(Striving to improve or meet a standard of excellence)*

1. Are you results-oriented?
2. Do you set challenging goals and take calculated risks?
3. Do you pursue information and learn how to improve your performance?

B. Commitment *(Aligning with the goals of the group or organization)*

1. Do you make personal or group sacrifices to meet a larger organizational goal?
2. Do you find a sense of purpose in the larger mission?
3. Do you actively seek out opportunities to fulfill the group's mission?

C. Initiative *(Readiness to act on opportunities)*

1. Do you pursue goals beyond what is required or expected of you?
2. Do you cut through red tape and bend the rules when necessary to get the job done?
3. Do you mobilize others through unusual and enterprising efforts?

D. Optimism *(Persistence in pursuing goals despite obstacles and setbacks)*

1. Do you persist in spite of setbacks?
2. Do you operate from hope of success rather than fear of failure?
3. Do you see setbacks as circumstance rather than a personal flaw?

SOCIAL COMPETENCE
(How we handle relationships)

I. EMPATHY (Awareness of others' feelings, needs, and concerns)

A. *Understanding others (Taking an active interest in others' perspectives and concerns)*

1. Are you attentive to emotional cues and do you listen well?
2. Do you show sensitivity and understand others' perspectives?
3. Do you help out based on understanding other people's needs and feelings?

B. *Developing others (Sensing what others need in order to bolster their abilities)*

1. Do you acknowledge and reward people's strengths and accomplishments?
2. Do you offer useful feedback?
3. Do you mentor and give timely coaching?

C. *Service orientation (Anticipating, recognizing, and meeting the needs of others)*

1. Do you understand needs and match them to your services and products?
2. Do you seek ways to increase satisfaction and loyalty?
3. Do you offer appropriate assistance?

D. *Leveraging diversity (Cultivating opportunities with diverse people)*

1. Do you respect and relate well to people from varied backgrounds?
2. Do you understand diverse views and are you sensitive to group differences?
3. Do you create environments where diverse people can thrive?

E. *Political awareness (Reading a group's power relationships)*

1. Do you accurately read key power relationships?
2. Do you detect crucial social networks?
3. Do you understand the forces that shape people's views and actions?

II. SOCIAL SKILLS (Adeptness at facilitating desirable responses in others)

A. *Influence (Using effective tactics for persuasion)*

1. Do you fine-tune presentations to appeal to the listener?
2. Do you use strategies to build consensus and support?
3. Do you orchestrate events to effectively make a point?

B. *Communication (Sending clear and convincing messages)*

1. Do you listen well, seek mutual understanding, and welcome shared information?
2. Do you foster open communication and stay receptive to bad as well as good news?
3. Do you deal with difficult issues straightforwardly?

C. *Conflict management (Negotiating and resolving disagreements)*

1. Do you handle difficult people and tense situations with diplomacy and tact?
2. Do you spot potential conflict and help de-escalate?
3. Do you orchestrate win-win solutions?

D. Leadership (Inspiring and guiding groups and people)

1. Do you arouse enthusiasm for a shared vision and mission?
2. Do you step forward to lead as needed, regardless of position?
3. Do you lead by example?

E. Change catalyst (Initiating or managing change)

1. Do you recognize the need for change and remove barriers?
2. Do you enlist others in the pursuit of change?
3. Do you model the change expected of others?

F. Building bonds (Nurturing instrumental relationships)

1. Do you cultivate and maintain extensive informal networks?
2. Do you seek out relationships that are mutually beneficial?
3. Do you build rapport and keep others in the loop?

G. Collaboration and cooperation (Working with others toward shared goals)

1. Do you balance a focus on task with attention to relationships?
2. Do you share plans, information, and resources?
3. Do you spot and nurture opportunities for collaboration?

H. Team capabilities (Creating group synergy in pursuing collective goals)

1. Do you model team qualities like respect, helpfulness, and cooperation?
2. Do you build team identity and commitment?
3. Do you protect the group and share credit?

REFERENCES

Goleman, D. (1998). *Working with emotional intelligence.* New York, NY: Bantam Books.

Papir-Bernstein, W. (2001, November). *Creating the perfect fit: Merging personal competence with program effectiveness.* Presented at ASHA Convention, New Orleans, LA.

Index